Is It in Your Genes?

The Influence of Genes on Common
Disorders and Diseases That Affect
You and Your Family

Is It in Your Genes?

The Influence of Genes on Common
Disorders and Diseases That Affect
You and Your Family

www.is-it-in-your-genes.org

Philip R. Reilly, M.D.

Fellow, American College of Medical Genetics

COLD SPRING HARBOR LABORATORY PRESS
Cold Spring Harbor, New York

Is It in Your Genes?
The Influence of Genes on Common Disorders
and Diseases That Affect You and Your Family

©2004 by Cold Spring Harbor Laboratory Press, Cold Spring Harbor, New York
Printed in the United States of America

Publisher and	John Inglis
Acquisition Editor	
Editorial Development Manager	Jan Argentine
Image and Permissions Coordinator	Maria Falasco
Project Coordinator	Mary Cozza
Production Editor	Patricia Barker
Desktop Editor	Susan Schaefer
Production Manager and	
Interior Designer	Denise Weiss
Cover Designer	Mike Albano

Library of Congress Cataloging-in-Publication Data

Reilly, Philip, 1947-
    Is it in your genes? : the influence of genes on common disorders and diseases
that affect you and your family / Philip R. Reilly.
        p. cm.
    Includes bibliographical references and index.
    ISBN 0-87969-719-9 (hardcover : alk. paper)—ISBN 0-87969-721-0 (paperback : alk.
paper)
    1. Medical genetics--Popular works. I. Title.
    RB155.R42 2004
    599.93'5--dc22
                                    2004002458

10 9 8 7 6 5 4 3 2

For Nancy and the children

Contents

Preface

Most people think of genetic diseases as rare conditions caused by mutations in a single gene that generally afflict children. This impression is 20 years out of date. It's simply no longer accurate. Extraordinary advances in our understanding of human genetics are changing how physicians think about the causes of disease. Today, we know that virtually *all* the diseases and disorders that afflict humans are influenced by the genes with which they were born.

We have entered the era of Genetic Medicine. It is a new field, still in its infancy; but over the next couple of decades, thanks to the success of the Human Genome Project and countless other research efforts, it will substantially change the nature of health care. We already know a great deal about the role of genes in many health problems ranging from the beginning of life (infertility and miscarriage) to infancy (birth defects and deafness) to childhood (autism and asthma) through adulthood (heart disease, cancers, and Alzheimer's disease). In many cases, our knowledge is not yet refined enough to use in the clinic, but we are rapidly advancing to the point where we will be able to translate these discoveries into new tests, new treatments, and new prevention strategies. As we cross that boundary, we will enter a new world which some scientists and physicians are already calling Personalized Medicine.

To successfully move genetic knowledge into mainstream medicine, both physicians and the lay public must be educated about the influence of genetic variation on human health and disease. Despite more than a decade of efforts to educate physicians, there has not been much progress. Indeed, it is often patients worried about their family history who drive physicians to think genetically.

I wrote this book to help people of all backgrounds understand the role of genes in health and disease. I hope it stimulates readers to ask physicians, nurses, and others involved in health care whether a problem in their family might be more strongly influenced by genes than the professionals might at first think. The countless conversations I have had with people over the years have convinced me that it is time for such questions. If we pursue the path to Personalized Medicine, we will travel to a new world of health care—one in which, ultimately, prevention will dominate therapy.

The core idea in Personalized Medicine is that both the maintenance of optimal health and the defeat of disease depend on understanding an individual's genetic makeup. Current knowledge suggests that at least 10% of the people who develop common chronic disorders do so in large part because of a genetic liability. This is a vast number of people. Just think. More than 60 million Americans have heart disease; more than 17 million have diabetes, more than 5 million have cancer, and at least 4 million have Alzheimer's disease. If we could avert or substantially delay the onset of these diseases in just 10%, we would be helping more than 8,500,000 people.

Over the past 25 years, I have had the privilege and pleasure of talking with hundreds of audiences about how a better understanding of the DNA molecule will change our world. Almost without exception after my lectures, a few people wait to speak privately with me. Invariably, they want to tell me about an illness or condition in their family and ask me about the risk they or their children face. They want to know whether they or their children are at increased genetic risk for a disorder their doctors do not think of as having a hereditary component. They want to know, "Is it in my genes?" In asking the question, they are more in tune with modern genetics than are many of their doctors.

I wrote this book to help people answer some of the more common versions of that question. "My 22-year-old daughter was recently diagnosed with manic-depressive disorder. What are the risks to my other kids?" "My father died of a heart attack at 45. What's my risk?" "My sister has just been diagnosed at age 35 with multiple sclerosis. What does that mean for me?" These are three of the questions I have recently been asked most often recently. They are not easy to answer. However, in each case the person asking the question correctly guessed that family genes are important. Imagine, for example, that you have just learned that your sister has been diagnosed with multiple sclerosis (MS). What, if any, evidence is there that MS arises in part due to the genetic background of the afflicted individual? It turns out there is much reason to suspect that a few genes play a major (however murky and complicated) role in predisposing people to MS. Indeed, as I write this, several leading research groups have joined forces to track down the MS genes. Is this because they think that MS is a single-gene disorder that obeys the Mendelian rules of inheritance (like Huntington's disease and cystic fibrosis)—rules that are taught in high school about the transmission of traits from one generation to the next? No. MS is not a single-gene disorder. However, several facts, especially that relatives of people who develop MS are at increased risk for the disorder, provide powerful evidence that certain gene variants (alleles) increase one's risk. In a few years, we will probably know a lot about these variants, and a few years beyond that, we may have some new medicines to treat the disorder. And we will also have discovered other interventions to reduce risk among those born with predisposing genes. Today, in counseling persons with an affected relative, we can provide empirical risk figures based on studies of hundreds of similar families.

The questions about a serious disorder like MS resemble questions about scores of other disorders and conditions in which genes are important. This book is based on my review of what we know today about the role that genes play in common conditions, disorders, and diseases that occur throughout the human life cycle. From nearly 200 candidates, all of which I chose because I'd been asked about them, I selected nearly 100. Together they account for about 95% of the non-traumatic causes of death and disability in the United States. I then investigated what experts have learned to date about the role that genes play in their origin and how that knowledge can be translated into statements about risk. For each condition, I briefly summarize what is known; for some conditions, I discuss where the research is headed. Where possible, I offer the best current estimates concerning risk to relatives. In some cases, the best I could do was to comment in the most general way about the genetic contribution; in other cases, I was able to draw on family history to offer helpful empirical risk estimates.

A word of caution. This book is no substitute for good medical care or sound genetic counseling. I hope it will stimulate people to ask questions of their doctors that they might not normally ask. I also hope it will provoke physicians to think in new ways, to ask new questions of their colleagues, and to value the role of genetic risk assessment and genetic counseling in modern medicine.

Acknowledgments

In this book I have taken on an extraordinarily broad field, fully recognizing that I can provide only a superficial discussion of its many topics. No person can rationally claim a deep familiarity with the full range of information encompassed by genetic medicine.

As is so often the case when one distills information from a grand field and offers it to the general reader, I frequently consulted leading texts for guidance. I want to recognize the superb resource that they provide, and urge physicians (in particular) to use them. I have been greatly helped by the massive and superbly constructed text, Emery and Rimoin's *Principles and Practice of Medical Genetics* (Fourth Edition; Churchill Livingstone 2002), edited by David L. Rimoin, J. Michael Connor, Reed E. Pyeritz, and Bruce R. Korf. The scores of scientists who contributed chapters also deserve my thanks. I owe another note of thanks to Richard A. King, Jerome I. Rotter, and Arno G. Motulsky, the three editors of *The Genetic Basis of Common Diseases* (Second Edition, Oxford University Press 2002). Both books often pointed me to primary sources that I read in an effort to distill the many brief sections in my book. Given the nature of my text and mission, it seemed pointless to cite each time I relied on a text that itself was a collection of superbly synthesized chapters.

The staff at Cold Spring Harbor Laboratory Press, led by the able and erudite John Inglis, have with this book (as with an earlier work of mine) been tremendously supportive. Naming names risks omission. Nevertheless, I owe my thanks to Pat Barker, Mary Cozza, Denise Weiss, Jody Tresidder, and Susan Schaefer, and it is a pleasure to say so.

My wife, Nancy, a nurse and a biologist, lent a helpful ear and gave good advice on how to communicate certain ideas. Thomas, Sarah, and Christopher occasionally did the same. Sarah, in particular, thought hard about cover art.

A Note about Technical Terminology

In this book, certain technical terms occur frequently and by necessity. What follows is intended to clarify their meaning.

A chromosome is a thread-like structure in the nucleus of a cell that anchors genes and other DNA. Human cells contain 23 pairs of chromosomes, one pair of which is the sex chromosomes that specify the gender of the individual concerned.

An autosome is a chromosome that is not concerned with determining sex.

Concordance is a measure of comparison used frequently in studies of the rates of disease in identical (monozygotic, MZ) versus fraternal (dizygotic, DZ) twins in order to assess the extent to which genetic factors are involved in the genesis of the disease.

Haplotype refers to a combination of two or more DNA variations which indicate that a block of DNA has been inherited as a unit.

Heritability is a measure of the degree to which the presence of a biological condition can be attributed to genes rather than to the environment. Heritability ranges from 0 to 1, and a measure of 0.5 or higher suggests a fairly strong genetic influence.

Heterozygosity refers to the common situation in which a person has inherited two different variations of a gene at some particular location.

Penetrance refers to the likelihood that an inherited mutation will produce a specific effect in its carriers.

Single-nucleotide polymorphisms (SNPs) are one-chemical-letter variations in the DNA sequence at a particular spot in the genome. There are several million of them, and they are valuable "flags" in finding genes and in indicating genetic differences between populations.

Is It in Your Genes?
Companion Web Site

Genetic medicine is advancing at high speed, with new findings appearing in the medical and scientific literature every month. To inform readers of this book about these advances, Dr. Reilly will contribute articles to the freely available Web site www.is-it-in-your-genes.org. The site will also contain links to other online resources of value to people seeking information about genetic influences on diseases and disorders. The site is planned to become available by August 2004.

Introduction: Genetic Medicine

Despite the immense amount of public interest in genetics, information about the role that genes play in common conditions and illnesses is not easily accessible to the average person. I wrote this book to build a bridge from the nation's molecular biology laboratories, research wards, and medical textbooks to its living rooms. Knowledge about the role of genes in health and disease need not be esoteric. Anyone who wants to can visit the world of genetic medicine. Those who do will discover that their suspicions are correct. Even complex conditions with obvious and important environmental factors do tend to cluster in families. This book is constructed in a manner that allows a reader to begin anywhere he or she wants. However, for those who know little about genes, it should be helpful to read the introductory material straight through.

How do genes shape risk for disease long before it occurs? There are several different ways in which genes can influence risk for and severity of chronic disorders. First are the *germ line* variants in the DNA of the egg, the sperm, or both, that are present from the moment of conception. The genes you are born with may include a variant of a gene that vastly increases your risk for disease. A dramatic example is breast cancer. About 5–10% of all the women who will develop breast cancer are born with a mutation that increases their lifetime risk for the disorder from about 10% to as high as 85%. These women have an alteration in a protein that in some way helps to maintain orderly cell division. As these women grow older, the risk that some of their aberrant cells will escape this protein monitor and become cancerous rises faster than it does in persons who do not have such mutations. In addition to two genes that strongly predispose individuals to breast (and ovarian) cancer, we know of six that predispose to colon can-

1

cer, more than a score that predispose to heart disease, a rapidly growing number that predispose those who carry one or more of them to diabetes, three that cause rare forms of Alzheimer's disease, and one common variant that significantly increases the risk for the garden-variety form of this disorder. Overall, we know of scores of genes with variants that increase risk for dozens of diseases most people do not think of as genetic. The list is growing steadily and will continue to do so for many years.

A second way that genes increase risk for disease is *somatic* mutation—changes in genes that develop during an individual's lifetime. During its life, any cell with a nucleus (i.e., all the cells in the body except red blood cells) can acquire mutations that are passed on to daughter cells when it divides. If a certain group of mutations accumulates in a cell, the cell can become cancerous. *All* cancers are genetic disorders. They are clonal in origin; i.e., they start from a single cell that no longer obeys the fundamental rules concerning orderly cell division. As somatic mutations accumulate over the years, a cell may escape its natural growth controls and become cancerous. In general, one can think of cancer as the end result of the accumulation of somatic mutations in a particular cell. During the 1990s, Dr. Bert Vogelstein and his colleagues from Johns Hopkins University figured out the mutational events that transform a normal cell in the colon into the founder of an aggressive bowel cancer.

A few "strongly predisposing" genes dramatically increase the risk for many different diseases, but there are many more (most still not yet identified) gene variants that more modestly increase the threshold of risk. It is sometimes hard to draw a clear distinction between these groups. The latter, which is the most difficult to study, is almost certainly the more important because the gene variants are common. Indeed, it is virtually certain that all of us are born with some of these variants. They are the most difficult to study because the contribution of each one to disease risk is relatively small. That is, it is exceedingly difficult to tease out and quantify the risk associated with them. It will also be difficult (but not impossible) to devise ways to curtail the specific risk that each confers.

Common variations in thousands of different genes can shape the manner in which the body functions in many different situations. Gene variations can sharply affect one's fertility, a woman's risk for miscarriage, a baby's risk for heart malformations, a toddler's risk for recurrent severe ear infections or asthma, a child's ability to learn to read, a middle-aged adult's risk of sudden death from a disordered heart rhythm, or an elder's risk of stroke. In most instances, these genes are involved in a complex minuet. Interacting over time with other genes and environmental factors, predisposing genes (depending on their level of influence) can act as minor or major risk factors. They can raise or lower a person's risk of disease, alter the trajectory of disease, influence its severity, and shape the response to treatment. Let me give an example.

Most people today are aware of the major risk factors for coronary artery disease. They realize that male gender, a positive family history, diabetes, high blood pressure, high blood lipid levels, smoking, and a sedentary life style are all important risk factors. What comes as a big surprise is that about 40% of all the people who will die in the United States this year of a heart attack do not (except for gender, which is, of course, determined by genes) have any of the major risk factors. Put another way, despite all the research devoted to understanding the causes of coronary artery disease, the risk factors we know apparently contribute to only about 60% of the heart attack deaths that occur each year. Although there are as-yet-undiscovered environmental risk factors, a rapidly growing body of evidence suggests that much of the risk that is still to be determined will ultimately be attributed to gene variants. A prime example of this is that, thanks to work led by Dr. Paul Ridker at Harvard, we now understand that chronic low-grade inflammation is a major contributor to risk for heart disease. Ridker has shown that levels of a protein called CRP strongly correlate with risk for heart attacks. Production of that protein (which is made in the liver) differs substantially among people, depending on which versions of several genes they inherited.

A powerful example of how a small variation in a single gene can dramatically affect human health involves a cancer drug called 6-mercaptopurine, which is used to treat acute lymphoblastic leukemia in children. Some children who develop the disease happen also to have been born with a variation in the gene that codes for an enzyme called thiopurine methyltransferase, which metabolizes that medicine. In some people, the variant profoundly reduces the body's ability to break down this dangerously powerful drug. For those patients, a normal dose of the drug can so depress bone marrow function that it is itself life-threatening. It is now a standard of care to perform genetic testing on individuals to look for this variant before administering 6-mercaptopurine.

How do geneticists discover genes that increase the risk for disease? There are several different approaches, and new variations are being invented all the time. Three kinds of gene-sleuthing studies dominated research during most of the 20th century: twin studies, adoption studies, and family studies. Twin studies take advantage of the fact that identical (monozygotic or MZ) twins have identical genomes (sets of genes) whereas fraternal (dizygotic or DZ) twins share only half their genes. Thus, assuming relatively similar environments (an assumption that may not always be appropriate), if both members of many MZ twin pairs develop a disease more often than do both members of many DZ twin pairs, one can infer that genes explain the higher concordance rate. For example, several different studies showed that on average when one identical twin developed schizophrenia, in 40% of the cases the other identical twin did, too. But when fraternal—nonidentical—twins were studied, only 10% developed the disorder along with their sibling. Under these circumstances, one could draw a strong inference that there is a significant genetic component to this disease, even though the gene or genes involved might be unknown. On the other hand, because only 40% of the co-twins in the MZ group became ill, environmental factors, also unknown, play an important role, too. When the concordance rate for a disease among MZ twin pairs approaches 100%, the role of environmental factors diminishes and the putative role of genes soars.

Adoption studies (historically often done in Scandinavia because of relevant record-keeping) compare the presence of disease in adopted individuals with the prevalence of the same disorder in their rearing parents and their biological parents. Higher prevalence among the biological parents strongly implies a genetic contribution to the risk. If diabetes is found in 20% of the birth parents of adopted individuals who developed diabetes in mid-life, but in only 5% of the adoptive parents, one can infer that heredity has played an important role in setting the threshold of risk.

Family studies compare the prevalence of disease among first-degree relatives of a group of affected persons with its prevalence among first-degree relatives of a control group. If the disease is much more common among the first-degree relatives of those with disease than among the equivalent relatives of the control group, one can infer that genes are an important risk factor. In this book, I often mention such studies because they yield important clues about the role of genes in diseases that have not yet been widely recognized by physicians as having a genetic component. I also discuss newer approaches to understanding the role of genes in disease that have been made possible by extraordinary advances in molecular biology during the last 20 years.

How do geneticists prove that certain genes are risk factors in complex disorders like diabetes or heart disease? One of the major dividends of the Human Genome Project is the development of powerful methods we now have for hunting genes that influence risks for disease at a level much too subtle to discern 25 years ago. Prior to the advent of molecular biology (about 40 years ago), geneticists could use the kind of empirical studies discussed above to establish the heritability of diseases and conditions. That is, they could amass evidence to rule genetic factors in or out. If they were ruled in, their likely overall significance could be estimated, but the predisposing gene or genes could not be identified. Today we have the tools to track the genes down, clone (isolate and copy) them, and, eventually, study how the proteins made by those genes affect risk for a particular illness or even unusual wellness. For example, scientists are currently studying the DNA of hundreds of persons who have lived 100 years to see whether they can isolate longevity genes. One way to do this is to find out whether there are gene variants that are much more (or less) common in centenarians than in a group of people in their seventies. There are many reasons why these gene *association* studies are difficult to conduct, and the early efforts sometimes were too small to yield robust evidence. However, the research community is now conducting much larger, statistically more powerful studies.

This book is organized according to the human life cycle, from conception to death. In each part—pregnancy, infancy, childhood, and adulthood—I talk about the most important health problems and discuss what we know about the role played by genes. I start almost every section of this book with a question like one of the hundreds that I have been asked. Where it is possible to do so, I have provided some firm data on risk within families. It is important to remember that *Is It in Your Genes?* is a work in progress. It includes speculations about the prospects for new discoveries and guesses about what we can fairly infer from the current state of knowledge. Also, even if I rewrite this book just a year from now, I will have to make significant revisions in many sections.[1] That is great news! There is a vast amount of clinical genetic research under way, and there is no chance that it will soon decrease. More importantly, this book is a dialog with interested persons about the role genes play in health. I hope for many readers this book will stimulate an ongoing interest in this subject.

[1]*Publisher's Note:* See page xvi for information on a Web site that will provide Dr Reilly's updates on the material discussed in this book.

Genes and Mutations

Each human begins life as the union of a sperm cell with an egg. The single fertilized cell contains two sets of genes, one from each parent. In the language of genetics, the two haploid cells—egg and sperm, each with only half the number of chromosomes found in a normal cell—fuse to create a diploid organism; one with the full number of chromosomes. Humans and almost every other creature have two copies of each gene. The genome contains the full set of instructions on how to organize a human, to order fetal development, to reset major physiological pathways at birth, to control all aspects of growth, to orchestrate the changes of adolescence, and even to program the descent into old age. My favorite example of the power of the genetic software is that in the course of just a few months in the womb, genes direct the organization of trillions of cells into the some 300 tissues and a dozen organ systems that will constitute a new baby.

What is a gene? For years it was conceived of as an abstract unit of information that was transmitted faithfully through the germ—or reproductive—cells. This concept was first grasped in the 1860s by Gregor Mendel, a monk whose painstaking study of the transmission of certain traits in peas led him to the basic laws of inheritance. Although Mendel published his discovery, its revolutionary nature was not initially appreciated. It was not until 1900, when several European scientists, working independently, rediscovered Mendel's laws, that modern genetics was born. Even so, for the next 30 years the concept of a gene remained abstract, for we knew nothing about its physical structure. In 1927 the great geneticist, H. J. Muller, discovered that X-rays could create mutations in fruit flies. This work (which earned him a Nobel Prize) was a big step toward understanding the physical reality of genes.

In the 1940s, the meaning of the gene was refined, based on the discovery (made originally in fruit flies and yeast) that every gene codes for (provides the blueprint for the construction of) a protein. This was called the "one gene–one enzyme" theory and earned its inventors, George Beadle and Edward Tatum, a Nobel Prize. In the late 1940s, it was settled once and for all that genes are composed of DNA (deoxyribonucleic acid). In 1953, James Watson and Francis Crick elucidated the double-helical structure of the molecule, another Nobel-winning discovery that has been ranked as the leading biological event of the 20th century. In the 1960s, we learned how DNA, which has an alphabet of only four letters—four kinds of chemical components named adenine (A), guanine(G), cytosine(C), and thymidine (T)—was able to write the genetic text for all organisms. Nature could use such a puny alphabet because the text is composed in triplets. Four letters can be used to construct 64 separate triplets (AAA, AAC, etc.). This is more than enough information to provide the instructions for the 20 different amino acids (protein building blocks) that are assembled in different sequences (often hundreds of amino acids in length) to make the thousands of different proteins that, quite literally, run our lives.

Today, thanks to the work of many researchers over several decades, we know the physical structure of a gene in intimate detail. All human genes are composed of DNA sequences containing stretches called "control elements" and others called "exons." Enzymes within the cell act on the control elements to determine the timing and level of gene activity. An active gene permits the DNA in its exons to be transcribed (read by a set of enzymes) to form a molecule called messenger RNA. Messenger RNA, once formed, moves from the nucleus to the cytoplasm—the jelly-like part of the cell that surrounds the nucleus—where it provides the template for making the specific protein the DNA encoded. Proteins are vital to cell function, and many of the most important human diseases may arise because key proteins are made in such a way that they do not organize themselves into the proper shape.

In the late 1960s and 1970s, molecular biologists discovered ways to cut DNA with extreme precision. Almost overnight these chemical tools (called restriction endonucleases) permitted scientists to conduct studies that would have been impossible even to contemplate a few years earlier. The tools revolutionized the ability to figure out the location of a gene on a chromosome—the science of gene mapping—but did not tell us anything about what a gene does.

In the 1980s, new tools that permitted scientists to discern the letter-by-letter sequence of genes (thanks to advances made in the mid 1970s that garnered Nobel Prizes for Frederick Sanger and Walter Gilbert), made it possible to dream about decoding the complete genetic text of humans or any other organism. However, the dream only became even remotely possible after the discovery and development in the mid 1980s of a technique called the polymerase chain reaction (PCR), a method of making copies of segments of DNA billions of times over, which made analysis much easier. This led to a Nobel Prize for its inventor, Kary Mullis. The ambitious decision to launch the $3 billion Human Genome Project was in large part based on the scientific consensus that a sustained application of these tools could achieve the goal. Among other things, its successful completion permitted the studies that have stimulated me to write this book.

It is now possible to track down the mutations in the genes that are the direct cause of single-gene disorders or which significantly influence risks for the more complicated diseases of adulthood and old age. The Human Genome Project has moved genetics from the study of rare diseases of childhood to center stage in the understanding of virtually every disease. By the 1990s, scientists were able to cut and paste genes, even to move them from one species to another. Such transferred genes still direct the construction of the same protein, but they work in a different factory and their products may be used for different purposes. Although still in its infancy, genetic engineering will one day lead to gene therapy—the delivery of new genes to counter the action of those with harmful mutations.

What is a mutation? Simply put, a mutation is any change in the DNA. What causes the change? Mutations can arise due to the action of some physical agent such as radiation (all life in earth is constantly bombarded by various forms of radiation, mostly from outer space), a chemical, or a virus. They can also occur because of some failure of the enzymatic machinery in the nucleus that is responsible for copying the DNA before the cell divides. There are many kinds of mutations. A single change in a DNA letter (say from A to T) may alter the coding instruction for an amino acid and possibly render the protein dysfunctional, resulting in a potentially fatal genetic disease. Segments of DNA may also be deleted, duplicated, inverted, inappropriately silenced, or even moved to a new location within the genome. Mutations can also arise because of copying errors. In the last decade, scientists have discovered that a dozen brain disorders arise because a DNA triplet in a particular gene is copied too often, an event that results in a dysfunctional protein.

Most DNA mutations are not harmful. There are two basic reasons for this. Mutations can occur anywhere in the genome, but only a small percentage of our DNA actually codes for proteins. DNA changes in the noncoding regions are usually innocuous. Even when they occur in the coding regions, many single-letter DNA changes are not harmful. This is either because the mutations do not alter a protein's structure or because they cause a change that does not significantly affect how it performs its work in the cells. If they are common enough, these variants are called polymorphisms.

Mutations can be either dominant (producing a condition even if inherited from only one parent) or recessive (producing a condition only if inherited from both parents). A single dominant mutation (or a recessive mutation in the same gene in both the egg and the sperm) can be the cause of devastating disease. Just a tiny error in the genetic code, a change in one or a few nucleotides out of the roughly 3,100,000,000 nucleotides in each sperm and egg, can lead to the birth of a child who might (for example) be born with severe mental retardation. Geneticists have identified several thousand disorders caused by such single-gene mutations. Fortunately, all but a few are quite rare. In this book, I do not discuss these disorders. Rather, I focus on the influence of gene variants on the common disorders, ranging from those that affect human development to those that influence common childhood disorders to those that will debilitate or kill most of us unless we learn new ways to prevent or treat them.

The genes, acting through the proteins for which they code, interact with many other proteins inside a cell. These interactions are in turn influenced by the cell's larger environments—organ, organism, home, family, climate, and the like. Together, they shape the course of our lives in trillions of unknowable interactions that result in health or disease. In any given cell at any given moment, in response to the many influences, a particular permutation of genes is "on," producing proteins that operate the cell. We share many of our genes with other people, but individual variations in the expression of our genes affect our risk for disease as well as (in some cases) the course taken by a disease once it develops.

How many genes does it take to make a human? For more than five decades, the working estimate was 100,000 genes per sperm or egg cell. However, as we have drawn near to completion of the sequence of the human genome and as the rules for defining the physical nature of the gene have become firmer, it appears that 26,000 is much closer to the facts. That is still a pretty big number. On the other hand, a mouse has about the same number of genes. Even more disconcertingly, humans appear to have only about twice as many genes as does a fruit fly, even though our physiology is so much more complex. The explanation probably lies in how our gene function is regulated and how our proteins interact rather than in the absolute number of genes with which we are endowed. Recent comparisons of chimpanzee and human genomes suggest that over the last 1,000,000 years, some human genes have changed much more rapidly than have their chimp counterparts.

After reading this brief introduction to genetics, you are ready to explore the role of genes in your risk for disease throughout your life. Although it is organized to track the human life cycle, this book need not be read from start to finish. There is no family on earth that is not touched by at least several of the nearly 100 conditions, disorders, and diseases that I discuss. Depending on your family history, some disorders will interest you more than others. It makes sense to read about them first.

PART 1

Pregnancy

My sister and her husband are infertile. They have seen several experts and spent a fortune on fancy tests that have not provided an answer. Am I at increased risk?

Infertility is defined as the lack of pregnancy after one year of unprotected intercourse. There are many known causes of infertility and, almost certainly, there are many more not yet elucidated. Infertility is an all too common problem. In the developed nations it is estimated that about one couple out of six is either infertile or subfertile. Over the last 20 years, there has been a dramatic increase in our knowledge of the causes of infertility, especially in men. Currently, experts think that female factors cause about 45–50% of cases, male factors cause about 30–35%, and in about 20% of infertile couples, both individuals have reduced fertility.

Infertility is an extraordinarily complicated subject. There are literally dozens of known causes of female infertility, but the most important is also the most simple—age. Women in their late thirties are only about one-fifth as fertile as they were in their mid-twenties. The reasons for this are not clearly understood. Among the obvious, relatively common, physical causes of infertility are anatomical abnormalities, pelvic inflammatory disease, and endometriosis (discussed separately). In this section, I briefly discuss only some of the genetic causes. Individually, most of these are uncommon. However, it is likely that among the many women for whom there is

13

not yet a satisfactory explanation for infertility, it will turn out that as-yet-undetermined genetic factors are a significant cause.

Perhaps the best known (but by no means common) chromosomal cause of infertility in women is the absence of all or part of a sex chromosome or the disruption of a sex chromosome through translocation of part of it to some other chromosome (a condition known as Turner syndrome). The severity of the clinical syndrome varies with the precise nature of the chromosomal loss. For example, some women have mosaics of two cell lines, one of which has a normal X and one of which lacks all or part of the other X. Such unusual situations will only come to light as part of a full workup of infertility. Turner syndrome is present in about 1 in 2500 women.

At least four single-gene disorders are known to cause infertility through inhibiting normal production of hormones from the hypothalamus, a region in the brain that controls the production of sex hormones. Two of these involve genes that, when impaired, cause severe obesity. Together the four account for less than 1% of infertility. Similarly, about 10 rare single-gene disorders have been described that, among other things, cause infertility by impairing ovarian function. For example, about 1 in 300 women carries a mutation in a gene that can cause their sons to have a form of mental retardation called Fragile X syndrome. For unknown reasons, some of these women have reduced fertility.

Perhaps the most prevalent heavily genetically influenced cause of infertility is polycystic ovarian syndrome (PCOS). This condition is common, complicated, and confusing. By some estimates, PCOS is found in 4% of women of reproductive age. It is definitely associated with reduced fertility as well as with a significantly increased risk (up to 7 times the general risk) of type II diabetes. The disorder varies greatly in severity. The classic physical features are irregular periods, extra body hair, acne, and ovarian cysts. Excess male hormones are often present in the blood. The condition tends to worsen with weight gain.

There are several rare single-gene causes of PCOS, such as a condition called 21-hydroxylase deficiency. Together these account for only about 5% of cases. It has long been known that essential PCOS (the 95% of cases of uncertain cause) clusters in families. In the original genetic study (1968), a researcher found that irregular periods were far more common in sisters of patients than in an age-matched control group of women. The few twin studies carried out have shown more concordance among identical than nonidentical twin pairs. A large Norwegian study in 1989 found that 15% of the sisters of affected women had irregular periods.

The genetics of essential PCOS has been hard to study for two main reasons: (1) The presentation of the disorder is so variable that it is hard to agree on a diagnosis and (2) there are probably many causes. Nevertheless, the best guess is that there is at least one highly penetrant, dominantly acting gene that accounts for a significant fraction of all cases, which neither genetic linkage studies nor candidate gene studies have yet found. The best overall guess is that sisters of affected individuals have a 10% risk of also being affected. However, family history-taking can greatly modify such risk estimates, for there are surely some women whose risk is much closer to 50%. For all at-risk persons, maintaining a healthy weight is important.

Until recently, the most common cause of genetic infertility in men was thought to be Klinefelter's syndrome, a disorder characterized by the presence of an extra X chromosome in all the individual's cells, that is present in about 1 in 600 boys. Teenagers and young men with Klinefelter's syndrome have a variety of problems, the most severe of which are a tendency toward the body shape of a woman, lack of muscle mass, abnormal breast development, behavioral problems, and, in some cases, reduced intelligence. When those with Klinefelter's syndrome are excluded, studies of men with extremely low sperm counts have found chromosomal abnormalities in about 4% of cases.

The discovery that deletions in the Y chromosome were associated with infertility was made in 1976. Over the last decade, researchers have demonstrated that about 5–10% of all infertile men are missing a portion of their Y chromosome. It seems the more they look, the more scientists find Y deletions in infertile men. In 2003, a research group led by Dr. David Page at the Whitehead Institute reported that about 2% of men carry a 1.6 million base-pair deletion that is transmitted from father to son, but is also associated (at the population level) with reduced fertility!

Such microdeletions cannot be seen with a microscope, but they can be defined through DNA analysis. Multiple clinical studies have established that microdeletions (the loss of hundreds of thousands of DNA base pairs) in the region called Yq11 are common among men with little or no sperm production. DNA analysis is fast becoming a routine part of the evaluation of infertile men. If a man is found to be infertile due to a deletion of part of the Y chromosome, there is little reason to suspect that his brothers will be similarly affected. With the exception of the deletion described at the Whitehead Institute, such deletions are usually new mutations.

In the mid-1990s, infertility researchers developed a new technique called intracytoplasmic sperm injection (ICSI) to help men with very low sperm count become fathers. With ICSI, a single viable sperm can be injected directly into an egg, which can then be placed in the uterus. Unfortunately, ICSI creates the disconcerting situation in which clinicians assisting infertile men in the conception of children foster the births of sons who will also be infertile.

Another important development has been the finding that men whose infertility is caused by congenital absence of the vas deferens (CBAVD) often carry two mutations in the pair of genes responsible for cystic fibrosis. Current estimates are that a gene variant known as the 5T allele, with which about 1 in 10 persons is born, and other mild alleles of the cystic fibrosis (CF) gene are present in 80% of men with CBAVD. This form of infertility is now regarded as an incomplete form of CF.

Unhappily, for many (perhaps 20–25%) couples, the cause of infertility still goes unexplained. Advances in genetics, especially concerning the study of the Y chromosome, have begun to provide answers for a small, but steadily growing, percentage of couples. We can expect genetic research to identify many more causes.

For obvious reasons, infertility is not usually found to run in families. However, if one has a brother or sister who is infertile, it is certainly possible that if a genetic cause is identified, it could be relevant to other family members. A thorough infertility workup must include a search for causes such as those enumerated here. The simple answer to the question posed at the top of this section is that we lack sufficient knowledge to provide much guidance. Given that a thorough workup was non-diagnostic, it is highly unlikely that there is a significantly quantifiable increased risk to the closely related couple.

ENDOMETRIOSIS

My mother and one of her sisters have endometriosis. How big is my risk?

Endometriosis is the presence of endometrial (uterine) tissue outside the uterus. Although it can be found almost anywhere in the pelvic space, it is

Table 1. *Endometriosis: Studies showing genetic influence*

Study	Mothers (%)	Sisters (%)	Controls (%)
Simpson 1980	5.9	8.1	0.9
Lamb 1986	6.2	3.8	2.0
Moen/Magnus 1993	3.9	4.8	0.6

Incidence of endometriosis among first-degree relatives of patients compared to control groups. Adapted, with permission, from King R.A., Rotter J.I., and Motulsky A.G., eds. 2002. *The genetic basis of common diseases*, 2nd edition. Oxford University Press, United Kingdom.

especially common to find endometrial tissue growing on the ovaries, behind the vagina, and on the pelvic wall. It is difficult to tell what percentage of women with endometriosis experience discomfort. However, for many affected women endometriosis is a cause of chronic, often significant, pain. At least 1% of adult women have endometriosis, and it is likely that the real prevalence is closer to 3%. It is about as common in blacks as it is in whites. For a long time endometriosis was thought to be unusually prevalent among white, upperclass, compulsive women. Today, a more objective statement would be that it is found more commonly among women who delay childbearing. The consensus risk factors for this problem are age, increased exposure to menstruation (due to more frequent, shorter, cycles), lack of childbearing, and retrograde menstruation. In addition to chronic discomfort, endometriosis can cause pain during intercourse. It may be the single most important cause of infertility, by some estimates accounting for 40% of female cases. Some experts have estimated that it is a (sometimes) reversible cause of infertility or subfertility in up to 10% of all women.

Endometriosis has long been known to cluster in families. At least four studies since 1980 have found that first-degree relatives of affected women are about 5–6 times more likely to report that they too have endometriosis than are first-degree relatives of the affected women's husbands (who were used as control groups). The few twin studies of endometriosis have been highly concordant. In a study in Iceland, of 18 women with endometriosis who were identical twins, 16 of the co-twins also had the disorder. The relative risk of endometriosis to a first-degree relative is sufficiently strong that in some families the disorder could be due to the action of a single dominantly behaving gene.

The search for gene variants that predispose to endometriosis began in earnest in the late 1990s. The most important effort was spearheaded by the Oxford Endometriosis Gene Study (OXEGENE). Researchers at Oxford University gathered hundreds of families with two or more sisters, both with surgically proven endometriosis. They collected DNA samples from the women and their parents and looked for DNA markers that appeared more often in persons with the disorder. In 2001, the Oxford group joined forces with an Australian research group that was pursuing the same quarry to launch the International Endogene Study (IES). By mid-2002, the IES had recruited more than 1100 families with two affected sisters and more than 1200 triads (affected women and both their parents) for gene-hunting studies. The research team has found evidence that there are several major predisposing genes in the human genome, but it has not yet cloned (isolated) any. In the meantime, other groups using a candidate gene approach have found impressive evidence that may lead to the indictment of several genes. In 2002, a Japanese group showed that a variant of a gene called CYP19 was more prevalent in a group of affected women than in a healthy control group. These and several similar reports need to be replicated. In 2003, a Finnish group performed a genome scan on 31 families with multiply affected women. They found evidence for predisposing loci on 7q, 8q, and 1p, although these data must be regarded as preliminary.

Currently, it is difficult to quantify how individual risk is altered by a positive family history. The Iceland study suggests that sisters of affected women have a fivefold greater risk for developing endometriosis than do women without a positive family history. If one has an affected mother and an affected sister, one could impute an even higher risk figure. It is likely that a decade from now there will be a genetic test to predict risk for endometriosis. In the meantime, what practical action should a woman consider based on a positive family history? If she has an affected sister, she may wish to have her children earlier than she might have otherwise considered.

UTERINE FIBROIDS

My sister has uterine fibroids. Am I likely to develop them?

Uterine fibroids, noncancerous tumors arising in the smooth muscle cells in the uterine wall, are common. Although they may be benign, they also can cause a host of problems, ranging from uterine bleeding to infertility. As many as one in ten adult women in their twenties has at least one fibroid. That percentage increases with age until menopause. African-American women are more than twice as likely to develop fibroids as are white women. A small percentage of women with fibroids have many, large tumors, the sheer mass of which can cause infertility.

Several epidemiological surveys agree that close female relatives of women with uterine fibroids are two to three times more likely also to develop them than are women who do not have affected mothers or sisters. Since fibroids are in general quite common (found in about 8–10% of the population), this suggests that a sister of an affected woman may have a lifetime risk of about 20–25%. This does not necessarily mean that she has an equivalent risk of infertility.

Although there are reports that fibroids run in families in a manner that suggests the action of a single gene, so far scientists have found only one gene that definitely can predispose women to this uncomfortable condition. One of several important genetic studies of uterine fibroids is being conducted by the Center for Uterine Fibroids at Brigham and Women's Hospital in Boston. In 2003, the center was about halfway to its goal of enrolling 600 families in which at least two sisters were diagnosed with this condition. By screening the DNA from affected individuals (using a statistical analysis called the sib-pair method), the researchers hope to find stretches of DNA that are present in both sisters more often than expected by chance. Depending on the strength of the association, this could pinpoint a small region in which a predisposing gene lies.

Another approach that some of the scientists in Boston are taking is to intensively study the genes in a region of the long arm of chromosome 7. Deletions of that region are unusually common in the tumor tissue. Yet another group is studying the DNA of similar tumors, focusing on a region on chromosome 12 that is often abnormally rearranged.

In 2002, a group of scientists from the Multiple Leiomyoma (the medical name for fibroids) Consortium reported that through detailed genomic screening of 22 families in England and Finland in whom uterine fibroids were part of a dominantly inherited condition, they had discovered a causative gene on the long arm of chromosome 1. The gene, called FH, codes for a protein called fumarate dihydratase (FH) that is important in a key energy pathway. The scientists sequenced (read all the DNA letters in) the FH gene in 42 patients and found a mutation in 25. In comparison, the gene sequences of 150 normal controls had no mutations. There is strong evidence that FH is one of many genes that act as "tumor suppressors"; i.e., they maintain order in cell division and growth. Thus, prevalence of fibroids in women in whom the gene is dysfunctional makes sense. Although it is highly unlikely that defects in this gene cause any more than a tiny percentage of fibroids, this advance may provide a new avenue for therapeutic research.

CONSANGUINITY

Do marriages between first cousins face a greater chance of having babies with genetic disorders?

Consanguinity is the term used to define marriage between blood relatives. Until relatively recently, consanguineous matings were common among humans, and in certain cultures, they remain so today. For most of the thousands of years of their evolution, the ancestors of modern humans existed as small groups. Mate choice must have been highly limited. Beginning slowly about 10,000 years ago, coincident with the rise of agriculture and the growth of larger, stable communities, non-consanguineous mar-

Table 2. *Consanguinity: Two studies showing high mortality in offspring of cousin marriages*

Region and outcome	First-cousin Marriage	Second-cousin Marriage	No Consanguinity
Morbihan			
Stillbirth/neonatal death	51/461	23/309	72/1628
	11%	7.6%	4.4%
Death in early childhood	64/410	32/286	138/1556
	15.6%	11.2%	8.9%
Loir-et-Cher			
Stillbirth/neonatal death	18/282	11/240	36/1117
	6.4%	4.6%	3.2%
Death in early childhood	32/264	17/229	60/1081
	12.1%	7.4%	5.6%

These studies were conducted many decades ago. Today the mortality rates would be lower. Adapted, with permission, from Morton N.E., Crow J.F., and Muller H.J. 1956. An estimate of the mutational damage in man from data on consanguineous marriages. *Proceedings of the National Academy of Science* **42**: 855–863.

riages, mostly in a pattern in which young women left their village of origin, became dominant. However, even as recently as 200 years ago, before the advent of modern transportation, most marriages occurred between individuals who had been born within a few miles of each other, and many of whom could trace a biological relationship.

Today, there are still large groups of people living in cultures that encourage consanguineous marriages. This is especially true in certain parts of the Middle East and the Indian subcontinent, where both uncle–niece and first-cousin marriages are viewed as preserving and strengthening family structure. In the United States and Europe, first-cousin marriages are discouraged by religious dogma and rule of law. In the Netherlands, Brazil, and the United States, the frequency is less than 1% of all marriages. Second-cousin marriages are generally accepted. Extensive studies dating from the 1950s demonstrate the wide range of cultural attitudes about first-cousin marriages. For example, not so long ago in rural Japan, about 16% of marriages were between cousins. Among the Andhra Pradesh people in rural India, the frequency was 33%. Today the rates in Japan are much lower. However, in rural Pakistan, first-cousin marriages are still common.

Consanguinity is important because the odds that first cousins (because it is the most common, the example I shall use) share the same allele (form of a gene) at any particular location in their two genomes is 1 in 8. Put another way, if one cousin carries an ancestral mutation, the odds that the other also does is 1 in 8. Assuming the mutation is found on only 1 in 50 chromosomes in a population, 1 in 25 persons will be a carrier (remember, chromosomes come in pairs). The risk of first cousins both having the mutation if one does is roughly three times higher than if a cousin with such a mutation marries outside the family. In fact, the risk appears to be lower than that, probably because a fair number of the mutations cause such early pregnancy loss that the pregnancy is not even recognized. Because the mutations in question are rare, even among first-cousin marriages the risk of having a child with a genetic disorder on this basis is in absolute terms quite low. The risk of a first-cousin marriage resulting in the birth of a child with a recognized genetic disease or congenital malformation is about 4–5%, while the risk to the general population is about 3%.

The general approach today in genetic counseling clinics is to characterize cousin marriages as carrying only a small degree of increased risk.

Nevertheless, it is important that cousins contemplating marriage have a thorough evaluation of family history to search for signs of risk of a single-gene disorder. Usually no such evidence can be found, a fact that does not, unfortunately, rule out the very small possibility that each pregnancy in their marriage will be at 1 in 4 risk for a rare recessive disorder.

RACE AND ETHNICITY

Is the risk for certain genetic disorders more common in certain ethnic and racial groups?

Here we confront two terms that defy precise definition. The concepts of race and ethnicity became scientifically important with the rise of physical anthropology in 19th-century Europe, coincident with the high water mark of colonialism. Although scientifically unsupportable assertions about the genetic inequality of the races largely dissipated by the mid-20th century, the concept of race has remained. Although it uses many fewer subdivisions than a century ago, physical anthropology still teaches that there are several major racial groups (Caucasoid, Negroid, Mongoloid, and Australoid), each in turn with subgroups.

Over the last several decades, advances in molecular biology have challenged racial typologies. Studies of how genes vary among racial groups have repeatedly found that there is much more variance within groups than among groups. Put another way, most of the genetic variation in our species seems to be contained within any identifiable subgroup.

The fact is that if we randomly obtain DNA from any two people on the planet, molecular analysis will show that their DNA sequence is 99.9% the same. On the other hand, given that the human genetic code is more than three billion letters long, these two persons will have several million differences. In the world of DNA, we both are profoundly alike and have easily recognizable differences. Perhaps someday widespread understanding of the similarity of our DNA sequences will help to quench the last embers of harmful racial typology.

The frequency of important genetic variants differs substantially among racial and some ethnic groups. It would be foolish to ignore that fact, for it sometimes leads to clinically important discoveries. Genes do not work alone. Their action occurs in the environment in which the individual lives. There has to be a good reason why a mutation known (when two copies are present) to cause a severe genetic disease is common in a particular racial group. One in 10 Africans carries a single mutation for sickle cell anemia because its presence protects the individual from malaria. Over the generations, the sickle cell mutation has become more common in the gene pool. In essence, nature has allowed some children to die of sickle cell disease so that many more would not die of malaria. From a population perspective, the trade-off worked.

The major reason that couples should be concerned about their racial or ethnic background is because of historic patterns of intermarriage. Couples who are both members of the same ethnic group may, because of history, be at higher risk for having children with one or more recessive disorders. Although the numbers and kinds of disorders vary by ethnic group, the issue of risk is almost universal. A full compilation of ethnic groups and the disorders for which they are at risk is beyond the scope of this book, but some examples will suffice.

Ashkenazi Jews (the heritage of more than 90% of the Jews in the United States) are at increased risk for bearing children with Tay-Sachs disease, Canavan disease, Gaucher disease, Nieman-Pick disease, adrenoleukosystrophy, familial dysautonomia, and Bloom syndrome. In addition, they are more likely to carry genes that predispose to breast cancer, a form of colon cancer, and inflammatory bowel disease. A cohort of French-Canadians is also at increased risk for Tay-Sachs disease. The Amish people of Pennsylvania and Ohio who have intermarried for many generations are at increased risk for a number of rare genetic disorders including glutaric academia, bipolar disorder, and a liver disease called Criggler-Najjar syndrome type 1. Several other disorders that affect the Amish have not yet even been characterized. Among the Finns, another historically inbred population group, there is an increased risk for a form of kidney disease called congenital nephrosis, a brain disease called neuronal ceroid lipofuscinosis, a lipid disorder that greatly increases the risk of heart disease, and many more. In the southwestern United States, the Pima Indians have what is probably the highest risk for diabetes in the world. Many ethnic groups whose geographic origin lies in the tropical climes are at increased risk for sickle cell anemia and β-thalassemia (another genetic disorder in which carriers are less vulnerable to malaria and affected persons have a severe blood disease). Across Asia, a severe blood disorder called α-thalassemia is far more common than in Europe. This is merely a sampling of the many ethnic groups known to be at increased risk for one or more disorders that are much less common in the general population.

Ethnicity is important to consider in counseling about reproductive risk. In the United States, couples of African-American background should be offered a screening test that detects the roughly 1 in 10 who are carriers of the sickle cell (and related) mutations. In addition, the woman should be offered a test for a genetic condition called G6PD deficiency. This X-linked recessive disorder (which usually does not cause medical problems for women because they have a second, protective X) can under certain circumstances cause red cells in men to break down, which leads to anemia. In severe forms of the disorder, men who are exposed to chemicals, including some that occur naturally in certain foods (fava beans), can experience sudden, severe red cell breakdown. G6PD deficiency is also common in people of Middle Eastern background, especially in Saudi Arabia.

In the last decade, the approach to screening Ashkenazi couples to see whether they carry a mutation for a recessive disorder has become quite advanced, with clinics offering a so-called Jewish panel of tests for the diseases named above. The list of ethnic groups does not end here. For example, Asian couples should be counseled about the risk of α- and β-thalassemia. Mutations in the gene responsible for cystic fibrosis are present in about 1 in 28 white persons (even higher among northern Europeans), a fact that has recently prompted suggestions for a new standard of care in the United States based on offering a CF carrier test regardless of the absence of a positive family history.

Overall, the basic genetic advice is straightforward. If two persons of the same ethnic background are planning to marry, they should ask a physician whether there are recessive genetic disorders for which they have an increased risk of carrying one allele and whether he or she recommends any genetic tests. For certain groups, like the Ashkenazim, there is a clear answer. For others, such as the Irish, there is not. In the end, it depends on the history of intermarriage.

RECURRENT PREGNANCY LOSS

My sister has had three miscarriages in three years. What are my risks?

Pregnancy loss (spontaneous abortion, SAB) is the death of an embryo or fetus before 20 weeks of gestation. SAB is a common event. A large num-

Table 3. *Pregnancy loss: Terms used to describe loss at different times*

Biochemical pregnancy: Positive maternal β-HCG test within 10 days of ovulation, but no further evidence of pregnancy.

Preclinical abortion: Abortion prior to 6 weeks due to failed implantation or disruption after implantation.

Blighted ovum: Empty gestational sac (usually diagnosed at 5–7 weeks).

Missed abortion: Fetal parts without heart activity in uterus beyond time of fetal death.

Intrauterine fetal death: Fetal demise after 20 weeks gestation, but before labor.

Adapted, with permission, from Rimoin D.I., Connor J.M., Pyeritz R.E., and Korf B.R. 2002. *Emery and Rimoin's principles and practice of medical genetics*, 4th edition. Churchill Livingstone, London; © Elsevier.

ber of studies have reported SAB rates ranging from 10% to nearly 50% of all pregnancies. However, if the definition of SAB is limited to clinically (as opposed to biochemically) recognized pregnancies, then only about 10–15% of pregnancies end in SAB. About 45% of these occur between 7 and 11 weeks. Thus, after week 12 the risk of SAB is closer to 5–7%. Fetal loss after 20 weeks, but before labor, is not viewed as an abortion; it is called an intrauterine fetal death.

The most common cause of miscarriage is chromosomal abnormalities in the embryo. Taken together, the many different kinds of chromosomal disorders cause more than half of all losses before the 12th week. Some studies suggest that they account for at least 60%, and a few suggest that they account for a much higher percentage. Studies of abortus material have shown that most of these abnormalities are due to an extra chromosome (a condition called trisomy), of which number 16 is the most common (chromosomes are numbered from 1 to 22 in descending order of size). Lack of an X chromosome is also a major cause. About 10% of early abortuses are triploid (they have an extra one of every chromosome).

Recurrent pregnancy loss is defined as the spontaneous loss of three pregnancies. Given how common the event is, about 2% of couples would be expected by chance to experience two losses, and about 1 in 300 couples would be expected to experience three. The fact that 1–2% of couples lose three pregnancies suggests that genetic or other risk factors may sometimes be at work. The two risk factors for pregnancy loss that are well recognized are a history of pregnancy loss and maternal age. By her early forties, a woman's risk of pregnancy loss approaches 50%, which is about 5 times higher than that faced by a woman in her mid-twenties.

Despite extensive study, there is no clear explanation for SAB in most couples. A relatively common cause is chromosomal. In somewhat less than 5% of these couples, one person has a "balanced translocation." In essence, this means that the individual has a normal amount of chromosomal material, but that two (or, rarely, more) chromosomes have been broken and rearranged with each other. The consequence of this is that the individual is at high risk for producing germ cells with an abnormal set of chromosomes. In 2003, a team of researchers reported that in a study of women who had lost three pregnancies, they had identified five who were missing a tiny piece of a chromosome near its center. The deletions are so small that they could not be uncovered with standard chromosome studies. If replicated, this discovery may represent a significant advance in identifying causative factors. There are a few rare single-gene disorders (for example, the neurogenetic disease, Rett syndrome) that are associated with SAB or intrauterine fetal death, but together they cause less than 1% of all SAB.

For some years, experts have thought that mild disorders in the body's blood-clotting pathways, variants that cause little harm to women, could increase the risk of miscarriage because of their impact on maternal–fetal circulation. In 2002, Dr. Raj Rai, an expert in reproductive medicine who works at the Imperial College in London, announced the results of research that strongly reinforces that suspicion. About 5% of white women have a genetic variant called Factor V Leiden (FVL). Dr. Rai conducted some of the first prospective studies of the influence of FVL on miscarriage. He compared the pregnancy outcomes of 25 carriers to that of 198 noncarriers; all 223 had already had three documented miscarriages. Among noncarriers, the live birth rate for their next pregnancy was nearly 50%, whereas among carriers, the live birth rate was only 11%. The finding is important for two reasons. Because FVL is common, it may explain a small, but important, fraction of miscarriages. For FVL carriers, treatment with blood thinner may reduce the risk of pregnancy loss by countering the clotting tendency. Research to assess the benefits of blood thinners in such women is under way.

As pregnancy progresses beyond 20 weeks, the role of genetic disorders in fetal demise diminishes. The major genetic causes in these fortunately uncommon events are chromosomal abnormalities, with the most common being trisomy 13, 18, or 21, or the absence of an X chromosome.

In summary, the risk of loss in pregnancy is very high at conception but diminishes rapidly as gestation progresses. The major cause of early loss is chromosomal abnormalities that were present at conception. Absent a family history or other data to suggest risk for a single-gene disorder, there is little reason to assume a recurring genetic risk until a third loss. After a third documented loss, genetic factors should be considered. Testing for FVL probably should be part of the evaluation. However, the chance that studies will uncover a clearly genetic cause is currently less than 10%.

PREECLAMPSIA (PREGNANCY-INDUCED HYPERTENSION)

My mother spent the last two months of her pregnancy with me in bed because of preeclampsia. What is my risk?

Preeclampsia is a relatively common, potentially life-threatening, complication of pregnancy that is characterized by new onset of high blood pressure and protein in the urine. Experts estimate that up to 8% of pregnant women in the United States develop this condition (though not in its severest form) and that the risk is even higher in poor countries. Although the cause is not known, the dominant hypothesis is that the disorder arises due to some failure of the woman's body to adapt to the presence of the fetus. Many think the key lies in understanding the physiology of the placenta. Preeclampsia, which usually has its onset in the second half of pregnancy, can progress to eclampsia, which manifests as severe hypertension (higher than 170/110) and, in the most severely affected, seizures. Each year worldwide about 10,000 pregnant women die with eclampsia.

Preeclampsia is more common among women in their first pregnancies, especially if they are over 35. Women with diabetes and women who are overweight are also at increased risk for preeclampsia. Women who experience preeclampsia in their first pregnancies are about 12 times more likely to be affected in a subsequent pregnancy with the same partner than are other women. These second cases tend to manifest earlier and more severely than in the first pregnancy. A large study in Norway found that among women with preeclampsia who changed partners, the risk of preeclampsia was 8 times greater than background, but still much less than that of preeclamptic women who did not change partners. Men who have had a child with a woman who was preeclamptic contribute some of the genetic risk. For those men who took a new partner, her risk of preeclampsia was nearly double the background risk. Such findings have triggered HLA (immune system) gene studies of the fetus. At least one uncommon HLA haplotype (gene combination) is present three times more often than expected in the offspring of preeclamptic women. However, this would explain only a tiny fraction of cases.

Several studies have shown a significant correlation between risk for preeclampsia and a polymorphism for the angiotensin II gene, which plays a central role in regulating blood pressure. Other studies have shown that women who develop preeclampsia are more likely to carry the Factor V Leiden mutation (a common genetic variant that increases the coagulability of blood). Finnish scientists, studying a group of 15 families in which many women develop preeclampsia, have recently found strong evidence of a predisposing gene lurking in the region of 2p25.

Currently, efforts are under way to investigate whether some genes are improperly turned on or off in the placentas of women with preeclampsia. Several studies have found that the relatives of women who have had preeclampsia are at higher risk for preeclampsia than are women in the population at large. Preeclampsia is more common in women born to mothers with preeclampsia than it is in those sisters who were born after pregnancies that did not suffer this complication. Taken together, the studies suggest that a positive family history of preeclampsia increases a woman's risk from two- to fourfold over the background risk. Obstetricians should always ask about a family history of preeclampsia, and women should always investigate it.

TWINNING

My brother and his wife just had nonidentical twins. Does that mean I am more likely to have twins?

There are two kinds of twins. The more common are dizygotic (DZ) or fraternal twins. They are full siblings who were conceived because two eggs were simultaneously available for fertilization. Fraternal twins may be of the same or different sexes. On average, one-quarter of DZ twins are both boys, one-quarter are both girls, and one-half are of different sexes. About 1 in 88 births in the United States results in a set of DZ twins, so about 1 in 44 persons has a DZ twin. In Nigeria, the rate of DZ twinning is report-

Table 4. *Twin births: Evidence of genetic influence on DZ twinning*

Country	Years	DZ/10,000 births	MZ/10,000 births[a]
Spain	1951–1953	59	32
Portugal	1955–1856	56	36
France	1946–1951	71	37
Austria	1952–1956	75	34
Sweden	1946–1955	86	32
Italy	1949–1955	86	32
USA whites		67	39
USA blacks	1905–1959	110	39

Adapted from Propping P. and Krüger J. 1976. Über die Häufigkeit von Zwillingsburten. *Dtsch. Med. Wochenschr.* **101:** 506–512.

[a]The incidence of MZ twinning is essentially the same in all groups, whereas DZ twinning varies significantly by population.

ed to be much higher (1 in 22), whereas in Japan it is reported to be lower. There is reason to think that the frequency of twinning is at least 10% higher than is reflected by birth data because ultrasound studies suggest that in about 1 in 10 DZ pregnancies, a twin dies before the end of the second trimester. Some researchers have found that there is seasonal variation in the birth of twins, with peaks in the spring and late summer. Women who are in their late thirties, who have had many children, or who are large, are more likely to have twins than are younger women, those who have not yet had children, and those who are petite.

There are many reports in the scientific literature of families in which the women seem to be at very high "risk" for bearing DZ twins. This is thought to be because these women are much more likely to ovulate multiple eggs during each cycle, a phenomenon that may be due to the fact that they have higher levels of a hormone called gonadotropin. The best predictor of having DZ twins is a history of having DZ twins. A woman who has given birth to one pair is about twice as likely to have another pair as is a woman who does not have such a history.

The most astounding (admittedly unverifiable) report on familial twinning comes from Russia. In 1853, a peasant named Kirilov was presented to the tsar because he claimed to be the father of more than 70 children born in two consecutive marriages. His first wife had 57 children, including four sets of quadruplets, seven sets of triplets, and two sets of twins. His second wife had six sets of twins and one set of triplets. The record for twins in the United States may be held by a South Dakota woman who is reliably reported to have given birth to eight sets of twins, as well as 8 singletons!

The best evidence that the influence of a gene or genes on a woman's reproductive cycle is a significant factor in twinning comes from studies in Norway. Because of the well-established high incidence of twinning in the region, researchers exhaustively studied the birth records over more than two centuries in the Trondheim Valley. In one pedigree there was not a single pair of twins in 800 births; in another there were 101 twin pairs among 3,645 births. Overall there was a high rate of twins—3.25%. In extended families with more than one pair of DZ twins, the twinning rate was over 8%.

Monozygotic (MZ) or identical twins are much less common. These twins arise from the separation of the embryo into two cell masses so early that each has the capacity to develop normally. The incidence of MZ twins appears to be very similar across all human populations. About 1 in 300 births results in MZ twins, so 1 person out of 150 is an identical twin. The consumption of folic acid (which protects against the risk of bearing a child with spina bifida) may be increasing the rate of MZ twinning. MZ twins are not absolutely identical. When the embryo separates, there may be an uneven distribution of the mitochondrial DNA, the small circles of DNA that reside outside the nucleus and that contain genes important in maintaining the cell's energy levels. There have been a few case reports of families in which many women have had MZ twins, but these are far fewer than the reports of DZ twins. Thus, it appears that the vast majority of MZ twins cannot be attributed to a major predisposing gene or genes.

The answer to the question posed at the top of this section is that there is no firm evidence that a woman's chance of having DZ twins is higher if her brother is married to a woman who gave birth to DZ twins. However, the sister of a woman who has borne DZ twins has about a 70% greater chance of bearing twins than does a woman without a comparable family history.

PREMATURE BIRTHS

My sister, who I thought was in perfect health, gave birth to her first child 8 weeks early. Am I at risk for the same thing?

Prematurity is the birth of a baby prior to 37 weeks of gestation (3 weeks before the date of delivery predicted by menstrual history). In the United

States, about 10% of all babies (about 400,000 a year) are premature. The more premature the baby, the greater the chance that he or she will have health problems. Virtually all premature babies have low birth weights. Babies weighing less than five and one-half pounds at birth are at increased risk. Most of the severe morbidity and mortality is associated with birth before 32 weeks of gestation. Premature births account for 70% of all neonatal deaths. African-Americans are about twice as likely as whites to have very premature babies.

Risk for giving birth prematurely is associated with poverty and alcohol and drug abuse; it is mildly associated with tobacco use and exposure to some environmental toxins. Together, these and related factors are thought to account for about half of the increased risk that burdens African-American women. In addition, however, there is a growing interest in the possibility that there are gene variants which put some people at significantly increased risk for having premature babies. For example, one small study has shown that women who have had a premature birth are more likely than those who have had babies at the end of a normal gestation to carry a variant of the interleukin-1 gene, which has been associated with a hyperinflammatory response. This finding is compatible with (but does not prove) the idea that low-level chronic vaginal infection may trigger early labor.

Some research supports the hypothesis that genetic background, if not the cause of prematurity, may well determine the threshold of risk. Several small studies of pregnant women have shown that there are differences in the expression patterns of genes turned on during normal parturition compared to those women having a variety of problems in labor. In 2002, the National Institute for Child Health and Disease committed funds to support research focusing on the genetic risk factors for prematurity. Some of these funds will support research with powerful new tools that permit scientists to assess what genes are turned on or off in specific tissues. The hope is that they will be able to discern significant differences in expression patterns. In turn, this should show which genes play a particularly important role in the genetics of labor and delivery. For now, however, there is little genetic information that can help us to explain any more than a small fraction of premature births.

Without more information about whether there are identifiable risk factors in a particular pregnancy, it is not possible to assess risk to one person based on the fact that her sister gave birth prematurely.

PART 2

Infancy

CONGENITAL MALFORMATIONS (BIRTH DEFECTS)

My brother's wife just had a baby with a birth defect. I plan to have a baby next year. I know that every pregnancy carries some risk, but are my risks now higher?

Congenital malformations (birth defects) include a large number of different physical abnormalities that by definition are present at birth. These defects vary widely in severity from conditions that are incompatible with life (such as anencephaly, a closure defect at the back of the head causing a severe brain malformation and death, usually either before or just a few hours after birth) to defects that are of only cosmetic concern (such as webbed toes). About 3% of all children are born with one or more minor malformations, but less than 1% are born with a major malformation. Although the details vary with each case, the birth of a child with a physical defect often implies a recurrence risk in a subsequent pregnancy that is higher than that faced by the general population.

The causes of some birth disorders are well understood. For example, Down syndrome, which affects about 1 in 300 fetuses, is caused by the presence of an extra chromosome 21 (from either the mother or the father's germ cell). Other common disorders, such as spina bifida, which arise during the early life of the embryo when the spinal column fails to fold normally, appear to have both genetic and nongenetic causes. In this section, I briefly discuss some of the most common of the many different congenital

Table 5. *Common birth defects: Incidence in the general population*

Birth defect	Incidence per 1000 births
Anencephaly	1.6
Spina bifida	2.0
Heart defects	6.9
Cleft lip	1.2
Pyloric stenosis	3.5
Clubfoot	6.2

Adapted, with permission, from Rimoin D.I., Connor J.M., Pyeritz R.E., and Korf B.R. 2002. *Emery and Rimoin's principles and practice of medical genetics,* 4th edition. Churchill Livingstone, London; © Elsevier.

disorders. The birth of a baby with any serious malformation should always trigger a careful genetic evaluation to ascertain recurrence risk.

Down Syndrome

At age 40 my mom gave birth to my younger sister, who has Down syndrome. How does this affect my childbearing risks?

Because it is relatively common, Down syndrome is among the best known of birth defects, first formally described by a British physician about 150 years ago. Children with this disorder have dozens of minor physical anomalies that together constitute a distinctive look (phenotype). It has been recognized for more than 60 years that children with Down syndrome are born more often to older women than would be expected by chance. Indeed, the risk of bearing a child with Down syndrome increases about 20-fold from the maternal age of 25 to 45. Down syndrome is always due to the presence of extra DNA from chromosome 21. About 95% of the time, the cause is nondisjunction, the failure of chromosomes to separate properly in the formation of the germ cells (causing an egg or sperm to have two copies instead of one). In most other cases, one parent has a "balanced translocation" of chromosome 21 that predisposes him or her to form germ cells with an extra piece of that chromosome. A tiny percentage of all children with Down syndrome are affected because they are "mosaics"; they have both normal and abnormal cell lines in their tissues. These children tend to be less severely affected.

The key problem faced by children with Down syndrome is mental retardation, which varies widely in severity, but is usually significant. Congenital heart defects, an increased risk for leukemia, and an extremely high risk of developing Alzheimer's disease by about age 60 are other important problems. Except for the few cases that arise because a parent carries a balanced translocation, the recurrence risk to a couple who have given birth to a child with Down syndrome is largely determined by empirical figures based on maternal age. The younger the woman when she gave birth to an affected child, the higher her chances are of bearing another child with Down syndrome in the next pregnancy. At age 20 her relative risk is about fivefold greater than the standard risk; at age 40 it is about 30% greater than the standard age-associated risk. Today there is a biochemical screening test to identify pregnant women who appear to be at high risk of carrying affected fetuses. The gold standard for prenatal diagnosis is amniocentesis (the removal by needle of amniotic fluid) and fetal chromosome analysis.

Assuming that there is not a balanced translocation chromosome in the family, the risk to a sister of a woman who has given birth to a child with Down syndrome at age 40 of also conceiving an affected fetus is only slightly greater than the background risk associated with her age at pregnancy. The risk to a woman in her twenties who has a sister with Down syndrome (that is not due to an unbalanced translocation) is not materially different from the population risk.

Spina Bifida

My sister gave birth to a child with spina bifida. What are my risks?

Spina bifida (SB), also known as a neural tube defect (NTD), is the term used to describe birth defects affecting the region that runs from the base of the skull all the way to the base of the spine. It is caused by the failure of the neural tube to close properly at about the 21st day of fetal life. In general, the higher up the defect, the more severe the medical consequences. Anencephaly, the failure of the brain to develop properly because of a closure defect, usually leads to fetal death or death very shortly after birth. An encephalocele, in which the brain protrudes through the back of the skull, may be compatible with life, but affected children are profoundly retarded. Defects of the mid to lower spine vary hugely in their clinical severity.

The incidence of NTDs varies widely across the globe. Historically, it was quite common in England and Ireland (as high as 1 in 200 births) and rare in Asia (1 in 1500 births). In the United States, the incidence (before prenatal screening became common) was about 1 in 600. In addition to a few rare single-gene disorders, known risk factors include folic acid deficiency and exposure during the first trimester of pregnancy to valpoic acid, a drug used to treat epilepsy. Women who must take this medicine face about a 2% risk of bearing an affected child. In most cases, the precise cause of SB is not known, and counseling about the recurrence risk is based on a large amount of empirical data. If a woman has one affected child, the recurrence risk to the same couple for the next pregnancy is about 30-fold higher, about 1 in 20. If a parent was born with SB, the risk that his or her child might also be affected is about 1 in 25. The nieces of women with SB have about a 1 in 50 chance of conceiving a fetus with SB. The sisters of women who have conceived a fetus with SB face a risk in each of their pregnancies that is in the same general range, more than 10 times higher than the general population risk.

Two developments are dramatically reducing the incidence (new births) of SB in Europe and the United States. The supplementation of breakfast cereals with the vitamin, folic acid, cuts the background risk for this disorder in half. Furthermore, the widespread use of prenatal screening of the mother early in pregnancy with selective abortion (chosen about 75% of the time) of confirmed cases has cut the incidence of live births of affected children in the United Kingdom by about 90% in 25 years. The trend in the United States is similar, although the selective abortion rate is lower.

Congenital Heart Defects

My sister was born with a heart defect. Are the risks to my kids higher?

About 0.5% to 1% of babies are born with some form of heart defect, making it among the most common congenital malformations. In about one-third of these babies, the defect is moderate to severe, requiring one or more reconstructive operations. There are many kinds of heart malformations, and in most cases, the exact cause is not known. Rare genetic diseases, chromosomal disorders (including Down syndrome, DiGeorge syndrome, or a deletion of a tiny portion of 22q11), exposure to drugs (both medicinal and recreational), certain diseases in the mother (especially diabetes), and some infections are known causes, but together they account for less than 10% of cases. About 90% of the time the cause is thought to be multifactorial; that is, due to the combined action of several genes interacting with environmental factors.

As with many other birth defects of uncertain cause, one major risk factor for having a baby with a heart defect is simply that the mother herself was born with one. Absent any other known risk factors, such women have about a 3% chance of having a baby with a similar problem. For parents who have one child with a heart defect but for whom there is no other known risk factor, the risk to their next pregnancy is also about 3%. If a parent and one child were both born with a congenital heart defect, the recurrence risk for the next child is about 10%. The nieces and nephews of a woman who gave birth to an affected child have a 2–3% chance of being affected.

Cleft Lip and Cleft Palate

I was born with a cleft lip. What is the risk this will happen to my children?

Cleft lip (with or without cleft palate) is a quite common birth defect that appears to be caused by factors other than those that cause just cleft palate. Clefts occur relatively early in gestation at about week 7 or 8 during the embryological formation of the face. Although the primary cause is in most cases not known, the cleft is due to a reduction in size of certain tissue prominences that are supposed to migrate together and fuse. Cleft lip and palate occur together about 45% of the time.

Cleft lip (with or without cleft palate) is found more often in boys, who account for about 70% of cases. The incidence varies across racial groups. Cleft lip affects about 1 in 1000 whites, about 1 in 2000 blacks, and about 3 in 1000 Native Americans. Known risk factors include a prenatal history of alcohol abuse, cigarette smoking, and use of certain anti-epileptic drugs, but these explain only a small fraction of the cases.

The evidence that genes play a major role is strong. The concordance rate for cleft lip among MZ twins is 40%, which is about 10 times higher than it is for DZ twins. Although the inheritance patterns do not obey Mendel's laws, there are many families in which two or more people have been born with cleft lip, or cleft lip and cleft palate. Data generated from many family studies permit genetic counselors to offer fairly solid odds about recurrence risk. The parents of a child born with cleft lip have about a 4% chance that their next child will also be affected. A parent who was born with the defect also has about a 4% chance that his or her child will be similarly affected. If that individual does have an affected child, the risk in the next pregnancy rises to about 10%.

Isolated cleft palate is less common than cleft lip with or without cleft palate, occurring in only about 1 in 2500 births. There is relatively little variation in incidence across racial groups. Contrary to cleft lip, isolated cleft palate is more common in girls than in boys by about 3:2. The recurrence risk to unaffected parents who have had one affected child is about 2% (which is more than 20 times higher than the background risk). If either parent was born with cleft palate, the risk of bearing a similarly affected child is about 7%. If there is an affected child, the risk in the next pregnancy is about 15%. Children born with clefts usually do not have other physical problems, and their defects can be surgically repaired with excellent results.

Pyloric Stenosis

My first child was born with pyloric stenosis. What are the risks for my next pregnancy?

Pyloric stenosis is an enlarged ring of tissue at the site where the stomach joins the small intestine. When this ring of tissue is too large, it can obstruct the flow of food in newborns, a potentially life-threatening, but easily curable, problem. Once the diagnosis is made, a surgeon cuts the ring to relieve the obstruction. About 1 in 500 white babies is born with pyloric stenosis. For some reason, the condition is much more common in boys, who are affected five times more often than are girls. Another highly unusual aspect of pyloric stenosis is that it is far less common (less than 1 in 10,000) in African-Americans and Asians.

Careful studies by Dr. Cedric Carter in the 1960s demonstrated that the risk of pyloric stenosis in first-degree relatives of affected persons was far in excess (20- to 30-fold) of the risk to the general population. Another odd feature of the disorder is that the recurrence risk to relatives of affected girls is much higher than the recurrence risk to relatives of affected boys. This strongly suggests that genes play a larger role in causing the condition in girls than they do in boys. When a woman has given birth to a son with pyloric stenosis, the risk to the next child is 20% if it is a girl and 10% if it is a boy.

Clubfoot

I was born with a clubfoot. What is the chance that my children will have the same problem?

Clubfoot is the term used to describe two different birth defects involving the angulation of the foot. It occurs in about 1 in 500 births. Although scientists have studied clubfoot for decades, there is little knowledge about its cause. However, the data are most compatible with its being a polygenic disorder (due to the action of several different gene variants). Talipes equinovarus (TE) is the name given to the deformity in which the foot is adducted (pointed away from the body), the heel is inverted, and the ankle is flexed. It occurs in boys twice as often as in girls. About 20% of children with TE also have other subtle physical abnormalities. About 2% of first-degree relatives are also affected. For those couples with an affected child, but no other family history, the recurrence risk for the next child is about 3%.

In the other major form of clubfoot, talipes calcaneovalgus (TC), the forefoot is flexed dorsally and the bottom surface of the foot faces away from the body. About 5% of children born with this condition also have a dislocated hip. This defect is more common in girls (about 5:3) than in boys. After the birth of an affected child, the recurrence risk in subsequent pregnancies is about 4–5%.

NEWBORN GENETIC SCREENING

My sister just learned from her pediatrician that her daughter has a disease called phenylketonuria (PKU). How serious is this? What are the risks for my children?

Each year in the United States (and most of the western world) almost every newborn baby undergoes a heel stick to capture a few drops of blood that is subjected to biochemical testing to screen for a growing number of rare single-gene disorders. Phenylketonuria, to which I will return, was the first disorder around which screening programs were developed. Although the baby has an exceedingly remote risk of being affected with any one of these disorders, as the number of disorders for which screening is offered increases, the cumulative risk rises. In states with the most technologically sophisticated and comprehensive programs (states offer testing through their departments of public health), such as Massachusetts, a few drops of blood are enough to test for more than 30 disorders. The risk for having one of them is about 1:1500.

Newborn screening is inexpensive; one can test an individual for many different disorders for about $50 a sample. Untreated, many of these disorders can cause severe mental retardation. Fortunately, for most of the diseases there are clinical interventions that either dramatically improve the child's prospects or help the parents and physicians in their struggle against the disease. Newborn genetic screening provides an excellent return on the expenditure of public health dollars.

With a couple of exceptions, the genetic disorders that are tested for in newborn screening programs are autosomal recessive conditions for which there is rarely a family history. The babies who are born with one of the conditions have had the bad luck to inherit a mutant form of the particular gene responsible for a disease from each parent. There is no family history because being born with one mutation and one normal gene does not cause illness. Although the range varies, for many of these diseases only about 1 in 40,000 children is affected. The chance of a person being a carrier of a mutant gene for one of these disorders is about 1 in 100. This means the odds of both the man and the woman in a couple being carriers for the same disease is only 1 in 10,000. Furthermore, the odds that each baby born to them will be affected are only 1 in 4 (the chance that any particular baby will receive *both* mutant genes at the same time). Using these numbers as representative for the disorders screened for among newborns, it is easy to appreciate the cumulative risk. If each disorder independently is present in 1 in 40,000 newborns, and if there are tests for 40 diseases, the cumulative risk would be 1 in 1,000. (A few disorders covered by newborn screening are fairly common).

The conditions screened for are for the most part so rare that few physicians have ever cared for even one affected child. It is crucial that the babies who are discovered to have these rare disorders be referred to and monitored by the few specialty clinics with health care personnel who are familiar with their problems.

Most of the disorders that are currently screened for fall roughly into three groups: (1) those in which affected infants are unable to metabolize some particular component of a diet such as a particular amino acid or sugar (such as phenylketonuria and galactosemia) and who benefit greatly from being given a specialized diet that can prevent mental retardation and ameliorate other risks, (2) those involving disorders of the thyroid gland which, if severe and not promptly treated, will cause mental retardation, and (3) disorders of the hemoglobin molecule (such as sickle cell anemia).

Phenylketonuria is the disorder that stimulated the creation of newborn screening programs more than 40 years ago. The most common form of this recessive disorder occurs when a child has a mutation in each copy of the gene he or she carries for an enzyme called phenylalanine hydroxylase. An affected child cannot properly metabolize the amino acid phenylalanine, which is nearly ubiquitous in human food. Untreated, these children (about 1 in 12,000 white newborns) will be profoundly retarded and often have seizure disorders. However, if promptly diagnosed and placed on a low phenylalanine diet, affected children have a near normal life. It was the great success in preventing mental retardation in these children that fostered the growth of newborn screening programs in the 1960s and 1970s.

Currently, the United States is in a period of rapid expansion of newborn screening, thanks to the availability of a technology called tandem mass spectrometry (TM/TM). TM/TM provides a very low cost method for diagnosing more than 20 rare autosomal recessive diseases by looking for chemicals of certain molecular weight in a dried blood sample taken from ostensibly healthy newborns. These metabolic disorders fall into three groups: amino acid disorders, organic acid disorders, and fatty acid disorders. Each is a rare condition caused by an enzyme failure. Some states, led by Massachusetts, have moved aggressively to use TM/TM to expand the scope of newborn screening. Other states (for example, Mississippi) are beginning to follow suit, but some are not yet moving forward. This has created a shameful inequity. Depending on the state in which he or she is born, whether a baby affected with one of these rare disorders lives or dies (or becomes severely retarded) is determined by the scope of that state's screening program. Since the cost of setting up and running an expanded newborn genetic screening program is quite small, there is no excuse for not screening every baby born in the United States.

If a baby with any one of these rare disorders is born into a family, there is a 1 in 2 chance that the sisters and brothers of the parents carry one copy of the disease gene. This means their risk for bearing a child with the same disorder, although still comparatively low, is much higher than the population risk. For a disease with an incidence of 1 in 40,000 births, their a priori risk in each pregnancy is about 1 in 400 (1 × 1/100 × 1/4). In the case of a woman who has a sister with a rare recessive disorder for which the population risk of being a carrier is 1 in 100, the odds that she is a carrier are actually 2 in 3. This risk is calculated as follows. We know that both her parents have to be carriers and that she does not have the disease. Thus, she can either not be a carrier or be a carrier. There are two ways of being a carrier and only one way of not being a carrier (thus, the 2 out of 3). For her, the risk of bearing a child with the same disease is not 1 in 40,000, but about 1 in 600. That risk is calculated by multiplying her risk (2/3) times the general risk her husband has of being a carrier (1/100) times the risk to each pregnancy (1/4). Every person who learns that a close blood relative has a rare autosomal recessive disorder should receive genetic counseling about his or her reproductive risks.

DEAFNESS

> *My daughter just married a man who was born deaf. He has no other medical problems and no family history of deafness. What are the risks that they will have a deaf child?*

Hearing loss is a common problem, especially the impairments that come with age. More than 6,000,000 persons in the United States have significant hearing loss, including 400,000 children. Although the hearing impairments of adulthood and old age almost certainly have a genetic component, I focus here on deafness and severe hearing loss present at birth. About 1 child in 500 under the age of 3 has a severe hearing impairment, and about 1 in 1000 children is born deaf.

In developed nations, at least one-half and probably as much as two-thirds of all deafness in early childhood is genetic. It is not surprising, given the complexity of our auditory system, that more than 80 loci (locations) on the human genome have been identified as harboring genes that play a role in its development. Of the known genetic causes of deafness, about 60% are nonsyndromic, meaning no other organ systems are affected. Of that 60%, about two-thirds of cases are recessive and one-third are dominant forms of deafness. X-linked genetic diseases and mitochondrial gene disorders account for less than 5% of all childhood deafness.

In the last few years, the United States has wisely embarked on a pro-

Table 6. *Deafness: Causes*			
Genetic:	35%	Without other physical problems	60%
		recessive	60–70%
		dominant	30%
		X-linked	2%
		mitochondrial	1%
		With other physical problems	40%
Acquired:	35%		
		Prenatal	20%
		Infancy	20%
		Later	60%
Unknown:	30%		

Data from Rimoin D.I., Connor J.M., Pyeritz R.E., and Korf B.R. 2002. *Emery and Rimoin's principles and practice of medical genetics,* 4th edition. Churchill Livingstone, London; © Elsevier.

gram of universal screening of all newborns to identify infants with severe hearing impairment. There has been some controversy about the best way to conduct such screening. Most experts favor bedside otoacoustic emission testing (a brief exam of how the infant responds to tones) as superior to (although more expensive than) parental questionnaires. Despite the controversy, in the United States we are well on the way to standardizing a practice by which we identify the vast majority of deaf children in the first few days of life. This should provide for much earlier intervention, more informed and better adjusted parents, more accurate counseling about risk recurrence, and a more effectively educated and functioning deaf individual.

In the last decade, there has been extraordinary progress in understanding the genetics of deafness. By the close of 2003, at least 16 genes had been identified in which mutations cause recessively inherited (nonsyndromic) deafness. More than 30 genes have been identified that cause or are strongly associated with dominantly inherited deafness. Almost certainly, that list will grow substantially.

Despite the discovery of so many genes for deafness, just two mutations in a gene called connexin 26 (or GJB2) account for about 50% of all the mutations found in persons with hereditary deafness. These two mutations are 35delG and 167delT (del denotes loss of DNA; the number indicates the spot in the gene where the loss occurred). About 1 in 30 whites carries a single connexin 26 mutation. Persons born with only that one mutation are not hearing-impaired. As many as 4% of Ashkenazi Jews carry the 167delT mutation. Another mutation, R143W (the capital letters indicate that a DNA change leads to a particular change in the amino acid structure of the protein), is prevalent in blacks, and yet another (235delC) seems to be prevalent among Asians. One perplexing aspect in genetic counseling for deafness is that many deaf children have a mutation in only one copy of the connexin 26 gene. In 2003 a large consortium of European geneticists helped unravel this mystery when they reported that a mutation (deletion) in a nearby gene called GJB6 (connexin 30) is frequently the second mutation in those children. It must somehow affect the function of connexin 26.

Because these few mutations account for such a substantial fraction of hereditary deafness, and because hereditary deafness is relatively common, as the cost of DNA testing drops, it would make sense to add deafness to newborn screening programs.

A prompt genetic diagnosis in the infant is important for two reasons. It will inform the parents of affected children about their recurrence risk in future pregnancies (which is 1 in 4), and it will alert the brothers and sisters of those parents about the chance that they also carry one of these mutations. The full sibling of an obligate carrier (the parent of an affected child) has a 1 in 2 chance of also being a carrier. If a sibling finds out he or she is a carrier, his or her chance of having a similarly deaf child is about 1 in 120 in each pregnancy. This risk is calculated by multiplying the chance that one is a carrier (which is 1 in 1) times the chance of marrying a carrier (about 1 in 30) times the chance of having an affected child (1 in 4). Of course a 1% risk is low, but it is also almost ten times higher than the risk faced by a randomly selected couple.

As for the question at the beginning of this section, there is about a 1 in 2 chance that the man's deafness is genetic in origin and a greater than 1 in 2 chance that the causative mutations are recessive. The young woman has about a 1 in 30 chance of having a mutation for a recessive form of deafness. Thus, the chance that the couple is at 1 in 4 risk is about 1 in 100. Therefore, their risk of having a deaf child is quite low—about 1 in 400 in each pregnancy.

SUDDEN INFANT DEATH SYNDROME

My brother died of sudden infant death syndrome. Will my children be at increased risk?

Sudden infant death syndrome (SIDS) is a term that almost certainly includes several (perhaps many) mysterious disorders that take the lives of about 4000 babies in the United States each year. It is defined as sudden death in an infant less than the age of 1 year that remains unexplained after a thorough investigation, including autopsy. It causes about 40–50% of all deaths in the United States of children between 1 month and 12 months of life. In 1998, the SIDS death rate was about 1 per 1300 infants. The rate was more than twice as high in African-Americans as in whites.

Persuasive evidence that sleeping prone (face down) is a major risk factor for death in infants resulted in a massive public health campaign in the mid-1990s called "Back to Sleep" which has had wonderful results. Over an 8-year period, the percentage of parents reporting that they allow their infants to sleep face down has dropped from about 80% to about 10%. During the same time, the death rate from SIDS fell by 40%, clear evidence that sleeping face down is a major risk factor. However, this improvement does not help us understand why a small number of babies who sleep prone die of SIDS.

Despite immense efforts to identify the underlying biological risk factors for SIDS, progress has been slow. Some of the advances have been genetic. It has been shown that several rare single-gene disorders involving the metabolism of fatty acids are associated with risk for SIDS. Together, these could explain at best only a tiny percentage of cases, but they must always be considered in the differential diagnosis and, if the infant turns out to have died because of one of them, that fact is immensely important to relatives.

Another possibility is that a small fraction of the infants dying of SIDS have one of several genetically determined abnormalities of heart rhythm. The most prevalent of these may be Long QT syndrome, a term referring to a particular tracing on the electrocardiogram of affected individuals. Sudden death is the most common form of death in adults with this disorder. Some experts think that Long QT syndrome is subtle and far more common than has been thought, and that it causes a small fraction of SIDS. In 2001, a team at the Mayo Clinic exhaustively studied 93 infants who died of SIDS and found that two had mutations in a gene (SCN5A) that controls the movement of sodium ions in and out of heart muscle cell. Mutations in this gene are known to cause heart rhythm disorders. A group in Sweden found that mutations in a cardiac gene called HERG were present in 2 of 120 infants with SIDS. It is possible that rare mutations in many genes involved in cardiac function will each be responsible for a small percentage of SIDS.

There have been some reports of families in which two children have died of SIDS, a finding that raises the possibility of an autosomal recessive disorder. However, these are so few that it is also possible that the reports document the chance occurrence of two rare independent events in the families. In most cases, a thorough evaluation (including an autopsy) should permit physicians to reassure the parents of a child who died of SIDS that they do not face a high risk in subsequent pregnancies. In a few cases, physicians will discover the underlying cause of death, a discovery that will greatly help reproductive counseling.

It is not possible to give a firm answer to the question with which I opened this section. This is because the precise cause of death is usually not known. However, even if the cause was a rare recessive disorder, the risk to the *offspring* of persons who in childhood lost a brother or sister to SIDS is less than 1%. This is because even if the person carried a mutation, the chance that he or she will marry a person who is also a carrier of a mutation in the same gene is quite low.

PART 3

Childhood

CEREBRAL PALSY

My uncle has cerebral palsy. Does this mean my children are at increased risk?

Cerebral palsy (CP) is a term used to describe a group of disorders that affect the brain's ability to coordinate the body's muscles. The condition is present at or develops soon after birth. The amount of damage varies widely. Patients with CP have tight muscles, involuntary movements, difficulty walking, much trouble with fine motor tasks like tying shoelaces, and some problems with sensations. In addition, depending on the extent of the brain injury, they may have many other problems such as seizure disorders. Although some people with CP are also mentally retarded, many are intellectually normal. Unfortunately, because the brain injury often seriously impairs the ability to speak, people sometimes erroneously think that persons with CP who are intellectually normal are mentally retarded.

CP is often characterized by which large muscle groups are most affected. A person with hemiplegia is affected on one side only; a person with diplegia predominantly suffers from involvement of the legs; a person with quadriplegia has deficits involving the arms and legs. In addition, affected persons may have remarkably rigid muscles, resulting in clumsy or "spastic" movements, or they may be athetoid—burdened with involuntary, writhing movements. Unlike many other developmental disorders, CP is not progressive. Even so, the actual manifestations of the condition

Table 7. *Cerebral palsy: Some conditions associated with an increased risk of having an affected child*
Twin pregnancy
Damaged placenta
Sexually transmitted disease
Poor nutrition
Abuse of alcohol and drugs
Infections
Difficult labor
Premature delivery
Low birth weight
Breech delivery
Malformation in baby's brain
Chromosomal abnormalities
Many associations are weak. Most children with the risk factors do not develop CP.

can change over time depending on the nature of the original injury and the support and care given to the individual.

Since it was first described by an English physician named William Little in the 1860s, CP has been shrouded with mystery and complicated by misunderstanding. Over the last 50 years, researchers have identified many factors that are associated with an increased risk for bearing a child with CP, including multiple fetuses, a damaged placenta, exposure to toxic substances such as alcohol, chromosomal abnormalities, biochemical disorders, Rh or ABO incompatibility between mother and fetus, chance congenital malformations of the brain, prematurity, low birth weight, breech delivery, and a prolonged, difficult labor. Events in early childhood that can cause CP include meningitis, brain hemorrhages, head injury, and near drowning.

For many years, a major cause of CP was thought by physicians and lay persons alike to be difficult labor and delivery. The key idea was that these babies suffered brief, but devastating periods of inadequate oxygen, which injured critical regions of the brain. Over the last three decades, several large research studies have rejected that thesis, and the current thinking is that birth trauma accounts for probably no more than 10–15% of cases and, furthermore, that many of these infants were at risk for difficult deliveries because they had underlying problems. CP is all too common, affecting about 1 in every 400 babies born in the United States and Europe. In the United States about 10,000 children a year are diagnosed, and there are about 500,000 persons alive with the disorder.

How do genes influence risk for CP? No one really knows. In every study of large groups of children with CP, there is no clear explanation for most cases. There are almost certainly uncommon, even undescribed, disorders lurking among this group. A fair guess is that 2–3% of all cases will turn out to be due to a variety of relatively rare (perhaps not yet even discovered) single-gene disorders. This guess is based on large studies of recurrence risk to siblings of children with CP. For example, a study in England found a second affected sib in only 1 of 349 families. Similarly, a study in Sweden found only 30 families out of 3150 in which there were two affected sibs. For some subtypes of CP, the recurrence risk is higher. A few studies suggest that if a child has a form of CP called congenital ataxia and mental retardation, the genetic component could be so high as to suggest a recurrence risk of 25%, a level that suggests the action of a few or perhaps just one gene. Recently, a large epidemiological study in England that compared rates of CP among English and Asian (mostly Pakistani) children found that the rate was twice as high among Asian children. Since about one-half of the Asian families involved cousin marriages, the findings suggest that uncommon recessive genes are an important risk factor.

Unfortunately, geneticists know so little about the causes of CP that when they are asked about recurrence risk by the parents of an affected child, they are only able to say that it is probably very low (1–5%), but that there is a small chance that it could be as high as 25% (the figure one would quote if both parents carried a rare gene for a recessive disease).

MENTAL RETARDATION

My brother is mentally retarded, but the doctors have never been able to figure out the cause. Does this history mean my children are at increased risk?

During most of the 20th century, the term "mental retardation" was used to describe individuals who have intellectual abilities that are at least two standard deviations below the mean (below the third percentile) on any one of several standardized tests. Intelligence (IQ) tests were developed in France about 1905, not to sort those of normal intelligence, but to sort those with obvious intellectual impairment. The goal was to develop a tool

Table 8. *Mental retardation: Prevalence in siblings of mentally retarded persons*

Level of MR in first patient	Number of sibs	Above average (%)	Mild MR (%)	Severe MR (%)	Total retarded (%)
Mild MR	2321	1.2	19.5	2.5	22.0
Severe MR	2549	1.6	12.2	4.3	16.5
Totals	4870	1.4	15.7	3.4	19.1

After the Colchester Survey by Lionel Penrose. Virtually all research shows that mild MR clusters in families much more than does severe MR. Adapted, with permission, from Penrose L.S. 1962. *The biology of mental defect*, 3rd edition. Grune & Stratton, New York, © Elsevier.

that would assist psychologists in deciding who was educable. H.H. Goddard, a psychologist who studied mental retardation at a large state school called Vineland in New Jersey, was among the first Americans to use the IQ tests in the study of mental retardation. At the time, IQ testing seemed a major advance over the impressionistic diagnoses that had been used to categorize mentally retarded persons as either morons, imbeciles, or idiots.

Today, the American Association for Mental Retardation relies much more on the status of an individual's functional (daily life) abilities in defining his or her level of "mental retardation." Nevertheless, IQ score is still routinely used as a shorthand measure to describe a person's level of cognitive ability.

By the 1950s, researchers had carefully described the more obvious and identifiable forms of mental retardation such as Down syndrome, but the causes of this and many other types of cognitive disorders eluded them. One happy exception was the discovery that the mental retardation in persons then called "cretins" was due to inadequate thyroid function. Since the late 1950s, there have been some remarkable advances in understanding the etiology of mental retardation. We now know, for example, that Down syndrome is caused by the presence of an extra chromosome 21 in cells, usually due to an error in the separation of the pairs of chromosomes during the maturation of the egg. A stunning advance during the early1960s was the discovery that newborns could be screened for a rare genetic disorder called PKU (phenylketonuria) and that, in affected children, mental retardation could be averted by rigorously following a low-phenylalanine diet. Since then, many other disorders have been added to the list for which all infants in the United States are screened. During the

1980s, perhaps the most extraordinary advance was the elucidation of Fragile X syndrome, a relatively common genetic cause of mental retardation that was described clinically in 1943, but for which the causative gene was not found until 1993.

A general rule of thumb is that the more severe the mental retardation, the more likely that the cause will be identified. For example, in autopsy studies of children with severe mental retardation, from 35% to nearly 100% of the individuals had obvious structural abnormalities of their brains. In three large studies of children with severe mental retardation conducted by expert clinicians, a definite cause was found in 82–88% of cases. In sharp contrast are the results of three studies of children with mild mental retardation. In one, the scientists could only find a definitive cause in 17% of the children; in the other two studies, the researchers were certain of a diagnosis in about 40% of the cases. Fortunately, most children with mental retardation are only mildly to moderately affected. Unfortunately, these are the children in whom it is most difficult to discern the cause.

Except for the conditions that are clinically obvious at birth, such as Down syndrome, or those diagnosed through newborn screening programs, such as PKU, most children with mental retardation are not diagnosed until they are about 2 years old, often after a year of frustrating clinical evaluations. Typically, these children appear normal at birth and through the first few months of life. They come to the pediatrician's attention because the parents are worried that the child is not meeting his or her developmental milestones. When this pattern of delay is confirmed (often over a period of several months), it triggers an evaluation that (if complete) includes a careful family history, a detailed neurological examination, and a physical examination by a clinical geneticist. It should also include a hearing test, an eye exam, and chromosomal analysis. In addition, it is sometimes appropriate to screen for Fragile X syndrome, to perform brain imaging studies, and to conduct a variety of biochemical tests. This extensive effort concludes with a definitive diagnosis in little more than 20% of cases. Recently, it has been discovered that a significant number of children with unexplained mental retardation have a tiny deletion at the tip of one of their chromosomes (a region called the telomere). By routinely testing for these deletions, it may be possible to increase the diagnostic yield by 5–7%, a big advance in this difficult field.

Unfortunately, diagnostic advances have not been matched by therapeutic advances. Although much can be done to support the child with mental retardation and to maximize his educability, in most cases nothing can be done to undo the neurological deficit. Still, reaching the correct diagnosis is extremely important. It provides the parents with an explanation and sometimes with a clear picture of the recurrence risk. It also avoids further, unnecessary medical evaluation.

When parents learn that their suspicions are correct, that their son or daughter is mentally retarded, they usually ask two questions: (1) Why? and (2) What are the odds it will happen to the next child? Usually, if there is a definite diagnosis such as Fragile X syndrome, tuberous sclerosis (a single-gene dominant disorder), or Down syndrome, the recurrence risk is relatively straightforward to estimate. However, more often than not, the physician and the evaluating team cannot make the diagnosis. This means that the recurrence risk must be based on empirical studies of families in similar situations.

Providing an estimate of recurrence risk is a challenging task, the success of which is highly dependent on the level of knowledge about the affected child. If, for example, the child with mental retardation has microcephaly (a markedly small head) as his or her major distinguishing feature, empirical studies suggest a recurrence risk of from 6% to 20%. When the affected child has severe mental retardation of unknown cause, the recurrence risk varies with the gender. If it is a boy, future brothers are at 1 in 12 risk, and future sisters are at about 1 in 30 risk. If the affected child is a girl, the risk to future brothers is about 1 in 22 and to future sisters about 1 in 17. These estimates are only approximate.

In families with one child with mild to moderate mental retardation for whom a full evaluation has not provided a diagnosis, the recurrence risk for the next child is about 5%. However, the risk is higher for brothers of affected sons than for sisters. This is almost certainly due to the large number of genes on the X chromosome that have been associated with mental retardation. It is extremely important to remember that these risk figures are only as good as the diagnostic evaluation that the child underwent. Hidden within these empirical studies are families for whom the recurrence risk is 1 in 4 because the parents are carriers of an undescribed genetic disorder.

What advice can be given to a concerned young woman who has a brother with unexplained mental retardation? Assuming the brother has been competently evaluated, the best one can do is to advise that the risk that she will give birth to a similarly affected child is moderately greater than the background risk, but still quite low, probably on the order of 3–4%. The difficult task is to explain that for a few, unidentifiable, couples, the risk is much higher.

AUTISM

I have a son with autism. What is the risk in my next pregnancy? Is my sister at increased risk for having a child with autism?

Autism is the name given to a mysterious childhood neurological disorder first described by the German psychiatrist Kanner in 1943. The cardinal diagnostic features are significant abnormalities in use of language, markedly poor patterns of social interaction, and a preference for highly repetitive activities, with at least one of these deficits obviously present before the third birthday. The classic picture of a patient with autism is a normal-looking child (who may appear to have a large head) who rarely speaks, is anxious with any disturbance of a set routine, is extremely reluctant to interact with adults or children, and often has stereotypical behaviors, especially of the hands. The disorder used to be diagnosed in boys about three times more often than in girls, but this ratio is diminishing.

Table 9. *Autism and similar disorders: Diagnostic terms*

Autism: At least two deficits in sociability, empathy, and insight. At least one deficit in language and imagination. At least one deficit in behavioral flexibility. Onset before age 3.

Asperger's disorder: Usually much less severe than autism. Features include social ineptness and behavioral inflexibility with narrow interests. IQ is greater than 70 and often normal or even high. Speech emerges normally. Clumsiness is often a feature.

Pervasive developmental disorder: A term applied to less severely affected children who do not meet the criteria for autism or Asperger's disorder.

Disintegrative disorder: After a normal development in the first two years, severe regression affecting language, sociability, and cognition.

Rett's syndrome: Severe global regression in infant girls, resulting in lifelong mental retardation, lack of language, and little functional use of the hands. Condition is usually fatal in boys before birth.

Adapted, with permission, from Rapin I. 2002. Perspective: The autistic spectrum disorders. *New England Journal of Medicine* **347:** 302–304.

During the last half of the 20th century, it was taught that autism was a rare disorder affecting about 1 in 1500 boys and about 1 in 4000 girls. More recently, the diagnosis has been made about three times more often than in the past. There are several reasons for this, including the uncertainty about the clinical boundaries, the fact that a familiar diagnostic label sometimes helps families get better social and medical support, and widespread public interest in early intervention. Many parents and some physicians think there is an "epidemic" of new cases, presumably due to some environmental exposure.

In past decades, well over half of children diagnosed with autism were found to have an IQ below 70 (a number often associated with borderline mental retardation), but some have had relatively high scores, and more than a few seem to excel in specific areas such as music. Many studies have attempted to identify physical parameters that are associated with autism. One consistent finding is that about 25% of autistic children have a head size above the 97th percentile; another is that about 25% of patients develop a seizure disorder by young adulthood. Both percentages are far in excess of the risk to the general population. The large head size is of particular interest because most of the children are born with small heads. They experience rapid growth of head size between 6 and 15 months of life (either due to excess cell division or deficit cell elimination during the brain's persistent remodeling). Some brain imaging studies have suggested that the children have small cerebellums, but the evidence is contradictory.

No one knows what causes autism, but over the last four decades there has been a marked shift in suspicion. Fifty years ago much attention was focused on the influence of mother–child interactions, a view that doubtless led to much unnecessary guilt and sorrow in the mothers of affected children. Today, autism is widely viewed as a neurodevelopmental abnormality in which environmental and, almost certainly, genetic factors are of major importance.

Unfortunately, the search for environmental risk factors has been frustrating, sometimes leading to false hopes, dashed expectations, and bitter controversy. For example, in 1999 the Food and Drug Administration realized that toddlers who were being injected with several vaccines simultaneously might be receiving a dose of mercury slightly in excess of federal safety guidelines. This is because a mercury compound called thimerosal was then used as a preservative in many vaccines. Soon thereafter, a parent group called Safe Minds proposed that thimerosal might increase the risk for autism. A study conducted by the Institute of Medicine in 2001, another conducted in Denmark in 2003, and data from Sweden found no evidence to support that fear. But some parents, arguing that the studies are inadequate, continue to pursue the connection.

Support for genetic influences in autism come from two major sources: (1) twin and family studies and (2) the high prevalence of autism associated with certain single-gene disorders and chromosomal abnormalities. Several large studies comparing the concordance rate for autism in MZ and DZ twin pairs have found that MZ co-twins of affected children were far more likely (70–90%) to be diagnosed with autism than were DZ co-twins (0–10%). Family studies also strongly implicate genetic factors. In one study of 207 families in Utah with at least one affected child, 20 (about 10%) had *more* than one affected child. The authors of that study concluded that the risk of developing autism in children born after the first affected child was nearly 9%. They estimated that autism is about 200 times more likely among sibs of affected children than within families with no affected children.

About 3% of children first diagnosed with autism will later be found to have a genetic disorder called Fragile X syndrome (so-named because the X chromosome looks abnormal when the chromosome analysis is done on cells grown in a certain cell culture fluid). Making the diagnosis of Fragile X syndrome is very important because of the high recurrence risk in future pregnancies. The heritability of Fragile X syndrome is much like a sex-linked single-gene disorder; if carrier mothers bear a son, there is a 1 in 2 risk (depending on which of the two Xs he inherits) that he will be affected. In the past the diagnosis of autism has sometimes been improperly given to children suffering with one of several other uncommon single-gene disorders, including phenylketonuria and tuberous sclerosis.

In the last few years, scientists have shown that mutations in at least three different genes (called MECP2, NLGN-3, and NLGN-4) are responsible for a small percentage of autism. They have also proven that there must be a gene or genes on chromosome 15q11-13 that are causative.

Currently, an international consortium of scientists is conducting an intensive search of the human genome in the hope of finding other genes that predispose to autism. Much of their work involves studying families who voluntarily participate in the Autism Genetic Resource Exchange. In 2001, the scientists reported that among 110 families with two or more affected children, they had found evidence suggesting that there could be predisposing genes on chromosomes 5, 19, and X. In the fall of 2003, they reported a much larger study of 345 families in which more than 400 markers were used. This study replicated the evidence for a predisposing gene on the short arm of 5 and uncovered powerful data suggesting that there was an "autism gene" on chromosome 17q. However, as often happens in this work, the larger study also eliminated some of the other suspect regions from consideration. The linkage to 17q is tantalizing because the marker is very close to a gene that codes for a neurotransmitter that is a plausible culprit. In 2003, the scientific literature was bursting with reports from efforts to use genetic markers in family studies of autism. Suffice it to say that well over 10 suspect loci have been identified, but we must wait for further work to be completed before the search can be narrowed.

Unfortunately, it is difficult to offer much firm guidance to the couple who have a child diagnosed with autism or to their siblings. The best estimate is that if the first affected child is a boy, the risk to the next child of either gender is 7%; if the first affected child is a girl, the risk to the next born child may be as high as 14%. The risk that aunts or uncles of children with autism will also have an affected child, although low, is still higher than the background risk. Here, too, it is impossible absolutely to rule out the risk that in a few (rare) families the disease is due to an undiagnosed single-gene disorder (making the recurrence risk 25%).

DEVELOPMENTAL DISABILITIES

Specific Reading Disability (Dyslexia)

As a child I had a lot of trouble learning to read. Will my children be at similar risk?

Often still called dyslexia, specific reading disability (SRD) is defined as an unexpected difficulty in learning to read in a child who has no known neurological problems, adequate intelligence, and appropriate opportunities to learn. SRD is a diagnosis of exclusion. For example, the child must not be suffering from severe emotional problems that could be temporarily blocking his ability to read. Unfortunately, there is not unanimous agreement about when to apply the SRD label. Some government programs allow children who are just one standard deviation below the mean in reading scores to qualify for services for SRD, whereas research groups typically prefer to study children who are two to three standard deviations below the mean (a much smaller and more severely impaired group). Some experts reject the notion that SRD is a discrete entity, thinking of it instead as occupying one end of the spectrum of children who are (unlike those with serious mental retardation) ultimately capable of reading.

Any estimate of the prevalence of SRD depends on the diagnostic criteria used. By any measure, it is a common disorder, affecting up to 10% of all children. SRD may be the diagnosis in as much as 80% of all learning disabilities. There is uncertainty about the sex ratio of children with SRD. For a variety of reasons, clinicians of all types tend to make the diagnosis more quickly in boys, resulting in a sex ratio of 3:1 or higher. However, in tightly controlled research studies, fewer children are diagnosed and the sex ratio is not as skewed, more like 3:2. Many more children are diagnosed with SRD in first grade than in third grade, a finding that suggests a catch-up phenomenon. This supports the views of those who argue that many kids with dyslexia will be adequate or even strong readers.

The causes of SRD are not known. Some research groups have looked for subtle anatomical differences in the brains of affected children, and others have sought evidence of subtle biochemical differences. There have been some tantalizing findings, but no consistent associations have emerged. Dyslexia has long been recognized to run in families. In the few studies that have prospectively followed very young children who have a positive family history, researchers have frequently found early warning signs. In one study of 34 children in families at high risk, 22 eventually were diagnosed with dyslexia, whereas the same diagnosis was given to only 2 of 44 control children.

One of the most important genetic studies is the Colorado Twin Study of Specific Reading Disability. Among a large number of twins, it found a concordance rate for dyslexia in MZ twins of 68% compared with 38% in DZ twins, a result which suggests that genetic and environmental factors are both at work. In studying a subset of twins who were labeled as having "phonological" dyslexia (trouble making sounds from letter groups), the role of genes appeared to be substantially more important than that of environment. Over the last 20 years, there have been many studies of multigenerational families in which dyslexia was common. Statistical analyses that search for a best-fit model have repeatedly found most support for the action of a single (unknown) gene that contributes about 50% of the overall risk.

Using the tools of molecular genetics, scientists have conducted many linkage studies of SRD. Some have been too small to be really helpful, and others have yielded results that have not been replicated. However, at least nine studies suggest there is a predisposing gene on the short arm of chromosome 6 (region 6p21.3). Unfortunately, this region is where the HLA genes are located, a fact that complicates the hunt for the hidden gene. In 2002, a group at Yale reported that in a study of 104 families with SRD, it had found very strong evidence that a gene in the 6p21.3-22 region was highly associated with a particular subtype of dyslexia called orthographic choice. In 2001, Finnish researchers working with 140 families found strong evidence for a predisposing gene on chromosome 3. In the autumn of 2003, a research team in Finland reported that a boy with SRD also had a chromosomal abnormality in which parts of chromosomes 15 and 2 had been translocated (switched). The chromosomal event had disrupted a gene called DYX1C1 on chromosome 15. This serendipitous discovery could mean that we have found an SRD gene. There are almost certainly more than a few genes involved in the risk for dyslexia. We will soon find them and they will help us to refine our understanding of the disorder, which will ultimately be seen as a collection of disabilities.

What can we say to parents concerned about SRD? The most important question to answer is whether or not there is a positive family history and, if so, how many relatives have been so diagnosed. Some of the research suggests that there are subsets of SRD that are due to the influence of a single gene that acts as a dominant. This knowledge forces counselors to err on the high side of risk. For example, if a man clearly had dyslexia as a child, it is necessary to counsel that any of his sons may have a 50% risk of being so affected, and any daughter may have a risk of 25–30%. The best current data suggest that if it is the woman who was affected in childhood, both her sons and daughters face about a 30% risk. These figures are soft and depend in part on assumptions about sex ratio that may not be correct.

Specific Language Impairment

As a child my husband had trouble learning to speak. Now my son has been given the diagnosis of SLI. What is the risk that my 6-month-old daughter will also have this problem?

Like SRD, specific language impairment (SLI) is primarily a diagnosis of exclusion, the boundaries of which are much debated by experts. The child with SLI has normal intelligence but fails to develop normal expressive and/or receptive speech despite the lack of any obvious neurological, emotional, or environmental problems. Children with SLI seem not to be "wired" for proper use of the inherent rules of language. Of course, any effort to understand their problems must be infused with full awareness of the complexity of human language. Workers in this field currently posit five separate language domains: phonology (the analysis of sound), morphology (word formation), syntax (word order), semantics (meaning), and pragmatics (word choice to express meaning). Children with SLI may have a range of deficits from mild to severe across each domain. For example, some children may have serious problems understanding speech and yet have relatively normal expressive speech. As with SRD, each child is unique; the magnitude of SLI reflects the subtle interactions of his or her genes with the ever-varying environment.

The research literature suggests that as many as 8% of school-age children in the United States have SLI, but prevalence data depend on the diagnostic boundaries used by the investigators. My guess is that 8% is too high. In one study that applied the label only if a child's score was more than 1.2 standard deviations below the mean score, just over 5% of the children were ultimately diagnosed with SLI. As the diagnostic criteria are tightened, the prevalence declines. Furthermore, the number of children labeled with SLI declines with age. As with SRD, the older literature suggests that far more boys than girls have SLI, but more recent studies suggest that the excess of boys is only about 1.3 to 1.

Although much research has been done, the cause of SLI is not known. Most experts agree that the most likely cause is one of several subtle prenatal injuries that harm language centers in the brain. Yet, careful study with advanced neuroimaging techniques has revealed no clear anatomic deficits (although there is some evidence of involvement of the left frontal and/or temporal areas). Various studies of auditory processing have also been inconsistent.

There is solid evidence that SLI is familial and heritable, but no one knows how many or which genes are causative. Several twin studies have found that concordance rates for SLI among MZ twin pairs are significantly higher than for DZ pairs. Most experts seem comfortable with the notion that genetic liability accounts for about half the risk for SLI, with environmental factors accounting for the balance. It appears that the more severe the impairment, the greater the role of the as-yet-unknown genes.

During the 1980s and 1990s, family studies consistently found that first-degree relatives of affected children are more likely also to have children with SLI than are first-degree relatives of unaffected children. For example, one study of 87 preschool children with phonological disorders found that 27% of their first-degree relatives also had a history of speech or language problems. Another study found that risk for SLI was associated with a region of chromosome 7 known to harbor a gene which, when mutated, causes Williams syndrome, a disorder that includes language problems.

Recently, a consortium of researchers completed a whole-genome scan of a large number of SLI families that uncovered evidence of predisposing genes on chromosomes 16 and 9. In 2002, a group at Rutgers University studying five extended Canadian families of Celtic origin found strong statistical evidence that associated SLI with a gene on the long arm of chromosome 13. The findings are particularly impressive because of the great care with which the scientists used diagnostic criteria. In June of 2003, a group of researchers at the University of Iowa reported on their genetic studies of 600 children with SLI and their parents. They found powerful evidence for an SLI gene on chromosome region 7q31. This region is close to a gene called FOXP2, mutations in which are known to cause a rare form of delay in speech acquisition. Incidentally, it appears that evolutionary changes in FOXP2 played a key role in the ability of humans to develop the capacity for speech. The DNA in the human FOXP2 gene differs far more from the comparable chimpanzee gene than do most other human genes.

What can family history tell us about the risk in the next generation? Unfortunately, not a great deal. SLI almost certainly encompasses several different conditions, each with its own cause. After reviewing most of the published studies, one prominent researcher suggested that the children of affected individuals are at about 20% risk. If the newborn child is of the same sex as the affected parent, the risk is closer to 30%.

Attention Deficit Hyperactivity Disorder

It seems as if there is a child labeled with ADHD in every classroom in my son's school. How common is it? How much of it is genetic?

Attention deficit hyperactivity disorder (ADHD) is the most commonly described mental disorder in children. In essence, it is defined as an impaired ability in maintaining attention to tasks and an associated marked impulsivity that cannot be easily explained by any medical disorder or by environmental factors. Child psychiatrists recognize two subtypes of ADHD, one in which inattention dominates and another characterized by hyperactivity. However, most affected children exhibit features of both types.

Debate rages about the prevalence of this disorder, and many researchers think that clinicians over-diagnose the condition. Several surveys in the United States found a prevalence of 4–8% of the school-age population. However, in Europe, where clinicians employ more stringent criteria, the prevalence is 1–2%. As with other learning disorders, the diagnosis is made more often in boys than in girls. The sex ratio is about 3:1. Children with ADHD often turn out to have other problems; in particular, depression is all too common.

Although the cause of ADHD is unknown, the dominant theory attributes the condition to some subtle impairment of the frontal lobe of the brain. However, although there are many hypotheses, little is known about what actually causes the impairment. There are several genetic diseases (including Tourette syndrome and Fragile X syndrome) in which affected children have some of the same problems as do children with ADHD. However, these disorders explain only a tiny fraction of all cases. Several family studies conducted in the 1990s found that 30–40% of children diagnosed with ADHD had family members who also had been given this diagnosis. Other family studies have demonstrated that families in which there are persons with ADHD also often have members who have been diagnosed with specific reading disability (SRD). Some think that many children with ADHD actually are dyslexic and that their behaviors grow out of the frustration they have with learning to read. Twin studies routinely find a greater concordance for ADHD in MZ than DZ twins. This has led some geneticists to attribute these findings to the effects of one or more dominant genes that are not completely penetrant (i.e., do not always manifest). One study concluded that the penetrance was about 45%, which implies that it causes ADHD in about half the individuals who carry it.

Because methylphenidate (Ritalin), which is known to affect the actions of the neurotransmitter dopamine, has been shown to be an effective treatment of many children with ADHD, interest in the genetics of this disorder has long focused on "candidate" genes—those that code for proteins which, if dysfunctional, could cause the disease. An increased risk for this disorder has been associated with variants in two genes (called DAT1 and DRD4), both of which are involved in dopamine metabolism, but the evidence is not compelling. Many people with these variants do not develop ADHD.

In 2003, scientists at UCLA completed a genome scan of 270 pairs of sibs with ADHD and identified candidate regions. They promptly conducted a second study in another group of 306 pairs of affected siblings. This allowed them to narrow their focus to just three regions common to both studies, but the data they generated are not sufficiently strong to constitute a high degree of certainty. With time, the focus will sharpen.

Although the numbers are soft, a fair guess is that for couples with no family history of ADHD on either side, the risk of bearing a child who will develop this disorder is probably 2–3%. When counseling parents or families with an affected child about recurrence risk, the best one can offer are figures based on empirical studies. Summarizing a number of studies, the recurrence risk in this situation is anywhere from 16% to 25%.

Stuttering

I stuttered as a child. What are the risks to my children?

Stuttering is a relatively common disorder of speech caused by spasm of the muscles involved in the production of word sounds. The affected individual cannot properly control the flow and timing of speech. Specific deficits include being unable to make a desired sound, repeating sounds, prolonging sounds, interjecting inappropriate sounds, and breaking up words improperly. In severely affected persons, stuttering disrupts at least 10% of speech efforts and can last up to 30 seconds at a time. Understandably, the affected child typically feels much frustration and stress.

Stuttering afflicts about 1% of children, with boys being affected about four times more frequently than girls. It is most prominent between ages 2 and 4 and again between ages 6 and 8 (a time in which reading aloud is a prominent feature of grammar school education). In most individuals, stuttering fades with age, although it may recur in adults under stress. Oddly, people who stutter can be quite fluent when they sing, whisper, or are unable to hear their own voice. People who stutter are of normal intelligence. Winston Churchill and James Earl Jones are just two of untold numbers of stutterers who have been wonderfully successful in their careers.

The once-common view that stuttering reflected underlying emotional problems has been abandoned. Today, there are nearly a dozen theories competing to explain the etiology of stuttering. Most are based in neuro-psychology and focus on trying to understand the neurological triggers that disrupt the normal flow of speech formation. Many experts view stuttering as the common endpoint resulting from any one of a clutch of developmental problems (much as anemia can be the result of many different blood disorders). In the search to understand the biological events that cause a child to stutter, there is currently much interest in brain imaging. One recent brain imaging study of a small group of adults who stutter found that a portion of their temporal lobe was larger on average than that of a control group. This finding has not been repeated, nor has it been found to be the case in children.

It has long been known that stuttering is highly familial, and the dominant view is that as-yet-unexplained genetic factors play an important role. A number of studies have shown a high concordance rate for stuttering among identical twins (ranging from 25% to 80%). Adoption studies have shown that if a child of biological parents, neither of whom ever stuttered, is adopted in infancy by a parent who stuttered, the adopted child will not stutter. This suggests that it is not a learned behavior. Family studies have shown that first-degree relatives of persons who stutter are 5–20 times more likely to stutter than are first-degree relatives of individuals who have never stuttered. The biggest risk factor for stuttering is simply having a parent who stuttered. (There are a number of scientific reports of families in which stuttering is caused by a single, dominant gene.) If a child stutters, the chances are about 1 in 10 that his brother will stutter as well.

Since the mid 1990s, there has been a surge of interest in finding the genes that predispose to stuttering. In 1996, a group of scientists at the Stuttering Research Institute at the University of Illinois began studying the DNA of the extended families of 66 children who stutter. Their results suggested that a single, relatively common gene variant was a major contributor to risk for stuttering. With colleagues at the University of Chicago, they are now conducting another study to see whether they can isolate the causative gene.

For parents who stuttered as children and who are worried about the risk to their young children, the best course of action may be to make sure that the pediatrician knows the family history, to monitor the development of speech in their sons and daughters, and to act sooner rather than later to obtain speech therapy if early signs of stuttering emerge.

EPILEPSY (SEIZURES)

My mother has seizures. What are my risks?

Epilepsy is the name given to a large collection of disorders of the brain, the hallmark of which is recurrent, unprovoked seizures. A seizure is the physical consequence of a sudden abnormal electrical discharge of brain cells. Depending on the location of the electrical events in the brain, a seizure can take many forms. To most people unfamiliar with the various forms of epilepsy, the term seizure evokes images of an unconscious person thrashing about on the ground. This is but one type, the "tonic-clonic seizure." Space permits only a superficial description of some of the many types of epilepsy.

One standard way to categorize seizures is as generalized or partial. Partial seizures involve only a region of the body. As a rule partial seizures are more likely to be due to specific brain injuries (such as a history of head trauma) and less likely to be under substantial genetic influence. There are many different partial seizure states. They can be limited to the abnormal motion of a single arm or leg, or they can be experienced as a sudden, overpowering odor. They can be auditory, hallucinatory, or they can present as sudden sweating. The possibilities are many, and the details are almost as varied as the number of patients.

As a rule, persons with generalized seizures have otherwise normal brain function and usually do not have a history of brain injury. Generalized seizures start in both sides of the brain at once. The two major types are absence and tonic-clonic seizures. Childhood absence epilepsy, which begins at about age 5, is characterized by many brief periods during which the affected person ceases all activity and stares into space as if in a trance. This can happen dozens of times a day. Absence seizures usually last for only a few seconds, but the child can also have generalized seizures that may last longer. Although the cause of absence seizures is unclear, much evidence suggests it is due to a defect in the circuitry connecting the thalamus to the cerebral cortex.

Generalized seizures are a common manifestation of many different uncommon brain diseases, several of which are caused by single-gene disorders. For example, benign neonatal convulsions, which usually begin in the third or fourth day of life and resolve within a few weeks, are caused by a defect in either one of two genes (KCNQ2 and KCNQ3) that control the

Table 10. *Some seizure syndromes caused by single genes*

Syndrome	Gene	Activity
Epilepsy with febrile seizures	SCN1B	sodium channel
	SCN1A	sodium channel
	SCN2A	sodium channel
	GABRG2	neurotransmitter receptor
Benign familial neonatal seizures	KCNQ2	potassium channel
	KCNQ3	potassium channel
Nocturnal frontal lobe epilepsy	CHRNA4	acetylcholine receptor
	CHRNB2	acetylcholine receptor
Absence epilepsy and febrile seizures	GABRG2	neurotransmitter receptor
Partial epilepsy with auditory features	LGI1	transmembrane protein

flux of potassium ions in and out of cells. Nocturnal frontal lobe epilepsy, a dominant disorder that produces shaking movements mostly during sleep, is caused by mutations in either of two genes (called CHRNA2 and CHRNA4) that make part of the cell surface receptors for a chemical messenger called acetylcholine. These two forms of epilepsy have distinct phenotypes and are comparatively easy to diagnose. However, most generalized forms of epilepsy are probably caused by the interaction of several genes with environmental factors, which makes it extremely challenging to understand their cause.

The medical evaluation of an individual with generalized epilepsy is lengthy and can be frustrating. It typically involves electroencephalographic (EEG) analysis, brain imaging, extensive biochemical studies, chromosome analysis, DNA studies, and sometimes lengthy videotaping so that doctors can observe an actual seizure. Even after extensive workup, it is often not possible to make a firm diagnosis and, therefore, difficult to offer any but the most general kind of genetic counseling.

Currently, genetic factors are thought overall to play an important role in about half of all cases of generalized epilepsy. Given the pace at which new genes that define particular forms of epilepsy are being discovered, that fraction is almost certain to increase. Although even experts have great trouble agreeing about the cause of some cases of epilepsy, they eventually make the correct diagnosis in those children affected by a recognized single-gene disorder. The correct diagnosis leads to relatively straightforward counseling of patients, their parents, and close relatives. However, for a large fraction of children with epilepsy, perhaps 40%, the reason for the disease is elusive.

About 5–10% of all seizures are cases of juvenile myoclonic epilepsy (JME). This seizure disorder typically has an onset in adolescence, but it can appear in younger children. The seizures, which usually involve the arms, typically occur in the mornings, especially on awakening. Lack of sleep and use of alcohol increase the liability to these seizures. The condition requires lifelong use of anti-seizure medication. JME has long been known to cluster in families, and it is widely believed that there is a significant genetic predisposition to the disorder.

During the 1990s, several research efforts compiled strong statistical evidence that a gene predisposing to JME (and dubbed JME1) is located somewhere in a region on the short arm of chromosome 6 called 6p21. In the summer of 2003, a team at Columbia University reported that they had identified the culprit. In studying a cohort of 20 JME families, they found that affected individuals had two DNA variations (SNPs) in the promoter region of a gene called BRD2 that is known to make a protein involved in the development of the central nervous system. These variants were not found in two control groups. This is the first study to identify a gene involved in a common form of epilepsy. The data suggest that the SNP variants do not cause, but rather, increase the susceptibility to JME, perhaps by altering the activity of the corresponding protein. Most likely, JME is a term that is being applied to several different disorders, each with its own genetic risk factors.

Another seizure pattern, "benign childhood epilepsy with centrotemporal spikes" (BCECTS), is a relatively mild disorder that has a characteristic EEG recording. Studies have shown that the families of affected persons have a much higher than normal history of seizure disorders, and that many of those without a history of seizures still have EEG abnormalities. The search for the predisposing gene has not yet yielded results.

There are at least three types of "absence seizure disorders of childhood." They are subdivided by age of onset, the presence of certain signature patterns on the EEG recordings, and whether or not myoclonic jerks (sudden involuntary movements, typically of the arm, that can be elicited by fatigue or drinking alcohol) occur. In each case, twin studies have suggested that predisposing genes are an important part of the syndrome, but in no case have we yet cloned the culprit gene.

The most common form of seizure disorder among children is strongly associated with high fevers. This diagnosis is made when the seizure occurs in a child under age 5 who has no signs of meningitis or serious neurological problems. About 3% of children born in the United States suffer a febrile seizure. In Japan, the incidence approaches 8%, and in Guam, it is even higher. Febrile seizures are highly familial. The odds of a brother or sister of a child with a history of a febrile seizure also being affected are high. Family studies have found concordance rates ranging from 10% to 40%. There is also an especially high concordance rate for EEG recording patterns, but so far, EEG patterns have not been helpful in predicting who will have a febrile seizure. The data are compatible with different modes of inheritance, but the best fit seems to be with one or more dominantly acting single genes, each with incomplete penetrance.

Thus far, gene-mapping studies have identified five susceptibility loci. In 2003, researchers in Japan found a sixth (on chromosome 18) and provided preliminary evidence that the causative gene is IMPA2, which makes a protein involved in brain cell metabolism. Fortunately, most children who have a febrile seizure have no more than two more during their childhood, and few develop a chronic seizure disorder.

What can we advise people who have a family history of epilepsy, but

Table 11. *Epilepsy: Risk in offspring and siblings of persons with epilepsy*

Type of epilepsy	Affected parent (%)	Affected sibling (%)	Children (%)	Siblings (%)
Childhood absence	7	5–10	6–7	5–10
Juvenile myoclonic	5–15	4–7	5–14	4–7
Photosensitive	7 females 2 males	6.5 females	2–7	6–10
Infantile spasms	unknown	1–2	unknown	1–25

Adapted, with permission, from Rimoin D.I., Connor J.M., Pyeritz R.E., and Korf B.R. 2002. *Emery and Rimoin's principles and practice of medical genetics*, 4th edition. Churchill Livingstone, London; © Elsevier.

for whom there is no strong evidence to suspect a single-gene disorder? The most common inquiry comes from a young couple planning a family when one parent has an idiopathic (a doctor's word for "unknown cause") seizure disorder. If the disorder is idiopathic, the recurrence risk in offspring is 5–10%. If the disorder in question is either JME or childhood absence epilepsy, the risk to each child of being similarly affected is about 5–7%. For unknown reasons, the risk is somewhat higher in the children of affected mothers than it is in the children of affected fathers.

Another common situation is when a couple with no family history of seizures has a child with a seizure disorder. The parents want to know the risk to their next child. For both JME and absence seizures, the recurrence risk is between 5% and 10%. When the disorder is idiopathic, the lifetime risk is closer to 10%, about fivefold higher than the risk in the general population. The younger sisters and brothers of a first child with febrile seizures have a 10–15% chance also of having such seizures. If a parent and one child are affected, the risk to other children is about 30%.

What is the risk of seizures to the son or daughter of a woman who has generalized seizures of unknown cause? Empirical data put the lifetime risk at about 10%, but there is little that can be said about age of onset.

JUVENILE DIABETES

> *My 12-year-old son has juvenile diabetes. What is the risk that his younger sister will also develop it?*

The classic presentation of juvenile diabetes (diabetes type I) is the relatively sudden onset in a previously healthy child of weight loss, increased urination, persistent thirst, and dehydration. By the time the child is brought to the emergency room, where the diagnosis is often made, he or she has a high blood sugar and a metabolic imbalance (ketoacidosis). The child and/or his parents usually recall that in actuality the signs of the illness had been becoming more apparent over several weeks.

The biochemical hallmark of juvenile diabetes is very low or absent levels of insulin. This is caused by auto-antibodies that destroy the insulin-producing β cells of the pancreas. About 15 out of every 100,000 children aged 0–14 in the United States have type I diabetes. Worldwide, the prevalence ranges from as low as 1/100,000 in Asia to as high as 40/100,000 in Sweden. The incidence of the disease appears to be on the rise, which suggests that more people are being exposed to environmental risk factors.

Juvenile diabetes is an autoimmune disease. Although it presents suddenly, there is good evidence that for months or even years prior to the diagnosis, circulating antibodies have been killing the cells in the pancreas that make insulin. Studies of the healthy identical MZ twins of children diagnosed with juvenile diabetes have found β-cell antibodies in their blood years before they too develop the disease. This is possible because about 90% of β cells must die before a child becomes sick.

As with other autoimmune disorders (those characterized by persistent attacks by the body's immune system upon itself) there is unequivocal evidence that genetic risk factors play an important role in the onset of this disorder. Still, the pathway to disease is complicated and not yet well understood. Studies of MZ twins have long shown moderately impressive concordance rates. One prospective study found that among MZ twins in which a first child was diagnosed, 36% of the second twins developed the disease. This suggests that only one-third of persons with genes "for" juvenile diabetes develop the disease. In the language of genetics, the predisposing genes have reduced "penetrance."

Table 12. *Juvenile diabetes: General population risk and risk to first-degree relatives overall and by DR gene pattern (haplotype)*

Population risks	Overall—1/500
	HLA-DR related
	0 high-risk allele 1/500
	1 high-risk allele 1/400
	HLA-DR3/3 or DR4/4—1/150
	HLA-DR3/4—1/40
Risks to siblings	Overall—1/14
	HLA haplotypes shared with diabetic siblings
	0 haplotypes shared—1/100
	1 haplotypes shared—1/20
	2 haplotypes shared—1/6
	2 haplotypes shared and DR3/4—1/5 to 1/4
Risks to offspring	Overall—1/25
	offspring of affected woman: 1/40
	offspring of affected man: 1/20
Monozygotic twin	Overall—1/3

Adapted, with permission, from King R.A., Rotter J.I., and Motulsky A.G., eds. 2002. *The genetic basis of common diseases,* 2nd edition. Oxford University Press, United Kingdom.

Table 13. *Juvenile-onset diabetes: Risk by DR/DQ haplotype and family history*

Proband DR/DQ status	Risk to first-degree relative (%)	No other relative affected (%)
DR 3-4	20–25	7
DR 4-4	16	5
DR 3-3	10	2
DR 4-X	6	1
DR X-X	<1	<0.2

Adapted, with permission, from King R.A., Rotter J.I., and Motulsky A.G., eds. 2002. *The genetic basis of common diseases*, 2nd edition. Oxford University Press, United Kingdom.

About 30 years ago, the risk for juvenile diabetes was associated with two of the so-called Class I antigens B8 and B15 (two proteins involved in the immune defense system made by a special class of genes on chromosome 6 that are called the HLA genes). During the 1980s, even stronger risk was found in persons who carried a combination of two Class II antigens called DR3 and DR4. About 95% of all people with juvenile diabetes have one or both of these antigens, compared to 50% of the overall population. However, it is important to note that about 1–3% of individuals in the general population have DR3 or DR4 and that the vast majority of carriers do *not* develop juvenile-onset diabetes.

The best current estimate is that HLA genes account for about 70% of the genetic risk for juvenile diabetes. Over the past few years, there have been several large-scale efforts to search the human genome to find other genes that predispose to this disease. As of 2000, at least 16 locations had been found in the genome which appear to harbor alleles that may predispose to the disease. Unfortunately, it will be very difficult to parse the relative role of these genes once they are identified.

What can we tell family members, especially the brothers and sisters of persons newly diagnosed with diabetes? We have to rely on empiric risk data based on family surveys. For siblings of a child with juvenile diabetes, the risk of developing the disease is 5–10%. If the father is affected, his children have a 4–6% risk; if the mother is affected, her children have a 2–3% risk. By far the highest risk is in the siblings who have the same DR3/DR4 haplotype (a term used to describe a combination of genes) as the affected child. In such cases, the risk approaches 25%.

ASTHMA

So many kids have asthma! Isn't it mostly due to environmental factors?

Asthma is a disease of the airways characterized by chronic inflammation and periodic hyper-responsiveness of the bronchioles. It is a common, complex disorder that arises in genetically predisposed people who are exposed to any one of a variety of environmental agents that trigger the acute flares which lead to shortness of breath. The most widely recognized risk factor for asthma is atopy, defined as the tendency for the body's cells to release a substance called IgE that is at the head of the complex bio-chemical response which leads to the clinical signs of acute asthma. High serum levels of IgE are commonly found in children with asthma.

There is no question that the incidence of asthma is on the rise. Studies in Australia show that between 1980 and 2000, the rate in children doubled from 5% to 10%. Data from the United States show a similar trend. The death rate from asthma also is on the rise, but the reason is not clear. In a country where there is not equal access to health care, such a trend can be influenced heavily by socioeconomic factors.

Several well-planned studies have provided strong evidence for a major genetic component to asthma. For example, studies of IgE levels in MZ twins indicate a strong genetic influence (a heritability score of 0.6). Similar studies have also showed strong correlation between serum IgE levels and risk for allergy and/or asthma. A 1984 study in Arizona examined the risk of asthma in 344 nuclear families. There were 273 families in which neither parent had ever been diagnosed with asthma, 68 families in which one parent had been diagnosed, and 3 families in which both parents carried the diagnosis. In the 273 families in which asthma had never

---

Table 14. *Asthma: Familial risk—Key points*

A positive family history for asthma is found in over half of children who are diagnosed with asthma.

The risk of a child having severe asthma (requiring hospitalization) is higher if the *mother* has a history of the disorder than if the father does.

The risk to a sibling if at least one parent and one other child have been diagnosed is about 25%.

been diagnosed in the parents, 35 of a total of 538 (6.5%) children had asthma; in the families where one parent had asthma, 24 of 122 (20%) of the children had asthma; in the families where both parents had asthma, 7 of 11 (64%) children also had the disorder.

The risk of a child's being hospitalized for asthma is strongly influenced by a parental history of the disease. Several studies have found that maternal asthma is a much stronger predictor than is paternal asthma. In fact, in some studies when parental history of the disease is broken down by gender of parent, having a father who had asthma in childhood does not seem to influence the risk at all.

During the mid 1990s, several large studies were conducted to screen the human genome to identify regions that contain gene variants which confer risk for asthma. Several locations have been identified that appear to be highly associated with airway hyperactivity or IgE levels. In a Dutch study, the evidence is particularly strong for a region on the long arm of chromosome 5. A large study of Hutterites, a group of Americans of European descent who rarely marry outside their religious community, found strong association of atopy within a small region on chromosome 16. One gene known to be located there is the gene called IL-4, which is involved in causing inflammation. Unfortunately, there are many predisposing genes, and it will be hard to track them down.

In 2003, a group of UK researchers reported that they had shown that variations in a gene called PHF11 (located on the long arm of chromosome 13 in a region already suspected of harboring an asthma gene) were highly associated with having severe asthma. In a study of unrelated British adults, one particular SNP (polymorphism) was found four times more often in adults with severe asthma than in normal controls. It was also found about twice as often as in adults with mild asthma. This gene appears to significantly influence IgE, levels of which are correlated with risk for asthma and atopic dermatitis.

Empirical data provide fairly good estimates to prospective parents about the risk of asthma in their children. If one parent has a clear history of allergies, the risk that a child will be allergic may be as high as 60%; if both parents have allergies, the risk may be as high as 85%. If two normal parents have an affected child, the chance that the next child will also be affected is on the order of 9–13%. If a couple in which one member has asthma has a child with asthma, the risk to the next child may be as high as 25–50%.

ECZEMA

Both my brother and I had eczema as children. My wife did not. What are the risks for our children?

Eczema (atopic dermatitis) is an extremely common, chronic skin disorder, the hallmark of which is an itchy dry rash that is most often found in the creases of the arms and legs. Other commonly affected areas are the neck and the tops of the hands and feet. The term "atopy" refers to a condition in which the body overproduces IgE in response to exposure to some allergen. Typically, eczema develops during infancy, but improves as the child grows. There is a poorly understood, but close, relationship between eczema and asthma. As children who have had severe eczema get older, as many as 60% develop asthma. In many families in which one child has asthma, another may have eczema.

Although there must be risk factors that predispose to eczema, certain changes in our environment, especially since World War II, seem to have greatly increased the incidence of this disorder. Central heating, wall-to-wall carpeting, and, in particular, dramatic increase in the use of harsh skin and laundry soaps all track with the rise. The soaps are almost certainly contributing to the breakdown of the skin barrier, which is an essential feature of eczema.

Eczema is much more common in persons who have a family history of allergies. About one-third of the children who have severe eczema also develop food allergies. Consuming certain foods can cause the skin disorder to flare. Preventive treatment focuses on keeping the patient's skin moist and avoiding known triggers. Careful use of topical steroids on inflamed areas is warranted, as is close monitoring for, and treatment of, skin infections.

In Britain, researchers at the Wellcome Trust Center for Human Genetics have mapped genes for atopic dermatitis to chromosomes 1, 17, and 20. Each of these regions has already been associated with other skin diseases. Another ambitious effort is under way at the Karolinska Institute in Sweden, where Dr. Magnus Nordenskjold has enrolled 500 families in which at least 2 persons have eczema. He is using 400 DNA markers to scan the family genomes to find areas where a culprit gene may be hiding.

If one parent in a couple has a definite history of eczema as a child, the chance that any one of his children will develop eczema is about twice the background risk; if both parents have a positive history for this disorder, the chance that any one of their children will also have eczema is high—

between 30% and 50%. If the parents do not have a family history, but a first child is affected, the risk to the next child is between 10% and 25%. Parents of all children with eczema should be watchful for signs of respiratory distress, which signal the first flare of asthma.

SCOLIOSIS

My child's pediatrician told me that my daughter has scoliosis. What is the risk to my two younger kids?

Scoliosis is the term used to define a sideways curvature of the spine, a condition that is fairly common among children and adolescents. There are many uncommon causes of scoliosis, including neuromuscular diseases like muscular dystrophy and cerebral palsy, polio, spina bifida, and radiation to the spine. However, in the vast majority of cases, almost all of which occur in otherwise healthy individuals, the cause is unknown.

The two major categories of scoliosis are congenital and idiopathic. The congenital category is composed of children born with one or more malformed vertebrae. The treatment varies widely depending on the exact nature of the deformity, but surgery is necessary only in severe cases. Idiopathic scoliosis is subdivided by the age of onset. Most children with infantile scoliosis (age 0–3) have left-sided spinal curves. The children are observed closely, and a small fraction are treated with braces. In almost all these children, the scoliosis self-corrects over time. Juvenile scoliosis refers to children who manifest the spinal curve between 3 and 9 years of age. In some of these children, the scoliosis becomes markedly more severe with age, and braces are necessary. Surgery is not usually needed. By far the most common category is adolescent scoliosis. Mild cases are found in equal numbers of boys and girls, but girls account for the vast majority of severe cases.

Survey research has found idiopathic scoliosis in anywhere from 1% to 8% of the populations studied, with the rates varying according to the stringency of the diagnostic criteria. It has long been recognized that idiopathic scoliosis is familial, and researchers have argued in favor of a variety of single-gene models. However, because the condition is most commonly diagnosed in adolescent girls, it seems unlikely that a single-gene model will explain most cases. In adolescents with scoliosis, the same condition is found in at least one parent up to 30% of the time—far higher than would be expected in a randomly selected adult population. The more severely affected the child, the more likely that a parent also has scoliosis.

There have been few attempts to map genes responsible for idiopathic scoliosis. One empirical study by a Russian research group of 101 families concluded that for families in which the scoliosis is severe, the inheritance pattern best fit a single dominantly acting gene. In 2003, some researchers reported on a family in which the presence of scoliosis cosegregates with (travels with) an unusual structural change called a pericentric inversion on chromosome 8. Efforts to link mutations in the SNTG1 gene (which is disrupted by the chromosomal abnormality) with familial scoliosis have so far suggested it plays only a minor role.

Surveys of families indicate that the empirical risk to a younger sibling of a child with adolescent scoliosis is about 7%. This underestimates the risk in those few families in which the disorder may be due to an as-yet-unidentified, dominantly acting gene.

STATURE

My father's side of the family tends to be short; my mother's side seems to be about average. I am five foot, six inches. How tall is my son likely to be?

Geneticists have been interested in height for a century. A study published as long ago as 1903 correctly concluded that height is normally distributed (follows a bell curve) across ethnic groups, but is highly heritable within families. Over the last three decades, several large studies have led to the conclusion that even though adult height is the result of the interactions of several genes with environmental factors, it is far more influenced by genes than environment. True, there is evidence that over the last 100 years the average height of adults in a number of countries has risen steadily with the better nutrition that comes with a higher standard of living. However, there is also evidence that even in circumstances in which many children have endured severe calorie deprivation, the final adult height of those who survive is not discernibly affected. Today, in the well-fed United States, Europe, and Japan, most children grow up in an environment that permits the maximum expression of genetically driven height. On balance, the heritability of height appears to be between 0.7 and 0.9, making stature among the most genetically influenced of complex conditions.

During the last few years, several research groups have considered height as a trait for which it might be possible to track down the major genes, despite the challenge of not knowing how many there are or how they interact with the environment. In 2001, several groups, led by the

Whitehead Institute in Cambridge, Massachusetts, reported on their study of the genetics of height in four populations. The four groups were made up of 2327 persons in 483 families hailing from two regions of Finland, Sweden, and Quebec. Using genetic markers to identify blocs of DNA in the human genome that were found more often than expected in tall persons, the team identified four locations in which there was strong statistical evidence that a height gene is located. Of interest, another study in a different Finnish population independently found strong evidence for a height gene in one of those regions, the long arm of chromosome 7. Late in 2003, Australian scientists reported on their search for height genes in the nearly 800 families enrolled in the ongoing Victorian Family Heart Study. They found six promising leads, but the studies must be replicated before any region can be anointed as a true lead. The most impressive evidence to date is a Japanese study that found a strikingly high presence of a variation in a gene called FBN1 in men who are two standard deviations above mean height.

Just as there are genes that drive tall stature, there are genes that set children on a path toward short stature in adult life. One need only compare professional basketball players with jockeys to realize this. On a population basis, one can make the same observation by comparing Swedes to Greeks. Height, although highly genetic, has a wide base to its bell curve.

Short stature is a complicated topic for at least two reasons. First, there are many disorders in which poor growth is a feature (although together they account for only a small fraction of the children with short stature). Second, there are many societies that seem to favor height, which tends improperly to medicalize short stature. The vast majority of children brought to pediatric clinics that specialize in evaluating growth have either "familial short stature," "constitutional growth delay," or both. In essence, these are healthy children who are destined to occupy the left end of the bell curve or to reach a middling height a year or two after their peers.

What can be said to people who inquire about the likely height of their children? Barring serious prenatal insults, severe childhood diseases, and prolonged starvation, the single best predictor of final adult height in healthy children is a simple calculation based on the heights of both parents. For example, assuming a healthy family, a son born to a white woman who is five foot four inches tall and a white man who is five foot eight inches tall has nearly a 50% chance of reaching five foot nine inches. About two-thirds of similarly born children will be within two inches of that height, and 95% will be within four inches. Unusually tall children (who do not have one of several uncommon genetic disorders associated with extreme height) almost invariably are the offspring of tall parents. For them, too, the best predictor of final adult height is based on an assessment of parental heights.

The availability of human growth hormone (GH) (approved by the FDA for the treatment of the relatively few children with certain genetically caused growth disorders) has provoked much clinical and ethical debate about the proper use of this powerful drug (which is given by injections over several years). Although there is solid evidence that it improves final adult height for children who lack growth hormone and those with a few other disorders, there is still little firm evidence that GH much increases height in otherwise healthy, small children. Even if it does increase height by an inch or two, the cost (both economic and emotional) of taking growth hormone by injection for several years should give pause.

Returning to the opening question, assuming it was asked by a white man of European heritage (putting him at about the 10th percentile) and that his wife is of the same heritage (putting her at the 50th percentile for height), his son has a good chance of being an inch or two taller than the father, who is more than three inches below the mean for height. There are, however, fairly wide error bars on such estimates.

STRABISMUS

I had a lazy eye as a child. What are the chances that my children will have the same problem?

Strabismus (also called lazy eye or cross-eyed) is the result of an improper alignment of the visual axes of the eyes. It is a common problem of early childhood. Large population surveys have found that about 1–5% of all children are diagnosed with this condition. It has been known since ancient times that strabismus runs in families. The great physician, Hippocrates, is said to have noted the hereditary influence in his writings. Strabismus is subdivided into categories based on age of onset, the nature of the deviation (divergent or convergent), and whether or not it is present with both eyes uncovered or only when one eye is in use.

Although there has been much interest in the genetic influence on strabismus, it has been hard to perform good studies. This is in part because the condition varies widely in its severity, which suggests that it may be a collection of disorders with different causes. The siblings of an affected child are at significantly elevated risk. The many studies of this question quote risks ranging from 10% to greater than 50%, a variation so wide that it supports the hypothesis that there are multiple subtypes of strabismus. The risk for esotropia (inward deviation) appears to be higher in the sibs of an affected child than is the case with exotropia.

Many papers have described autosomal dominant forms of strabismus, but these account for only a small percentage of all cases. In one large study of the relatives of nearly 700 patients, it was found that the risk of being born with strabismus is about 25% if one sibling but neither parent was affected. The risk was about 35% if one parent is also affected, and 50% if both parents have been so diagnosed. Twin studies provide strong support for genetic factors. In one large study of MZ twins, if one twin had strabismus there was an 80% chance that the other twin was also affected. In contrast, the concordance rate in 101 sets of DZ twins was only 12%.

There has not yet been a genome-wide search for genes that influence isolated strabismus. There are few data to support answers to questions that the relatives of affected persons may ask. The best we can say is that the disorder is highly familial, and that the risk to their offspring appears to be substantial.

EYE COLOR

My husband and I have blue eyes. How can our child have brown eye color?

Despite long-standing interest, our knowledge of the genetic factors that determine eye color remains incomplete. In the early part of the 20th century, human geneticists thought that eye color was determined according to strict Mendelian rules of inheritance applied to a single gene. Charles Davenport, an early human geneticist who was a Director of Cold Spring Harbor Laboratory, was among those who asserted that brown was dominant over blue, essentially arguing that two brown-eyed persons could have a blue-eyed child, but that the reverse could not occur. One need only reflect on the many hues of human eye color to reject this thesis.

In the mid-20th century, the older view was superceded by the teaching that the genes for brown and blue eye color behave as codominant alleles, with the palette of eye color arising from stochastic events in the eye cells. Dr. Victor McKusick, the dean of human genetics, put the idea of strict codominance to rest. He wrote in his famous atlas, *Mendelian Inheritance in Man*, "My monozygotic twin brother and I, brown-eyed, had blue eyed parents and blue eyed sibs." By the 1970s, eye color was thought to be a phenotype that arose from the action of several different genes that influenced the production and transport of melanin.

During the 1980s, linkage studies were able to establish that there is a gene on chromosome 15 which codes for brown versus blue eye color. Similar studies also discovered evidence that there is a gene on the short arm of chromosome 19 that influences the spectrum from green to blue eye color. These studies are impressive, but not absolutely convincing. Furthermore, there are almost certainly other genes that influence subtle issues like depth of hue.

Eye color should be thought of as a polygenically influenced trait with at least two major genes. In some families and racial groups, particularly those that only produce brown-eyed children, it is easy to predict eye color of children. However, for most white populations, eye color cannot be accurately predicted merely on the basis of observation of the parents.

HANDEDNESS

Why are 90% of people right-handed and 10% of people left-handed?

As everyone knows, most people exhibit a strong preference to use the right hand early in childhood. A variety of evidence stretching back nearly 5000 years indicates that the vast majority of people (about 93% today) have always been right-handed. There is much folklore about handedness, some of it also dating back thousands of years. Consider that in the romance languages (those that derive from Latin) the word for "left" shares the same root as the word for sinister or evil. Until recently in human history, left-handed people were viewed as odd and, sometimes, even dangerous. The fact that the percentage of left-handed people in England today is more than double that of 100 years ago probably reflects the discrimination that society, consciously or not, directed against left-handed persons during the Victorian era. It is almost certain that in 19th-century England, many southpaws were forced by their parents to use their right hands. Even today, one still hears stories from older, left-handed folks who as children were forced to use their right hands.

Views about the role of genes in determining handedness have waxed and waned over the years. In the first decade of the 20th century, the years in which Mendel's laws were first applied to human inheritance, some thought left-handedness was an autosomal recessive (single-gene) condition, that left-handed children were so because they inherited an allele from each parent which in combination predisposed them to be so. The genetic argument was based on the fact that couples in which both parents are right-handed have the fewest left-handed children, and couples in which both parents are left-handed have the most left-handed children. Of course, this could almost as easily be explained by environmental factors, such as the way right-handed parents unconsciously teach infants to hold things. Although concordance for left-handedness is greater for MZ twins than it is for DZ twins, it falls short of supporting a major role for genes. On the other hand, adoption studies have shown that adopted children are significantly more likely to have the hand preference of biological parents than of adoptive parents, a finding compatible with genetic influence.

Of the many theories of environmental causation, the most appealing is that handedness is influenced by the tendency of mothers to hold infants in their left arms. This constrains the infant's use of the left hand, but allows him or her to be soothed by the sound of the mother's beating heart. Of course, this hypothesis would be impossible to test. In the 1980s, this may have led a neuroscientist named Daniel Geschwind to speculate that left-handedness is the result of a focal developmental problem in the brain which affects the relative influence of certain groups of cells that control motor activity. Interestingly, several studies have found that a childhood history of SRD (dyslexia) is more common among left-handed adults than among righties.

Currently, the role of genes in determining handedness is in ascendance. In 2002, Geschwind's team at UCLA reported on brain imaging studies that they had done on 72 pairs of elderly MZ twins and 67 sets of comparably matched DZ twins. They found that pairs of identical twins who were both right-handed had no structural differences, but that pairs in which one or both were left-handed did have measurable differences.

What is the bottom line on handedness? There is solid evidence that left-handed parents are more likely to have left-handed children than are right-handed parents, but most left-handed parents actually do have right-handed children. There is some evidence linking left-handedness to subtle developmental problems such as dyslexia. However, the vast majority of left-handed children do not have discernible developmental problems. Furthermore, there is no evidence that forcing them to behave as righties has any benefit.

PART 4

Adulthood

HEART DISEASES

Coronary Artery Disease (Atherosclerosis)

My dad died at 52 of a heart attack. What does that do to my risk?

Coronary artery disease (CAD) is the major killer in the western world. In the United States, some 529,659 people died of heart attacks in 1999. More than 25% of the people who die in the United States and Europe each year die of heart attacks. More than 1,100,000 persons have a first heart attack each year, and about 40% of them die. During the 1980s, the death rate from heart attacks (deaths per 100,000 citizens) declined by nearly 30%. From 1989 to 1999, it declined another 24%. However, because of the rapid growth of the elderly population, the absolute number of deaths only fell by 7%.

What are the reasons for this dramatic reduction in the death rate from CAD? Over the last 40 years, millions of Americans have quit smoking, started exercising, and started regularly taking medications for high blood pressure. More recently, widespread use of lipid-lowering drugs called statins has also helped to reduce the death rate from heart disease. Unfortunately, the rate of decline in death rate is slowing. This is in large part because so many Americans are overweight. Obesity is a major risk factor for adult-onset diabetes, and heart attack is the number one killer of diabetics.

A heart attack is the name we give to death of a portion of the heart muscle due to inadequate blood flow. This usually happens because one of the three main coronary arteries or their branches are blocked. Heart attacks (myocardial infarctions) are perceived to be devastatingly sudden, often occurring without warning in men and women who think they are healthy. Heart attacks are the result of a decades-long process during which various fats (lipids) are deposited inside the arterial wall. This deposition generates a complex set of biological processes that ultimately result in the formation of plaques. Recent research has shown that these plaques really are of two distinct kinds. Some are remarkably stable over many years. Others are fragile and prone to break loose and clog the vessel as they move downstream. As stable plaques build in size, they limit blood flow and cause angina, the chest pain typical of CAD. This "clogged pipe" image, which long dominated medical thinking, has recently been modified as we have learned about the dynamic biology of the arterial wall. We now know that many plaques are unstable. The sudden calving of a clot from the side of a vessel wall which suddenly blocks blood flow downstream is a major cause of death in older adults.

The latest report from the National Heart Lung and Blood Institute's Expert Panel on the Detection, Evaluation and Treatment of Cholesterol, the Adult Treatment Panel Report (usually called the ATP III) is unequivocal: The major culprit in CAD is inappropriately high levels of LDL cholesterol (a.k.a. bad cholesterol). The risk for death or severe illness from CAD is strongly correlated with the genetic factors that influence lipid metabolism. Many published studies demonstrate that by lowering LDL cholesterol, one reduces one's risk of having a heart attack.

CAD is a classic example of a multifactorial disease. Much evidence emphasizes the importance of environmental factors. Death rates from CAD vary widely among countries. The death rate from CAD is nearly six times higher in the United States than it is in Japan. However, when Japanese people immigrate to the United States, they develop a risk for CAD that is in between that of persons raised in Japan and that of those raised in the United States, strong evidence of the influence of diet and other environmental changes.

Study after study has implicated smoking, a high-fat diet, diabetes, high blood pressure, and a sedentary lifestyle as risk factors for CAD. Roughly speaking, persons who have smoked a pack of cigarettes a day for 20 years and persons who have had a high cholesterol level throughout their adult lives have about a threefold greater risk for a heart attack at age 60 than do nonsmokers who have reasonably good cholesterol levels.

Long-standing adult-onset diabetes, especially if poorly managed, is an even stronger risk factor for heart attacks. Unless it is unusually elevated, high blood pressure is not as dramatic a risk factor, although still quite important.

For more than a century, astute physicians have recognized that CAD clusters in families, often in an aggregation that is too dense to explain merely by the effects of a shared environment. Twin studies have repeatedly shown a higher concordance rate for heart disease among MZ twins than among DZ twins. The concordance rate for MZ twins is usually in the 50% range, which is high, but also supports a role for environmental factors. Among cohorts of men who are identical twins, if one dies of a heart attack before age 55, the relative risk to the other for the same death is more than tenfold greater than the risk in the general population for his age. Similarly, more than 30 years ago, researchers studying relatives of men who had heart attacks before the age of 55 found that first-degree male relatives had a fivefold higher risk of early death than did comparable relatives of unaffected men. Relatives of women who had a first heart attack before 55 had an even greater risk—almost sevenfold. The younger the age at which the heart attack occurs, the more likely that close family members carry an elevated genetic risk.

Table 15. *Heart attack: Relative risk of death by age of twin's death*

	Age at death	Relative risk	
		men	women
MZ Twins			
	36–55	13.4	14.9
	56–65	8.1	14.9
	66–75	4.3	3.9
	76–85	1.9	2.2
	>85	0.9	1.1
DZ Twins			
	36–55	4.3	2.2
	56–65	2.6	2.2
	66–75	1.7	1.9
	76–85	1.4	1.4
	>85	0.7	1.0

Adapted, with permission, from Marenberg M.E., Risch N., Berkman L.F., Floderus B., and de Faire U. 1994. Genetic susceptibility to death from coronary heart disease in a study of twins. *New England Journal of Medicine* **330:** 1041–1046; © Massachusetts Medical Society.

The challenge in understanding how genes confer a predisposition to CAD is that a heart attack is a "clinical endpoint" of a complex disorder that develops slowly due to the influence of many risk factors, some of which are in turn also under substantial genetic influence (e.g., cholesterol metabolism, diabetes, obesity, and blood pressure). There are several single-gene disorders that are highly associated with CAD. One of the more common is familial hypercholesterolemia (FH), an autosomal dominant disorder that affects about 1 in 500 persons. In 2003, researchers at the Cleveland Clinic proved that a 21-base-pair deletion in a gene called MEF2 was the cause of an autosomal dominant form of CAD. In the large family that was studied, everyone who inherited the deletion developed CAD, and 9 of 13 carriers had a heart attack, usually in their early 60s. Taken together, single-gene causes of CAD account for only a tiny percentage of all cases. However, such discoveries often lead to new insights about the more general causes of heart disease.

What do we know about the genetic contribution to the heart attacks that kill thousands of men and women in their fifties and sixties each year who are not suffering from some rare disorder like FH? The list of candidate genes that could be important risk factors is long, reflecting the complexity of the disease. It includes genes that affect blood pressure, glucose regulation, clotting, homocysteine metabolism, the inflammatory response, lipid metabolism, and body weight. Currently, more than 100 different genes are on the list, which is growing steadily. Many studies of the genetics of CAD are under way, but our knowledge of the relative importance of these genes at the population level remains rudimentary.

One of the most important developments in research involving the causes of heart disease has been the recognition that the human inflammatory response has a major influence on the dynamics of plaque formation and rupture, a main cause of heart attacks. Dr. Peter Libby and Dr. Paul Ridker, both of Harvard Medical School, are among those who have shown that excess LDL cholesterol in the blood leads to increased deposition of plaques, which in turn triggers inflammation in the walls of the coronary arteries, and that chronic inflammation increases the risk for plaque rupture. A few years ago, Ridker showed that, when measured along with cholesterol levels, a biochemical marker of inflammation called C-reactive protein (CRP) provides important added information about risk for heart attack. In 2002, he demonstrated that elevated CRP levels are an important, independent risk factor for heart disease. CRP testing is rapidly becoming as routine as cholesterol testing.

Table 16. *Coronary artery disease: Familial risk*

Prevalence:
>   In families of men who had a myocardial infarction (MI) before age 45: about 40% have first-degree relatives with early CAD (before 60).

High-risk families are characterized by:
>   Early onset (under 55 in males and 65 in females).
>   Multiple affected family members, especially women.
>   Involvement of several arteries.
>   Poor response to risk factor modification.
>   Several relatives with related disorders (diabetes, high BP, high cholesterol).

Risk:
>   Men with parental history of MI or death from CAD have 2-fold risk of CAD.
>   Women with a parental history of MI at or before age 60 have about a 2.4-fold risk of nonfatal MI and 4.9-fold risk for fatal MI.
>   Risk to first-degree relatives is 5-fold if patient is a man under 60 and 7-fold if it is a woman under age 70.

Adapted, with permission, from Rimoin D.I., Connor J.M., Pyeritz R.E., and Korf B.R. 2002. *Emery and Rimoin's principles and practice of medical genetics*, 4th edition. Churchill Livingstone, London; © Elsevier.

Few risk factors are more important than family history. A family history of significant CAD (two or more deaths among close relatives before age 65 and even one death before age 55) should be viewed as a red flag. To answer the question posed at the top of this section, an apparently healthy 45-year-old white man whose father died of a heart attack at age 55 has about a fivefold greater risk of dying of heart attack in the next year than other men the same age who have a similar health profile, but no comparable family history. Even though his absolute risk of dying remains low, his family history should prompt the man to seek regular medical checkups. At minimum, blood pressure, blood glucose, and lipid profile should be periodically evaluated. Depending on the circumstances, exercise stress testing might also be appropriate.

In time, it will become a routine practice to use genetic tests to assess risk for heart disease among apparently healthy people. In the meantime, fortunately, a great deal can be done to modify the risk of heart attacks in most people who are known to have a strong familial history (and, indeed, for everyone else). Smoking cessation, moderate regular exercise, sensible diet, low-dose aspirin, and the statin medications to lower cholesterol levels are all helpful.

High Cholesterol

How much influence do genes have on cholesterol levels? I eat a healthy diet, but my cholesterol is still well above 200.

The great interest in how our bodies metabolize lipids (fats) and recycle lipoproteins (molecules that transport lipids into and out of cells) is due to the excellent evidence that links certain abnormalities in cholesterol metabolism to increased risk for heart attack and stroke. A huge amount of research has gone into understanding the genetics of lipid disorders, and over the last 40 years, quite a few genetic disorders of lipid metabolism have been elucidated. For example, familial combined hyperlipidemia (FCH) affects about 1 in 100 people. It is a dominant disorder that is characterized by high levels of a protein called apoB and high levels of a combination of molecules called very low density lipoproteins (VLDL). In general, however, we do not yet know much about how common genetic variations influence blood levels of LDL (bad cholesterol) and HDL (good cholesterol).

Our bodies obtain lipids for use in providing energy (as well as for many other purposes) in two ways: dietary intake and manufacture in the liver. Dietary lipids enter the circulation from the intestines as complexes called chylomicrons, which are rapidly broken down to provide units of energy for cells. The liver makes fats that are secreted in particles called VLDL, which are quickly broken down to low-density lipoproteins (LDL) and high-density lipoproteins (HDL). HDL is called good because it transports cholesterol from cells to the liver where it can enter a pathway that eliminates it from the body.

It has been known for many years that, at any age, as serum cholesterol levels rise, so does the risk for mortality. One very large study involving over 300,000 men showed that those with cholesterols above 290 mg/dl had a mortality rate fourfold higher than men with a level of 150. More recently, it has been shown that the higher the good cholesterol (HDL), the lower the mortality rate. HDL actually has three subfractions, of which the two major forms have been shown to protect against heart disease. Independently of LDL, levels of another lipoprotein, Lp(a), have also been shown to correlate with risk of CAD.

Many family and twin studies support the thesis that lipid metabolism is heavily influenced by genes. Lipid metabolism, like so much else discussed in this book, is under the control of many genes, each one contributing a small fraction of the effect. Taken together, however, they set the rheostat for how our bodies deal with dietary fats. It is important to remember that the definition of what constitutes high and low levels of lipids is arbitrarily set. The guidelines used in the United States define those in the upper 10% as having elevated lipids. However, it should be kept in mind that most people in affluent nations consume a very high fat diet, and that the current norms reflect this. When compared with the lipid levels found in people living in poverty in much of Africa and Asia, most of us have very high levels of cholesterol. To the saying "You can't be too rich or too thin," one might add "or have too low a cholesterol level."

Lipid levels are significantly affected by other conditions, of which the most important are smoking, obesity, diabetes, alcohol abuse, thyroid function, and birth control pills. Obesity is associated with low HDL, diabetes with high LDL, alcoholism with high VLDL, hypothyroidism with high LDL, and birth control pills with high VLDL. The major cause of death among persons with diabetes is heart disease.

Although there is still much to learn about the role that genes play in influencing cholesterol levels, there is no doubt that their role is important. Fortunately, it is also clear that most individuals who tend to have a high level of cholesterol for genetic reasons can still significantly reduce it. Diet, exercise, and the use of cholesterol-lowering drugs almost always have a significant impact.

High Blood Pressure

My mother and her sisters are all being treated for high blood pressure. What are my risks?

High blood pressure (HBP, hypertension) is common. About 25% of the adult population in the developed nations meets the current definition for having an elevated blood pressure. Among people over 75, the number is over 50%. There is relatively little difference in its prevalence between men and women. At any age, African-Americans are about twice as likely as whites to have HBP, making it a very significant health issue for that population. Much effort has gone into trying to understand why HBP is more prevalent in American blacks than whites, but there is no clear explanation.

The evidence that a number of factors increase the risk for hypertension is well established. These are high-salt diet, high-fat diet, low-potassium diet, low-calcium diet, obesity, high alcohol intake, stress, and lack of exercise. The prevalence of hypertension varies widely across societies. In general, there is much less hypertension in less-developed nations. To explain this, researchers have suggested that such societies are less stressful places to live, that the people tend to be much more physically active, that there is much less obesity than in developed nations, and that their diets tend to have a lower fat and salt content. Until recently, given the magnitude of the problem, there has been relatively little research into the possibility that protective genetic factors also play a role.

In study after study, it has been shown that the risk for heart attack and stroke (the first and third leading causes of death in the United States) increases with increased blood pressure. This fact, combined with a steady improvement in our ability to reduce blood pressure, has resulted in periodic efforts to redefine the meaning of the term, high blood pressure. Between 1997 and 2003, the official definition of HBP was a systolic (the first number) pressure above 139 millimeters of mercury or a diastolic blood pressure (the second number) of more than 89 millimeters of mercury as measured with the same blood pressure cuff on three separate occasions.

In 2003, a panel of experts convened by the National Heart, Lung and Blood Institute issued new guidelines. Impressed by the growing evidence that people with blood pressures that had been defined as "high normal" were at increased risk for stroke and heart attack, the panel lowered the line between normal and abnormal BP. The new guidelines define a normal BP as a systolic that is less than 120 and a diastolic pressure that is less than 80. People whose numbers are above those, but less than 140 over 90, are defined as having "pre-hypertension," and advised to adjust their diet and increase their level of daily exercise. Those who have a BP between 140/90 and 160/100 have Stage I hypertension and are advised to add a medicine to lifestyle changes. People with numbers above 160/100 have Stage II hypertension and need treatment with two medications.

The new guidelines greatly increase the number of people who need treatment to lower their BP. About 50 million people in the United States now have a BP that has been defined as too high. Although it may seem that the new guidelines are too stringent, the experts assert that the dividend for lowering the nation's collective BP would be a 40% reduction in the incidence of stroke and a 20% reduction in the incidence of heart attack! Less than 5% of people who have HBP have an obvious reason for their condition. Less than 1% of people with HBP can attribute the problem to a single-gene disorder. Thus, the overwhelming majority of people with HBP have what is called essential hypertension.

It has been known at least since the 1920s that HBP often runs in families. Many studies have shown that monozygotic twins have a concordance for BP level that is about double that of dizygotic twins. Adoption studies have found that the BPs of biological parents of children given for adoption at birth correlate much more closely with those of their children than do the BPs of the rearing parents. A study of a Chilean village in which about 80% of the marriages are first-cousin unions strongly supports the role of genes in determining BP. Among the sibs in 12 of the large families, the correlation coefficient for BP was 0.6, which is quite high.

Armed with the tools of molecular biology, many scientific groups are searching for the many genes that must be important in determining both BP and the risk that HBP will lead to serious "end-organ damage" (mainly heart attack and stroke). In the period 1999–2000, at least seven groups published the results of their search for evidence that HBP is associated with particular regions of the genome. As of late 2003, the number of genome scans had jumped to 22. As might be expected for a trait (HBP) that can be influenced by many diverse factors (such as the structure of the arterial wall, smoking history, weight, and height), the results have been for the most part inconclusive.

There have been important developments, however. A study of the Amish (a particularly interesting population because they do not drink alcohol and few are obese, thus eliminating two confounding environmental factors) indicated that there might be an important predisposing gene on chromosome 2. Another study of 1,700 people in 332 families participating in the Framingham Heart Study gave very promising statistical evidence for a predisposing gene on chromosome 17, especially intriguing because an earlier study also implicated that region. A massive study in China involved subjects recruited from among 200,000 persons who underwent screening for HBP. By focusing only on persons with seriously high BP, the Chinese researchers found evidence of a predisposing gene on chromosome 15.

Taking a different tack, some scientists have posited that certain genes with known functions are likely to play important roles in determining BP. Studies of these "candidate" genes have been fruitful. For example, it has been shown that some variants of the gene that codes for a key hormone called angiotensinogen greatly increase the risk for HBP. In a review of 69 studies involving nearly 30,000 subjects, scientists concluded that a variant called AGT 235TT increased the risk for HBP by 30%. Studies of another gene called α-adducin have indicated that some of its variants may play a role in salt-sensitive hypertension. Given the large scale of the analysis, the finding was highly significant. Similar studies of more than a dozen other genes have identified several variants that increase the risk about twofold.

With rare exceptions (limited to persons at risk for certain single-gene disorders known to cause serious hypertension), there are no tests to predict risk of HBP. A positive family history of hypertension in a first-degree relative roughly doubles the risk that an individual will have HBP. The simplest advice is the best. If your parent or your sibling has HBP, you should be especially vigilant about checking your BP regularly. In fact, you should do so even if you have no known family history of HBP!

Cardiomyopathy

My father has cardiomyopathy. What is it? How much do genes influence the risk?

Cardiomyopathy is the word used to describe a number of disorders that cause heart failure, but for which the primary cause is not coronary artery disease, hypertension, or dysfunction of the heart's valves. In a nutshell, it can be thought of as pump failure due to causes other than heart attacks.

There are three broad categories of cardiomyopathy: hypertrophic, dilated, and restrictive. In hypertrophic cardiomyopathy (HCM), the ventricles (heart muscles) are unusually thick and can generate very high pressures when they contract. Severely affected patients are at risk for sudden death because the enlarged ventricles actually obstruct the outflow of the very blood they are trying to pump. The hearts of patients with dilated cardiomyopathy (DCM) look quite different. In the advanced stage of this disorder, the ventricles are thin and floppy and when they contract they generate relatively little pumping force. The third (and least common) group is the restrictive cardiomyopathies. In these patients, the ventricles contract poorly, either because of damage to muscle fibers that causes a loss of flexibility or because the fibers have been infiltrated with any of a variety of substances that limit contraction. Although most cases are due to environmental factors, there are several rare single-gene disorders that cause this form of heart disease. There are also at least six neuromuscular disorders (including muscular dystrophy) that cause cardiomyopathy. Each is caused by mutations in a particular gene, and once the first case is diagnosed, the risk to relatives is easy to calculate.

HCM is a highly familial condition. About 70% of patients have a positive family history, and a growing fraction of all cases can be traced to mutations in a few dominantly acting genes. Since the severity of the disorder, age of onset of signs and symptoms, and family history of heart failure or sudden death vary tremendously, HCM has often been diagnosed later than it should be or missed altogether. Tragically, HCM is an important cause of sudden death in teenagers and college-age individuals. Undiagnosed HCM may be the most common cause of sudden death in competitive athletics. Fortunately, the diagnosis of HCM is usually easy to confirm by undertaking an echocardiographic (ultrasound) study of the heart. Unfortunately, such studies are too often performed only after a family loses one of its members.

Over the last 20 years, there has been impressive growth in our understanding of HCM. Under the leadership of a group headed by Dr. Crickett Seidman at Harvard, several genes have been identified for which mutations have been shown to be causative. As of 2003, scientists had found at least ten causative genes, each of which has been studied extensively and for which there are more than 100 known mutations. Twenty-five years ago, most cases of HCM were said to be "sporadic" (a fancy term meaning "we don't know the cause"); today 80–90% of the cases are thought to be primarily genetic. As more and more attention has been devoted to studying HCM, there has been a steady increase in our estimate of its prevalence. A fair guess is that about 1 person in 3,000 has a severe form of HCM, roughly 100,000 persons in the United States. About 1 person in 500 has a milder (but still serious) form of the disorder.

There is fairly good evidence that some mutations in the HCM genes are much more highly associated with risk of sudden, early death than others. In the more severe cases (about 25%), the genetic defect causes outflow obstruction; the other 75% do not. The disease poses difficult counseling and management problems. In those families in which the HCM mutation is known to confer high risk for early, sudden death, parents and physicians have to weigh complicated preventive interventions (such as use of drugs to suppress abnormal heart rhythms and implantable defibrillators) in children who are affected. In the last few years, experts at a number of centers, notably the Baylor Heart Clinic in Houston, have had some success with a technique called ethanol ablation, which destroys hypertrophied heart muscle.

The diagnosis of hypertrophic cardiomyopathy in an individual, regardless of his age, should be assumed to have a genetic cause until proven otherwise. Furthermore, the suspect gene should be assumed to be acting as a dominant. The parents, siblings, and children of a newly diagnosed individual should be considered at 1 in 2 risk for having the same mutation and should be evaluated promptly.

Many cases of dilated cardiomyopathy (DCM) are due to nongenetic causes, the best-studied of which are viruses that attack the heart muscle, chronic alcohol abuse, autoimmune disorders, and multiple heart attacks (which can damage so much of the muscle that it is left scarred and floppy). Just 30 years ago, the textbooks asserted that no cause was known for the vast majority of cases. Since then, the fraction of DCM that experts attribute to mutations in genes has grown steadily from 1% to 30%, or even higher. The typical patient with DCM is a relatively young (40–50-year-old) man who tells his doctor that he is having unusual fatigue when he exercises. This is because his heart cannot respond to the increased demands placed on it by exercise. If there is no history of severe alcohol abuse, viral infection of the heart, or multiple heart attacks, a genetic cause is most likely.

DCM is less common than HCM. The current estimate is that only about 1 person in 10,000 is affected, but this is surely an underestimate. In one study of the families of 59 patients diagnosed with DCM at the Mayo Clinic, Dr. Virginia Michaels and her colleagues found that 18 of 325 (5.5%) relatives whom they examined were also affected. There was at least one affected relative in 20% of the families. Research in England and Canada has resulted in similar findings. DCM is often familial and frequently not diagnosed until the disease is far advanced in at least one person.

From 1995 to 2000, researchers studied many groups of families affected with DCM and identified ten separate regions within the human genome that appear to harbor predisposing genes. In addition, it has been shown that mutations in two genes (called LaminA and cardiac actin) may account for a small fraction of all cases. Unfortunately, the genetic aspects of DCM are not yet as well understood as are the genetic aspects of HCM. Despite our limited understanding, it is fair to assume that (absent other obvious causes like heart attacks or alcohol abuse) DCM is strongly influenced by genes, and that first-degree relatives are at significant risk of also becoming affected. Because DCM develops slowly over decades, a normal examination cannot be taken as a negative diagnosis. The most that can be said of first-degree relatives is that they are not yet affected. They should be reexamined every few years. Once the predisposing genes are cloned and the causative mutations found, it will be possible to offer pre-symptomatic testing.

A number of actions can be taken by people who learn that they carry a DCM mutation. These include strictly avoiding alcohol and cigarettes, maintaining a healthy diet, and lowering cholesterol, having regular checkups, and taking a medication to suppress a tendency to have an abnormal heart rhythm. If the patient with DCM has no medical history to suggest other causes, the odds strongly favor a genetic etiology. It is important to alert family members so that they can obtain an appropriate medical evaluation.

Pulmonary Embolism

My grandfather died of a pulmonary embolism while he was recovering from a broken hip. Is my risk increased?

Pulmonary embolism (PE) occurs when a blood clot breaks away from the veins in the legs or pelvis and travels through the right side of the heart to lodge in the trunk or a branch of the pulmonary artery and obstruct blood flow to all or (usually) a portion of the lung. The larger the obstruction, the more dramatic is the impact on lung and heart function. Deep venous thrombosis (DVT) refers to the condition in which an individual develops the clots that can cause PE.

PE is a leading cause of death, killing more than 50,000 Americans each year. Experts estimate that only about 10% of all patients who are afflicted with a PE die. This translates into an estimate that PEs occur in 500,000 Americans each year. This is probably about right, as we know that each year more than 300,000 people in the United States are afflicted with a PE of sufficient size that they require medical attention. It is quite possible that 200,000 other individuals have small PEs each year that are never diagnosed because they do not cause symptoms which are worrisome enough to make the person seek medical care. Because of the way they present, it is not uncommon for physicians to miss the diagnosis of even a fairly serious PE. In the past, autopsy studies of patients who died suddenly have reported that physicians correctly guessed that PE was the cause of death only about 30% of the time.

DVT afflicts about 1 in every 500 American adults each year. The three major factors that predispose to DVT (and, therefore, to PE) are poor circulation, abnormalities of the veins, and disorders of coagulation that make it easier for clots to form. The typical picture of a person who dies suddenly of PE is an older man with congestive heart failure who has been at bed rest (often in hospital) for a prolonged period of time. Pregnancy is a risk factor for DVT, but only very rarely does it lead to a fatal event. Use of oral contraceptives doubles the risk for PE in young women, but it is still very low, about 1 in 20,000. PE is more common in persons with metastatic cancer, usually because the disease has affected their coagulation system. PE is a feared complication of heart disease, emphysema, chronic venous problems in the legs, and some cancers.

The occurrence of DVT in patients younger than 45, recurrent DVT in any person, and a positive family history all suggest a genetic risk. Family history is positive in nearly half of the young patients. Three uncommon single-gene disorders collectively may account for only 5–10% of all DVT. These are known as antithrombin III deficiency, protein C deficiency, and protein S deficiency. Fewer than 1 in 1000 persons are born with one of these conditions.

The major genetic risk factors for DVT and PE are those that affect the coagulation system, mutations that create a "hypercoagulable state." Among them are deficiencies in one or more of the body's natural anticoagulants, especially a variant in clotting factor V called Factor V Leiden (named after the city in which it was described). There are also rare abnormalities of a protein called prothrombin. Because about 1 in 25 persons carries a mutation for Factor V Leiden, much attention has been paid to its role as a risk factor for PE. Genetic testing for this variant is widely available.

In the last decade, scientists discovered that Factor V Leiden mutations were present in about 20–40% of patients with DVT, about seven times the expected number, a finding that led some to advocate screening some groups (such as persons about to undergo surgery that requires prolonged bed rest) for common mutations in this gene. One of the most common mutations, called R506Q, is of interest because women who carry it and use oral contraceptives appear to be at risk for DVT and PE. During pregnancy, carriers have about a 1 in 500 chance of DVT. Women who have a mutation in the prothrombin gene (called G20210A) have about a 1 in 200 risk. The rare women who carry both mutations have about a 1 in 20 risk of having DVT while pregnant. So far, most experts have recommended against routinely screening pregnant women for Factor V Leiden deficiency, arguing that the expense does not justify the probable medical benefit.

However, a positive family history should stimulate the physician to order the test for his patient.

Any person who has a close (first-degree) relative who has had DVT for unexplained reasons prior to age 45 should consider the possibility that he or she is at genetic risk for a PE. Such a person should undergo genetic testing for Factor V Leiden and related defects. To return to the introductory question, the mere fact that a grandparent died of a pulmonary embolism does not (absent other predisposing facts) significantly increase an individual's risk, and it certainly does not suggest that one has a substantially increased risk for PE at a young age. If, however, one has lost a parent to a PE at a relatively young age (less than 65), there should be a higher index of suspicion that genetic factors played a role.

Sudden Death

My completely healthy 29-year-old cousin suddenly dropped dead. Is there a genetic risk to sudden death?

Each year in the United States, about 300,000–400,000 people die suddenly. By sudden, I mean death within a few minutes of the onset of illness. About 200,000 are young (less than 60).

The list of possible causes of sudden death in apparently healthy adults is quite long. In addition, the candidates for leading causes vary substantially with age. Above age 40, unsuspected CAD, manifesting as a catastrophically abnormal heart rhythm in a first heart attack, is the leading cause. However, below age 30, coronary artery disease ranks low on any list of causes. Since I have already discussed heart attacks, here I mention some other conditions that may have a substantial genetic risk factor—the ones that should always be considered in close relatives of a young man or woman who dies unexpectedly. It is in the best interests of their families that such unfortunate individuals undergo autopsy.

Some causes of sudden death occur due to abnormalities of the electrical system in the heart, causing catastrophic failure of its ability to pump blood. Among them is Long QT syndrome, a disorder sometimes, but by no means always, recognizable from the tracing on the electrocardiogram. We know of at least six different genes in which mutations can cause Long QT syndrome. Three of them, genes named KCNQ1, KCNH2, and SCN5A (and often called the LQT1, 2, and 3 loci), account for most cases. The first two regulate the flux of potassium ions across the cell membrane, and the third similarly regulates the flow of sodium ions. The smooth electrical operation of the heart depends on the orderly flux of these ions.

In 2003, cardiologists and molecular biologists in Pavia, Italy, published a major study of the risk of syncope (fainting due to an abnormal heart rhythm), cardiac arrest, and sudden death before the age of 40 among people born with mutations in one of these three genes. Among 647 patients, more than one-third (234) had suffered one of these events. Overall, about 10% of those with a mutation in LQT1 had had a cardiac arrest or died; about 20% of those with LQT2 and about 15% of those with LQT3 had suffered a similar fate.

Since one version of this disorder is dominantly inherited and several are recessively inherited, the diagnosis of Long QT syndrome in a patient should trigger careful medical evaluation in parents, children, and siblings. Since about one-third of persons with a mutation in one of these genes nevertheless have a normal cardiogram, DNA testing is a crucial part of the evaluation. Cardiologists who specialize in Long QT syndrome use medications to reduce the risk of electrical abnormalities in all those who are born with an LQT3 mutation and in everyone born with an LQT1 who also has a certain abnormality on the EKG. Among those born with a LQT2 mutation, treatment is based on sex (women are at higher risk) and the EKG data (men are treated if they have an abnormal EKG).

Another cause of sudden death, named for the two physician brothers who characterized it, is Brugada syndrome. This disorder also has suggestive findings on a routine electrocardiogram, including a condition called right bundle branch block and ST elevation on the ECG tracings from the right side of the heart. This syndrome is probably not as rare as was once thought. Throughout the nations of Southeast Asia there are widespread reports of a markedly similar disease. In the Philippines, it is called bangungut ("to rise and moan in sleep"), in Laos it is non-laitai ("sleep-death"), and in Japan it is pokkuri.

Even more important than primary rhythm disorders is hypertrophic cardiomyopathy (discussed earlier in its own section). This disorder is the leading cause of sudden death in young athletes, accounting for more than 25% of cases in the largest study ever undertaken of such events. In this condition, the walls of heart ventricles are markedly enlarged. During exercise, cardiac demand puts pressure on the outflow tract of the coronary arteries, the very vessels that feed the heart muscle and support the cells in its electrical circuits. This can cause lack of oxygen to those cells and lead to a fatally abnormal heart rhythm. A typical story involving death from hypertrophic cardiomyopathy might be one of a teenage boy or young man who, after playing tennis on a hot day, jumped into a swimming pool and died.

Second only to cardiomyopathy as a cause of sudden cardiac death in young athletes is blunt trauma to the chest that leads to a rhythm failure. This event is called commotio cordis and may be the cause of up to 20% of such (thankfully very rare) events. No genetic risk factors have been associated with these deaths. In a few families, there is an impressive history of sudden death that on autopsy turns out to be massive rupture of the abdominal aorta (discussed in the next section), the largest blood vessel in the body. These deaths tend to occur in the fifth and sixth decade. The evidence suggests that this rare familial syndrome is probably caused by a dominantly acting gene or genes.

In at least one well-known (albeit rare) form of sudden death in males called arrhythmogenic right ventricular cardiomyopathy (ARVM), cardiologists in Canada have shown that the placement of an implantable cardioverter defibrillator (ICD) is lifesaving. In one study of 11 extended families over 5 years, there were no deaths in patients with ICDs, while 28% of similarly affected relatives in a control group died!

The answer to the question at the top of this section is that any history of sudden, unexplained death in a close relative below age 60 should be considered as a possible warning of genetic risk, and should trigger a thorough medical evaluation. The younger the age at death, the greater should be the level of concern.

Aortic Aneurysms

My father died at age 65 from a ruptured abdominal aortic aneurysm. How high is my risk?

Aneurysms are bulges that occur in weakened areas of arterial walls. Although aneurysms can occur in any artery, except for the vessels in the brain (discussed under the section on stroke), the major site of concern is the aorta. Aortic aneurysms are classified by location. Those above the renal arteries are thoracic; those below the renal arteries are abdominal. There are a wide variety of causes of aneurysms, ranging from rare single-gene disorders which affect the structure of the collagen proteins that are key components of the vascular wall (such as Marfan syndrome) to chronic infections. Before the antibiotic era, thousands of people died each year from ruptured aortic aneurysms caused by syphilis.

Today, researchers working on this topic seem to agree that most aneurysms arise as the end result of many interacting factors that gradually erode the connective tissue in the arterial wall. For example, at least four enzymes that specialize in breaking down the collagen and elastin fibers which provide the structure to the arterial wall have been found to be elevated in people with aneurysms. Chronic inflammation, autoimmune factors, smoking, and hypertension all increase the risk for developing abdominal aortic aneurysms (AAAs). Aneurysms are surprisingly common. Each year more than 20,000 Americans die from ruptured aortic aneurysms, more than die from AIDS or many forms of cancer. About 7% of men over 60 have a clinically important aneurysm. The magisterial physicist, Albert Einstein, died of a ruptured abdominal aortic aneurysm.

Surgeons have long known that both thoracic aortic aneurysms (TAAs), which have been associated with several single-gene disorders, and AAAs, which are more common and seem to have a more complex etiology, run in families. Only recently, however, have there been efforts to define the familial risk. In 1999, Finnish researchers collected 241 siblings over age 50 of patients who had undergone surgical repair of an AAA. They performed ultrasound studies of their aortas and compared the results to a control group. Overall, the siblings of the affected persons had a 4-fold greater risk of having ultrasonic evidence of AAA. In particular, the brothers of affected patients had a 12-fold greater risk. Among the male siblings over age 60, nearly 1 in 5 was found to have an aortic aneurysm.

Geneticists have found three loci that are associated with an uncommon dominant form of TAA (on chromosomal regions 5q13-14, 3p24-25, and 11q23.3-11q24). Of great clinical importance is the fact that in the families in which this research was conducted, the disease showed a phenomenon called anticipation. In each generation, the age of onset was younger, moving from a mean of 61 in the grandparental generation to 22 in the grandchildren. Because many are due to dominantly acting genes, any person who had a parent die of a TAA should consider himself or herself at risk and seek medical evaluation.

Over the last decade, the evidence that a small number of genes predispose to AAAs has grown substantially. About 20% of persons diagnosed with an AAA have at least one first- or second-degree relative with an AAA. As with some TAAs, patients with a positive family history for AAA who also develop one tend to do so at a younger age than do those with no affected relatives. Sporadically arising aneurysms overwhelmingly affect men (6:1) over women. However, in affected families, many more women develop AAAs, and the sex ratio is closer to 2:1. In AAA families, the highest risk seems to be that faced by the sons of affected mothers.

A consortium of researchers led by a team at Wayne State in Detroit are intensively studying affected families with the goal of identifying predisposing genes. So far, there is little firm evidence to indict any particular gene as a risk factor for familial AAA. However, the clinical evidence strongly suggests that such a gene or genes will soon be found.

An inexpensive ultrasound examination of the chest and abdomen (as well as the more expensive MRI scans) is quite effective at finding silent aneurysms. Given that the test is noninvasive, inexpensive, and accurate, it is surprising that there is not more effort devoted to screening at-risk individuals in the population. Fortunately, interest in screening is on the rise. Currently, reasonable recommendations are that all men over 65, men over 50 who smoke, men and women over 50 with an affected parent, all first-degree relatives of persons diagnosed with a thoracic aneurysm, and anyone with two or more relatives who have had cerebral aneurysms or who died suddenly and were not autopsied should have an ultrasound screening test.

The answer to the question posed to start this section depends on the gender, age, and overall health of the person asking the question. A son of an affected father is at significantly higher risk than a daughter, especially after age 50, and the risk rises with each decade. Other factors, such as high blood pressure, further elevate the risk. Once identified as having an aneurysm, a person must be followed carefully. An individual with a serious aneurysm faces the daunting prospect of major surgery, an intervention that when undertaken by highly experienced surgeons has about a 2–3% risk of death. However, such folks will face a much higher risk of death—about 80%—if the vessel ruptures.

Atrial Fibrillation

My dad has been treated twice to convert his atrial fibrillation to a normal heart rhythm. Does this mean I am at increased risk?

In atrial fibrillation (AF), the most common abnormal heart rhythm in adults, the contractions of the small upper chambers of the heart are not synchronized with those of the larger ventricles. Electrical signals that originate in the atria must pass through an electrical substation called the AV (atrio-ventricular) node. When some of the signals do not pass smoothly through this junction, the individual experiences an irregular heartbeat. The biggest reason to be concerned about AF is that each year in the United States about 75,000 people suffer from strokes that occur because the irregular beats (fibrillation) cause small clots of blood to form. In some people they eventually break off from the atrial wall and travel in the arteries to the brain where they become lodged, cutting off the blood supply to the brain cells that are further downstream. AF accounts for about one-third of all strokes in people over 65. About 5% of people over 65 have AF, and up to 15% of people in their 80s are affected.

The treatment of AF varies with the nature of the condition and depends on a number of issues: How long has the AF been present? What symptoms does the patient experience? How fast is the ventricular heart rate? The key goals are to restore normal rhythm and to prevent recurrence. Generally speaking, cardioversion (the use of a mild electrical shock to convert the rhythm) is used only after the patient has been placed on anticoagulant medicine (to reduce the risk of embolic stroke) for 2–3 weeks. Various medicines are then used to prevent AF recurrence. The most recent study suggests that electrical cardioversion offers no long-term benefit over medical treatment. In untreated patients, there is about a 75% chance that AF will recur within one year; in treated patients it is half of that. In severe cases, surgery to disrupt the electrical focus is sometimes used, but there is disagreement among experts about whether the benefits justify the risks.

In a small percentage of cases, AF clusters in families. In even fewer families, it appears to behave as a dominantly inherited disorder. A team at the Baylor Heart Clinic in Houston has localized (but not yet cloned) genes associated with the rare dominant forms on chromosomes 3 and 10. Currently, there are several large studies under way to identify other genes that predispose to AF, but researchers have not yet captured a gene that is clearly causative.

What is the best course of action if there is a positive family history? If one has a parent or sibling with AF, especially if that condition was diagnosed before the age of 60, one should suspect a genetic risk factor. A physician can advise on certain preventive actions that may be mildly helpful in preventing AF, such as avoidance of coffee and alcohol, and in actions to reduce the risk of embolic stroke, such as regular use of low-dose aspirin.

Mitral Valve Prolapse

After a routine examination, my doctor told me he thought I had mitral valve prolapse. Is it genetic?

The mitral valve is a tough, fibrous ring of tissue located inside the left ventricle of the heart. It rings the opening through which blood flows from the left auricle into the much larger left ventricle that with each contraction sends newly oxygenated blood through the aorta out to the body. The opening and closing of the mitral valve, in concert with the contractions of the left ventricle, regulate blood flow from the heart to the body.

Mitral valve prolapse (MVP) is a common condition in which there is a billowing out of one of the leaflets of the valve, usually causing at most a slight, clinically unimportant, back flow of blood into the left atrium. MVP may arise in many ways, including as a consequence of several uncommon, but serious, forms of heart disease. It is most often diagnosed in healthy young women in whom it is an unexpected finding made after a doctor hears a small heart murmur, often with an accompanying sound called a "mid-systolic click" (caused by a snapping of the valve). As many as 10% of women may have MVP, and it is so highly familial that it is likely that one or a few dominantly acting genes cause most cases.

In some individuals, MVP is associated with chest pain, irregular (but not dangerous) heart rhythms, and with anxiety and fainting. In an exceedingly small number of affected persons, there may be increased risk for severe heart problems, including sudden death from rupture of the chords that attach the valve to the ventricle. However, this has never been proven. Expression of the symptoms associated with MVP is highly dependent on age and gender. In families where it appears to be an autosomal dominant condition, boys and men are still much less likely to express the condition than are women.

In 1999, a causative gene was mapped to a region on chromosome 16, but it has not yet been cloned. In 2003, a group of Harvard researchers reported persuasive evidence that they had mapped a second gene for a dominantly acting form of MVP to the short arm of chromosome 11.

Because MVP is also found as part of the many rare genetic conditions involving defects in the formation of connective tissue, it is likely that risk for MVP is due to one or more gene variants that affect production of collagen, the main structural protein of the valve.

In cases where people with MVP also have irregular heart rhythms, doctors sometimes use drugs called β-blockers to help maintain normal beats. This also often reduces the patient's understandable anxiety.

Longevity

What role do genes play in determining the chance that one will live to a very old age?

Perhaps the single most remarkable fact about the 20th century is that human life expectancy soared. Between 1900 and 2000, the median life expectancy of girls born in the United States rose nearly 40 years. Between 1950 and 2000, the chance of living to 100 increased 20-fold. White girls born in the United States today have an almost even chance of living past age 80; for white boys the life expectancy is approaching 76. This extraordinary increase is largely due to improvements in public health, particularly vaccines and antibiotics to defeat infectious diseases. In 1900, for example, tuberculosis, called the "white plague," was the number one killer in the United States. Today it is not even in the top 20.

The notion that there is a definite upper limit to the human life span was first proposed on scientific grounds by a demographer (expert on population) named Benjamin Gompertz about 1825. In essence, he proposed that the mortality rate increases exponentially with age to the point where it becomes infinite (meaning everyone of that birth cohort is dead). Whether true or not, Gompertz's theory does not address the question of what constitutes the upper limit of life span. Population studies dating as far back as 1840 reveal that record human life expectancy has increased on average 2.5 years every decade. For the last century, demographers have repeatedly asserted that the median age of life expectancy (the age which half of a cohort born in a certain year can expect to reach) would soon reach its limit. Largely because of advances in public health (clean water, access to better nutrition, and control of childhood diseases), they have been repeatedly proven wrong. Every major demographic study conducted in the last century has found an increase in median human life expectancy.

There is no evidence to suggest that the incremental advance in median life expectancy has slowed. With the horrible exception of Africa, where the AIDS epidemic will diminish median life expectancy until it is brought under control, the age to which humans can hope to live is rising steadily. There is strong demographic evidence that girls born in Japan today can expect to live past 85. According to James Vaupel, one of the world's experts on longevity, the overwhelming weight of the evidence argues against a biological limit to the human life span. He notes that for the last 20 years, life expectancy in Japan has been increasing every year by about 3 months. He further notes that death rates among people in their 80s and 90s throughout the developed world are steadily dropping! He predicts that by 2020 the median life expectancy in Japan may be 90 years.

Of course, as the median life expectancy rises, it must bump into any natural limits to longevity imposed by the human genome. Because the longest life span that we can irrefutably document is 122 years (the record is held by a French woman, Jeanne Calment, who died in 1997), many have argued that this age closely approximates our natural limits. Ultimately, the only way to determine the limit of the human life span is to monitor the lives of extremely old individuals. In 2003, authorities in Albania reported the death of a woman named Hava Rexha at 123 years and 2 months, perhaps adding a full year to the established record.

Over the last decade, there has been a huge growth in research on the genetics of longevity, almost all of which has been conducted with yeast, nematodes (tiny worms), fruit flies, and, more recently, mice. Among several approaches to promoting longevity in laboratory organisms, dietary restriction has been the most successful. The most recent news is that "It's never too late." In 2003, a team showed that when they sharply reduced the calories available to theretofore well-fed adult *Drosophila* flies, the insects' mortality rate quickly declined. Neither their age nor their dietary history seemed to be nearly as important as their current nutritional status.

Scientists have also successfully improved the median life expectancy of lab strains merely by selecting the most long-lived animals and using them as founders to create new strains. Some of these progeny strains have life spans that exceed the standard laboratory life span by 30% and more. Researchers are also investigating the impact of candidate genes for longevity. In 2003, a research team published convincing evidence that variants in a single gene that codes for an enzyme called dopa-decarboxylase have an important role in extending the life span of fruit flies.

Taken together, the research on lower organisms suggests that it may be possible to extend the limits of human life well beyond the current apparent limit of about 125 years. Indeed, some scientists are already claiming that some humans will survive to 150 during this century. One reason this may happen is that perhaps just a few genes greatly influence the upper limit of expectancy. If we identify them and learn to manipulate them, we may be able to chart a lifestyle path that redefines our conception of longevity. For example, some years ago, Italian researchers uncovered good evidence that a rare variant of a gene involved in metabolism of the "good" cholesterol (HDL) confers longevity.

Scientists have long wondered whether, and lay people have long sensed that, longevity is a familial trait. For many decades, it was thought that a fair predictor of life expectancy in an individual is the age attained by his or her parents. In the 1920s, Dr. Raymond Pearl, a geneticist and demographer at Johns Hopkins University, published several papers based on the study of birth and death records across generations that seemed to confirm this relationship. Starting with 2,319 people who lived past 90, Pearl sought to establish the age at death of their parents and grandparents. He succeeded in doing so in 365 cases. The sum of the parental and grandparental ages exceeded that of a control group. The study suggested that genes played a role in longevity, but it revealed neither how big a role nor in what way the genes operated.

Some recent research has cast doubt on the value of parental age at death as a predictor of life expectancy. The main reason for this is that there have been such dramatic changes in the forces that cause death over the last century. Use of parental age at death probably underestimates longevity in many people (for example, those who lost their parents to infectious disease, a world war, or the many diseases that are today so much more amenable to treatment). However, at least one recent study of longevity among Ashkenazi Jews supports the idea that parental age is a good predictor of extreme longevity.

Recently, gene hunters have started using new tools to search for genes that help one age long and well. There are major research projects under way in the United States, Italy, France, Denmark, and China that are studying the lives and probing the DNA of more than 10,000 people who have lived to be 100. In 2000, the New England Centenarian Project (which studies people who have reached age 100) teamed up with a biotech company called Centagenetix (now part of a company called

Elixir) to study the DNA of siblings who both had lived well into their 90s. Led by geneticist Dr. Louis M. Kunkel and gerontologist Dr. Thomas Perls, the team studied 137 sets of two or three siblings in which the older is at least 98 and the others were at least 92. They used 400 genetic markers to attempt to find some region of the genome that was present significantly more often than in control groups. In 2001, they reported that they had found such a region on chromosome 4, a finding which suggests that a gene variant highly associated with longevity is hidden therein. The scientists are currently replicating their studies in elderly populations in Italy and Okinawa.

The big surprise from the New England Centenarian Project research was that just one gene can have a major influence on longevity (perhaps by protecting against cancer or coronary artery disease). Prior to that publication, most scientists would have guessed that extreme longevity was a chance event due to a combination of fortunate environmental experiences and the protective effects of many different (perhaps hundreds) genes. In the fall of 2003, the scientists at Elixir published a paper identifying a variant in a single gene that makes a microsomal transfer protein which is strongly associated with human life span. In the autumn of 2003, a research team reported that homozygosity for a particular form of a gene that codes for cholesterol ester transfer protein (CETP) was dramatically more prevalent among more than 200 Ashkenazi Jews with a median age of 98 (that's right, 98) than among a cohort of 70-year-olds!

For my money, the most intriguing genetic research into human longevity is being conducted in several tiny, isolated, hilltop towns in Sardinia. Antonia Todde, a 114-year-old former shepherd who lives in the village of Tiana, is probably the oldest man on earth. What makes the Sardinian study so interesting is that so many of the centenarians are men. In general, for every one man who makes it to 100, there are in most studies five women. In the Sardinian hills, the ratio is much closer to 1:1. Demographers have verified records proving the birth claims of more than 50 people in Sardinia who claim to be over 100. Since many of these centenarians were born in tiny villages composed of the descendants of only a few families, genetic studies are unusually attractive. Generations of intermarriage may have selected for one or several genes that do much to increase the odds of making it past 100. Among the many speculations is that these folks have unusually strong immune systems. On the other hand, Mr. Todde acknowledges drinking some red wine every day, a disclosure that fits well with the current interest in reservatrol, a chemical in grapes that seems to protect against heart disease.

We will learn a lot more about the genetics of longevity in the next decade. For now, however, lifestyle (exercise and smoking history, type and amount of alcohol consumption, and diet) are better predictors of longevity than any knowledge we have of human genes. The best advice? Alas! Diet, diet, diet.

LUNG DISEASES

Chronic Obstructive Pulmonary Disease (COPD, Emphysema)

My father never smoked, but at age 55 he was diagnosed with emphysema. Was it caused by a gene? What is my risk?

Chronic obstructive pulmonary disease is a disorder of the lungs that causes obstruction of airflow, resulting in severely limited ability to obtain sufficient oxygen. People with COPD have chronic bronchitis and emphysema (abnormally large air spaces due to destruction of the delicate alveolar walls). The typical person with severe COPD is easy to recognize. He is in his 60s, wheelchair-bound or remarkably slow in his movements, and tethered to a portable oxygen tank. His lips are blue, his skin is severely wrinkled, and he is often so thin that strangers guess that he has advanced cancer. COPD is the fifth leading cause of death in the United States, taking more than 100,000 lives a year. It is the only major cause of death that is on the rise, having increased about threefold since 1964, the year that the Surgeon General unequivocally declared that smoking cigarettes caused emphysema.

If most cases of COPD are caused by smoking, why be concerned about genetic factors? There are at least two good reasons. First, there is a recessive genetic disorder called α-1-antitrypsin deficiency, which also causes emphysema. Although the disease almost always manifests in persons with two copies of the disease allele, the much larger number of individuals who carry one copy (roughly 3% of the population) may be at higher than normal risk for COPD if they smoke. They also may be at somewhat increased risk even if they do not smoke. Second, there is reliable evidence that risk for COPD (including its age of onset and severity of clinical course) is influenced by other genes. There are people who develop COPD despite the fact that they have never smoked.

No more than 5% of all cases of COPD are due to a deficiency of α-1-antitrypsin, a protein that in its normal form counters the action of other proteins that break down lung tissue. Although the percentage is low, the actual number of affected persons is high. Since AAT deficiency causes irreversible destruction of lung tissue, any measure to preserve lung tissue may extend life. It is important to identify people with AAT deficiency early, because they should never smoke. A screening program in Sweden has demonstrated that when informed early of their risk, persons with this genetic disorder are much less likely to start smoking and, if they do smoke, much more likely to stop. A purified form of α-1-antitrypsin (Prolastin) is available as an intravenous drug that is given monthly to help preserve lung tissue (but only to persons who have significant decrease in lung function).

What of the families in which there are several persons diagnosed with COPD despite the fact that they have never smoked? There is a growing body of evidence that lung function is significantly influenced by genes. For example, studies have shown that concordance rates for performance on spirometry (which measured the ability to move air against resistance) are higher for MZ than for DZ twins. First-degree relatives of persons diagnosed with COPD are much more likely to show signs of airflow obstruction than are first-degree relatives of their spouses (controlling, of course, for history of having smoked). A Boston-based study of patients with severe, early-onset COPD found that first-degree relatives who smoked were more likely to have reduced lung function at an earlier age than were the comparable relatives of age-matched controls. That is, these relatives appeared to be more vulnerable to chronic exposure to cigarette smoke.

There have been several efforts to find genes that predispose to COPD. In 2003, scientists at DeCode Genetics reported the results of a large linkage study. They found evidence that genes on 2p, 3q, and 10q may predispose heavy smokers to COPD, and a gene on 7q may protect heavy smokers from developing the disease. Given that only 15% of heavy smokers ever develop COPD, the discovery of protective genes will not be at all surprising.

What is the bottom line? The major cause of COPD is smoking, but about 3–5% of COPD may be due to AAT deficiency. A strong family history of COPD in nonsmokers is a warning (although not quantifiable) of genetic risk that merits investigation. It is difficult to assess the implications of the diagnosis of COPD in a close relative. If he or she is above age

50 and has a long history of smoking, there is little reason to think that genetic factors play a role. If the affected person is in his 40s or younger and/or he or she is not a smoker, there should be concern that genetic factors are at work. If the patient is diagnosed with ATT, first-degree relatives should be tested.

Sarcoidosis

My mother has sarcoidosis. What is my risk?

Sarcoidosis is a mysterious disease of uncertain origin that is characterized by the gradual development of granulomas (nodules composed of a variety of inflammatory cells) in many different organs, but especially the lung. Although the disease can present in a dozen different ways, the classic patient with sarcoidosis is a young to middle-aged black woman who reports that her capacity for exercise has fallen off. A physical examination may uncover nothing of note, but a chest X-ray often points to the diagnosis. It may show a sign called hilar adenopathy (the presence of enlarged lymph nodes).

Although it is found throughout the world, uncovering the causes of sarcoidosis would challenge Sherlock Holmes. The disease is three times more prevalent in Irish living in London than in English living in London. It is eight times more common in persons from Martinique living in France than in native-born French. It is extremely rare throughout Asia. In the United States, the disease is far more prevalent in the southeastern states than anywhere else. Sarcoidosis is about ten times more common in African-Americans than it is in whites. In whites the disease typically presents with a fairly sudden onset and resolves over 1–2 years. In blacks it develops insidiously and tends to progress slowly. Black patients are less likely to experience significant improvement.

Early epidemiological studies in the United States found that patients were very likely to have been raised in rural parts of the south. This finding generated many hypotheses about possible environmental agents, of which the most popular is a chronic hyperimmune reaction to pine tree pollen. Despite decades of study, there is not enough evidence to indict this or any other factor. Relatively few people die from sarcoidosis (if they do, the cause is respiratory failure), but tens of thousands of Americans are incapacitated by it. For example, sarcoidosis may also severely impair vision, and it is also a small (5%) but significant cause of chronic kidney failure.

The current leading hypothesis is that the disease arises when as-yet-unknown foreign antigen is recognized by a subset of T-lymphocyte (immune) cells that recognize it is an enemy and initiate a defensive cascade. This ultimately results in the formation of granulomas, cells that wall up the invader to protect the body from it. This hypothesis nicely accommodates environmental, immune response, and genetic factors as culprits.

The recognition that sarcoidosis can be highly familial dates back at least to a German study completed in the 1920s. A more sophisticated study by the British Thoracic and Tuberculosis Association in the 1970s provided unequivocal proof that in some families there is a strong genetic predisposition to developing the disease. A more recent study in African-American families attributed 70% of the risk to genetic factors but could not fit the data to a single-gene model. In a study of more than 1000 consecutively diagnosed patients in the Henry Ford Hospital in Detroit, researchers found that 14% of patients had at least one affected first- or second-degree relative. The rate was much higher in blacks, whose risk of having an affected relative was 17% compared to 6% in whites.

In 1999, the group at Henry Ford Hospital joined with seven other medical centers to form a consortium to untangle the genetics of sarcoidosis. The group acronym, ACCESS, stands for a case control etiologic study of sarcoidosis. In the fall of 2003, ACCESS presented the results of its genetic analysis of nearly 500 patients and an equal number of healthy controls. Their goal was to use newly available molecular techniques to compare the distribution of variant forms of HLA class II genes (which make proteins that are crucially important to the body's defense against foreign chemicals) in persons with sarcoidosis with the distribution in age-, gender-, and race-matched controls. They found that the prevalence of certain alleles called the HLA-DRB1 alleles was far greater than expected among patients with the disorder. One allele, known as HLA-DRB1*1101 was so strongly associated with disease that the odds of the association occurring by chance were less than 1 in 100. In addition, they found several alleles that seemed to confer protection from sarcoidosis. Finally, they also found somewhat less convincing evidence that the pattern of organ involvement in each patient was associated with particular alleles.

With this important advance in understanding risk factors for sarcoidosis comes the possibility that clinicians will soon obtain HLA typing on patients. The test results may turn out to be of value both in predicting how the disease is most likely to develop in a particular person and in ascertaining the degree of risk faced by relatives with the same HLA alleles. For now, however, the only risk information that is offered to relatives of a newly diagnosed individual is based on family history. If there is reasonably good evidence that one or more other relatives in prior generations also had sarcoidosis, suspicion that there is a genetic risk factor in that family should be high. Any relative who notices abnormalities consistent with sarcoidosis should be evaluated by a pulmonary physician.

GASTROINTESTINAL DISEASES

Inflammatory Bowel Disease

My sister has inflammatory bowel disease. What are my risks?

Inflammatory bowel disease (IBD) is a serious, noninfectious, chronic inflammation of the large and/or small intestines that is probably caused by an inappropriate activation of the mucosal immune system, that branch of our immunological defenses that protects our digestive tracts against a constant barrage of bacteria. There are two major forms of IBD: Crohn disease and ulcerative colitis. Patients with Crohn disease or ulcerative colitis have much in common, including abdominal pain, diarrhea, weight loss, bleeding, and anemia. During severe flares, they may be hospitalized for weeks. They have serious risk of infections and often require bowel surgery. In their full manifestations, both diseases are very debilitating. The major distinguishing feature of the two disorders is the distribution of inflammation in the intestines.

Despite years of intense study, experts are still not certain whether these are two separate diseases or two forms of the same disease. There are a variety of findings that are more characteristic of one form than the other, but in about 15% of cases, physicians cannot distinguish between the two. To complicate matters further, sometimes patients have an illness that over time manifests as both disorders! Besides being important for giving the best possible care, determining the proper diagnosis has important secondary implications. Furthermore, each diagnosis implies different risks for close relatives.

The cardinal features of Crohn disease are patchy (segmental) involvement of the colon with sparing of the right side, less involvement of rectal tissue, greater risk for fistulas (little tunnels inappropriately connecting tissues), inflammation that runs deeper into the intestinal tissue, granulomatous

Table 17. *Inflammatory bowel disease: Genetic evidence*

Prevalence varies among different populations.

Risk is increased among first-degree relatives of patients.

Greater concordance among MZ than DZ twins.

Frequent concordance in the type and site of disease among members of families with multiple affected members.

Variants of several candidate genes have been statistically associated with disease.

Screening with DNA markers has found linkage on chromosomes 16 (IBD1 locus; for Crohn disease), 3, 5, 7, 12 (linkage with ulcerative colitis), 18, and 19 and X.

Adapted, with permission, from Podalsky D.K. 2002. Medical progress: Inflammatory bowel disease. *New England Journal of Medicine* **347**: 417–429; © Massachussetts Medical Society.

(walled off) lesions, and a lower risk for bowel cancer. In contrast, the cardinal features of ulcerative colitis are inflammation that invariably involves the rectum and extends without interruption through part or all of the colon but spares the small intestine, very low risk for fistulas, less deep inflammation, absence of granulomatous lesions, and greater risk for bowel cancer.

The risk of bowel cancer to patients with ulcerative colitis grows slowly, but steadily, over the decades. Late in 2003, researchers at the University of Washington demonstrated that this cancer risk is strongly associated with a phenomenon called telomere shortening. Telomeres are structures at the very ends of chromosomes. Ulcerative colitis damages intestinal cells in a manner that causes the telomeres to shorten. This puts the chromosomes at greater risk for structural damage, which increases the risk that the cell will become cancerous. After 30 years of illness, the cumulative cancer risk is about 30%. Both disorders are diagnosed more frequently in whites than in other races. Ulcerative colitis is more prevalent—about 80 cases per 100,000 persons—compared to about half that for Crohn disease. The highest prevalence is in Ashkenazi Jews.

Today we know there is a significant genetic component to both disorders, confirming a suspicion that Dr. Crohn expressed when he first described the illness that bears his name. Shortly after reporting the features of a severe gastrointestinal illness in a 14-year-old boy, he diagnosed the same condition in the patient's 32-year-old sister! Typically, the age of onset is young adulthood.

Studies of the first-degree relatives of patients with IBD find a much stronger family history than one would expect by chance. Although the range is wide, in general it is about 10 times greater than would be found by randomly sampling families. Most studies find a moderately higher positive family history in patients with Crohn disease than in patients with ulcerative colitis. In particular, the concordance rate for Crohn disease among MZ twins is much higher than among DZ twins. For both disorders, the younger the age at which the index patient is diagnosed, the greater the apparent genetic load in the family—a phenomenon that, not surprisingly, characterizes many genetically influenced disorders.

During the late 1990s, the International IBD Genetics Consortium conducted a number of genome-wide scans searching for statistical evidence that predisposing genes were located within certain regions of chromosomes. By 2000, they had compiled solid evidence that a gene (called IBD1) on chromosome 16 predisposed to CD. Similarly, they uncovered evidence that there are genes on chromosomes 1, 3, 5, and 7 with variants that are found more commonly in patients with ulcerative colitis. Weaker evidence supported the case for predisposing genes on chromosomes 5, 12, and 19.

Because the statistical score associating the gene on chromosome 16 with risk for Crohn disease was so high and the math suggested it could account for 15% of all cases, several groups set out to find it. In 2001, two groups showed that a variant of a gene on 16 called NOD2 (sometimes called CARD 15) which makes a protein that is found on the surface of immune cells called macrophages is much more common in persons with Crohn disease. Persons homozygous (born with two copies) for this variant have a 20-fold increased risk for Crohn disease and have a marked tendency to have the worst manifestation of the disease in the last third of the small intestine. The discovery of the role of NOD2 in risk for Crohn disease is a remarkable advance, but because no more than 20% of patients have the variant, we still have much to learn about cause. Currently, one focus is on a region on the long arm of chromosome 5 where a gene variant seems to be associated with an early-onset form of this disorder.

In addition to genome scanning, scientists have done "candidate gene" studies, searches for associations of disease with the presence of certain gene variants more often than expected by chance. Such work is driven by a hypothesis about a known gene because it codes for a protein that, if dysfunctional, might be expected to cause the disease. This has led many researchers to study two genes that are central to marshalling the inflammatory response—tumor necrosis factor-α and interleukin-1 and its companion, the interleukin-1 receptor antagonist. Suspicion runs high. In particular, recent research on drugs designed to block the action of TNF-α seem to benefit patients with IBD.

The most impressive candidate gene study to date focused on a well-studied gene called MDR1. The acronym stands for multidrug resistance gene. Variants in its protein product are known to affect how readily various drugs are absorbed from the intestines. The scientists were drawn to this gene for two major reasons: (1) It is located on a region of chromosome 7 that has been linked to risk for IBD and (2) a strain of "knockout" mice (bred to lack the murine version of MDR1) spontaneously develop colitis. In a case-control study of 329 families with IBD, the researchers were able to show that a single amino acid change at position 893 in the protein was highly associated with risk for IBD, especially in those with Crohn disease. It is possible that the variant associated with IBD has this effect because it is less efficient in moving certain toxic substances away from the intestinal cells for detoxification in the liver.

There are, almost certainly, more genes to be found. In 2003, a team of researchers in the United Kingdom reported that in a study comparing the DNA variations in nearly 400 persons with Crohn disease to those in an equal number of controls, the risk for having the disease was strongly associated (odds ratio greater than 6) with having been born with a certain variant in the interleukin-10 gene. Another variant of the same gene seems to protect individuals from the disease. Since interleukin-10 is known to suppress the action of some inflammatory proteins, it is biologically plausible that a variant of it could play a role in the etiology of Crohn disease. An Italian research group has conducted two studies, both of which suggest there is also another risk gene on chromosome 16 located quite far from NOD2/CARD15.

The families of patients with IBD are at increased risk for two other uncommon disorders, ankylosing spondylitis (AS), a disease of the spine, and primary sclerosing cholangitis (PSC), a disease of the biliary tract. The first has long been associated with the presence of a gene called HLA-B27 that is also found more commonly in patients with IBD. It is not yet known whether IBD increases the risk for AS or whether patients with one are merely also at greater risk for the other. About half of all cases of PSC arise in patients with IBD, but the reason for this is not known.

When a patient is diagnosed with IBD, what is the risk to other family members? In one large study done at the Cleveland Clinic, the risk that at least one child of an affected parent would also develop the disorder was about 9%. The sibling of a person diagnosed with ulcerative colitis had about a 6% chance of becoming ill, whereas the sibling of a person with Crohn disease had about a 7.5% chance. Twin studies, although based on small numbers of patients, support an even greater role for genes in the onset of Crohn disease than in ulcerative colitis. Studies suggest that the MZ twin of an affected person has a 70% chance of also developing Crohn disease, whereas the MZ twin of a person with ulcerative colitis has about a 30% lifetime risk. Of course, that risk is still extremely high compared to the general risk of a randomly selected person. Studies of the spouses of persons with these disorders have not uncovered an increased prevalence of disease, a finding that argues against a strong role for common environmental factors.

Like many complex disorders with mysterious causes, the risk that a particular relative will develop IBD is, albeit much higher than the background risk, still low. Siblings of an affected person have about a 7% chance, whereas children of an affected person appear to have a somewhat lower risk. Thus, the answer to the question posed at the top of this section is about 5–10%.

Peptic Ulcer Disease

Both my father and one of his brothers have ulcers. Am I at increased risk?

Peptic ulcer disease (PUD) refers to common ulcerative conditions of the upper gastrointestinal tract, especially the stomach (gastric ulcer) and the part of the intestine to which the stomach connects, called the duodenum (duodenal ulcer). The problem arises in part due to an imbalance in the secretion and clearance of acid, and there is good evidence that chronic exposure to certain environmental factors and predisposing genes both play a role. Interestingly, problems associated with having an active ulcer differ depending on the anatomical location. Furthermore, it appears that a diagnosis of duodenal ulcer is not associated with increased familial risk for gastric ulcer, a finding that suggests different genes are involved in the risk for ulcers at each location. Various surveys have suggested that the lifetime risk for developing a peptic ulcer is between 2% and 10%. Historical data indicate that the diagnosis became steadily more common throughout the 20th century.

Each year, about 1 of 300 adults in the United States is diagnosed with

PUD. The disorder is about twice as common in men as it is in women. There is much variation in the prevalence of PUD between ethnic and racial groups. Native Americans in the southwest appear to have only 1/40th the risk for PUD as that of whites throughout the United States. In Japan, unlike the rest of the world, gastric ulcer is more common than is duodenal ulcer.

The classic sign of duodenal ulcer is the development of central abdominal pain about 1–3 hours after eating a meal. The individual often describes the pain as like the gnawing discomfort one can get on an empty stomach. The disease is chronic, but intermittent and relapsing. The key elements of medical treatment are diet, avoidance of cigarettes, regular use of antacids, and the so-called H-2 blocker drugs such as cimetidine (Tagamet and other drugs). In severe cases, the major complication is perforation of the intestine, which requires prompt surgery. Gastric ulcer most often occurs in the antrum, a portion of the stomach that is relatively close to the place where most of the acid secretion occurs. Gastric ulcers typically present in the sixth decade, on average about 10 years later than do duodenal ulcers. The approach to treatment is the same as for duodenal ulcers.

Much progress has been made in understanding the causes of PUD. Environmental factors are clearly important. Currently, the two most severe appear to be chronic infection with bacteria called *Helicobacter pylori* (*H. pylori*) and prolonged use of nonsteroidal anti-inflammatory drugs (NSAIDs). Other important environmental factors are smoking and heavy use of alcohol, caffeine, aspirin, or steroids. The best evidence is that chronic exposure to these agents creates a much higher risk for disease in those who are born with a genetic susceptibility.

Many studies have shown that PUD is a familial disease. The association of increased risk among close relatives of patients is consistent through the generations and across socioeconomic groups, facts that reinforce the probable role of genes. The risk of PUD is 2–3 times greater in first-degree relatives of patients than in first-degree relatives of unaffected persons. Multiple studies of PUD in MZ and DZ twins have shown that the disease has a much higher concordance rate in MZ than in DZ pairs.

There have been many efforts to determine whether PUD is associated with particular biomarkers or with risk for other diseases. It has been known for decades that PUD is about 30% more common in persons with blood group O than in those with other blood types. Their risk for duodenal ulcers in particular is even higher and seems to increase as they grow older. Studies of many other markers, especially the HLA system, have yielded contradictory results. PUD is a feature of about a dozen single-gene disorders (including cystic fibrosis and α-1-antitrypsin deficiency), but that explains only a tiny fraction of all cases. There are probably several paths to PUD, and each is associated with interaction of various environmental risk factors with a predisposing gene or genes. For example, levels of an enzyme called PG-I are consistently higher than normal in about one-half of the relatives of people with duodenal ulcers. These persons are themselves at increased risk

Epidemiological surveys have consistently found that the first-degree relatives of persons with PUD are two to three times more likely to develop the disease than are first-degree relatives of unaffected individuals. Because chronic infection with *H. pylori* is a risk factor with ulcers at both locations, it may be that part of this increased risk is due to the spread of the bacteria among family members.

To respond to the introductory question, about 20% of the first-degree relatives of persons with PUD will develop the same condition. Those with a positive family history should avoid the recognized environmental risk factors, especially cigarettes and anti-inflammatory drugs. They should tell their doctors about the family history and promptly report symptoms. In addition, they probably would benefit from being tested for *H. pylori* infection. Antibiotic therapy, which eliminates the infection, will reduce the risk of ulcer disease.

Celiac Disease (Gluten-sensitive Enteropathy)

I have been told that I have an allergy to wheat products. Is this genetic?

Celiac disease, also called gluten-sensitive enteropathy (GSE) or sprue, is characterized by the inability to digest properly foods made from wheat, rye, barley, and oats. In particular, patients have an allergy-like syndrome to gliadins, hordeins, and/or secalins, cereal proteins that have a high percentage of the amino acid glutamine. Seriously affected persons develop a chronic malabsorption syndrome characterized by diarrhea, fatty stools, bloating, and weight loss. The disease can manifest in children, but it is often not diagnosed until adulthood. This is in part because it has a wide range of expression from mild to quite severe.

GSE is an autoimmune disorder with a complex pathway. In genetically predisposed individuals, gluten proteins in the cereals stimulate the

Table 18. *Celiac disease (GSE): Association with HLA genes*

HLA haplotype	All children 3627	Affected children 56	Odds ratio
DR3-DQ2 (plus any other except DR4-DQ-8)	575 (16%)	46 (82%)	26.[a]
DR4-DQ8 (plus any other)	756 (21%)	6 (11%)	.5
DR3-DQ2 and DR4-DQ8	80 (2%)	2 (4%)	1.7
Any other	2216 (61%)	2 (4%)	.02

Adapted, with permission, from Mäki M., Mustalahti K., Kokkonen J., Kulmala P., Haapalahti M., Karttunen T., et al. 2003. Prevalence of celiac disease among children in Finland. *New England Journal of Medicine* **348:** 2517–2524.

[a]The DR3-DQ2 haplotype greatly increases the relative risk of developing celiac disease. Children born with other HLA gene combinations rarely have celiac disease.

production of a protein in the host, which, when overactive, impairs the integrity of the intestinal cell wall. This allows glutens to penetrate into a deeper tissue layer called the lamina propria, where they are broken down into fragments, some of which are interpreted by the body's immunological system as foreign, and attacked. The attack is carried out by cells known as CD8 and CD4 lymphocytes. Interestingly, these defenders are much more likely to be called into action if the individual has a particular set of HLA genes. In attacking the fragments, the CD4 cells also damage the cells that line the gastrointestinal tract, which leads to the chronic digestive disorder.

The prevalence of GSE varies across racial groups. It is most common in whites, and the highest reported prevalence is in Ireland and England. Because the phenotype can be so mild that affected persons do not come to medical attention, the more carefully one looks, the more cases one finds. Medical textbooks estimate that about 1 in 300 Caucasians is affected, but this number is probably too low. A major study of GSE in Finland recently found that at least 1%, and perhaps 1.5%, of the population has this disorder. On the other hand, GSE has not been reported in Japanese or Chinese, and it appears to be rare in African groups.

GSE is a familial disease. Large studies conducted in the 1970s, research that included intestinal biopsies (the gold standard for diagnosis), showed that GSE occurred in about 14% of siblings, 8% of parents, and

15% of the children of affected persons. Many of those with positive biopsies had not yet developed clinical signs of disease. The above numbers are the medians of several studies that yielded widely varying results. However, all showed a risk to relatives far higher than the general population risk. These early studies suggested that predisposition to the disease was linked to the inheritance of a dominantly acting gene with incomplete penetrance. There have been few studies of MZ twins with GSE, but there are reports of MZ pairs in which both have the disease.

Over the last decade, researchers have learned much about the genetic component of GSE. The haplotype (combination of genes) that confers the greatest risk is known as DR3-DQ2 (in addition, the person must not have another haplotype called DR4-DQ). At least 8% of all persons born with these autoimmune genes develop the disease. Put another way, such people have more than 20-fold the risk faced by the general population. The risk for disease in the siblings of affected persons varies tremendously, depending on what HLA genes they inherited. If an unaffected sibling has a different HLA pattern, his or her risk is only about 1%. However, if they share the same HLA pattern, the risk to the as-yet-unaffected sibling may be as high as 30%.

Currently, many physicians do not aggressively assess risk in the relatives of affected individuals. Since the disorder is comparatively benign if a proper diet is followed, the usual approach is to wait for telltale signs and symptoms and react at that time. This seems shortsighted. GSE is a common disorder for which there are highly accurate diagnostic tests and a clear therapy.

GSE may properly be thought of as one of the most common genetic disorders, affecting at least 1% of whites. Affected persons have a lifelong condition best treated by rigorous attention to diet. Even those with mild conditions should be careful to adhere to a gluten-free diet. Over time, the risk of certain cancers (including lymphoma) rises, and is almost certainly greater in those who have not followed dietary guidelines.

Pancreatitis

My uncle and his son have been diagnosed with pancreatitis. Can genes cause it?

The pancreas is a long, irregularly shaped organ (sometimes likened in shape to a dog's tongue) that lies just below the stomach and empties its myriad, powerful digestive enzymes into the small intestine. Pancreatitis (an extremely painful and debilitating condition brought about by acute or chronic inflammation of the tissue) is diagnosed in about 40,000 persons each year in the United States. People with acute pancreatitis are very sick indeed. They typically have a deep, steady, boring pain in the middle of their gut. They are anxious, dehydrated, feverish, and often on the edge of shock. Pancreatitis can be a true medical emergency that carries with it a risk of death.

There are many causes of pancreatitis, but the two most important are chronic alcohol abuse and gallbladder disease. Blunt trauma, infections, and side effects of medications are other fairly common causes. A significant fraction is called idiopathic because there is no obvious cause. In addition, there are more than a dozen rare disorders in which pancreatitis is a common complication.

Although the list of environmental risk factors is long, physicians have known for more than 50 years that some families are burdened with a genetic form of pancreatitis. In the mid 1990s, some astute clinical researchers, prodded by the father of a boy with the genetic form of the disorder, made a major advance in understanding this nasty disease.

In 1989, Kevin Slone, a member of a family in Kentucky burdened with an autosomal dominant form of pancreatitis that the town folk called Slone's disease, was admitted to the hospital with a severe attack. While the boy was being treated, his father showed doctors a detailed family history he had compiled that included 700 relatives over nine generations. A doctor–family research partnership blossomed. In 1994, Bobby Slone, Kevin's dad, organized a family reunion with a special twist. A key part of the party was blood drawing. About 90 relatives, some with the disease and some without, provided DNA samples.

By comparing the DNA from affected persons with the DNA of unaffected relatives, the researchers quickly found that the causative gene was on chromosome 7. Using a candidate gene approach, they were then, just 3 months later, able to show that the disease was caused by a mutation in the cationic trypsinogen gene, one of a group of related genes. This gene codes for a protein that is the precursor to one of the key pancreatic enzymes, so the association of the mutation with affected individuals made perfect physiological sense. The work has opened up new possibilities to understanding how the disease develops in the many people for whom it manifests sporadically with no clear cause. Perhaps many of them have mutations in this or related genes.

The elucidation of the gene that causes Slone's disease was important news for the Kentucky family and a few others that have the same problem. However, the vast majority of persons who develop pancreatitis do not have a family history suggestive of a dominant single-gene disorder. The fact that one has a relative or two with pancreatitis is much more compatible with a history of alcohol abuse or gallbladder disease than with strong genetic factors. This does not mean that there is no genetic susceptibility, only that it has not been found. After all, the majority of persons who are exposed to the major risk factors never develop pancreatitis. As-yet-unknown genetic risk factors probably determine the impact of the environmental risks.

Lactose Intolerance (Lactase Deficiency)

My husband cannot drink milk. Is this going to happen to our kids?

Lactose intolerance (LI) is the inability to digest a common sugar, lactose, found in milk, most dairy products, and foods made with them. For persons with LI, even one glass of whole milk can lead to bloating and flatulence, but usually not diarrhea. The disorder may not sound too serious, but in those parts of the world where malnutrition is common and poor children often depend on milk as an important source of calories, LI can greatly increase the risk for serious illness or even death. Indeed, our knowledge of LI grew out of research initiated in the 1960s after it was observed that a high percentage of African children had trouble consuming the milk products that were being donated by the United States and European countries.

There are several different types of LI. The most severe and the least common is congenital lactase deficiency (CLD), an autosomal recessive disease that occurs in less than 1 in 10,000 births. Affected infants who breast-feed begin to have severe watery diarrhea in the first few days of life. Unless the problem is recognized and they are switched to a non-lactose formula, they can quickly become severely malnourished. In 1998, a group of Finnish researchers showed that CLD is caused by a mutation in a gene on the long arm of chromosome 2. To their surprise, however, it turned out that the causative gene is located nearly 2,000,000 base pairs (DNA letters) from the gene known to code for the enzyme used by adults to metabolize lactose.

The common form of LI, although sometimes called adult-type hypolactasia, often begins in late childhood. Affected people can digest milk in infancy and early childhood, but lose that ability over time. The age of onset of the disorder varies widely among different populations. Researchers at the NIH have estimated that more than 30,000,000 Americans have LI. This seems like a lot, but persons of northern European descent actually have the *lowest* prevalence of LI of any part of the human family. Whereas only about 2% of Swedes have LI, 23% of the Fulani people in Africa and 89% of the Bantu are born without the ability to digest lactose. Nearly 100% of Native Americans have LI, as do nearly 75% of African-Americans. Nearly 90% of the people in China and Southeast Asia are lactose intolerant.

In 2002, the same group of researchers who had mapped the gene for CLD unraveled the genetic cause of the more common form. It was already known that the onset of symptoms was highly correlated with the decline in activity of an enzyme called LPH. They showed that LI is an autosomal recessive disorder, but that it is not associated with mutations in the LPH gene. Instead, it is associated with a change in a single DNA letter located nearly 14,000 base pairs away from the gene. For reasons not yet worked out, in persons with two copies of this variant, the activity of LPH is less than 10% of normal. The team quickly checked to see whether this variant also caused LI in other human population groups. Checking more than 1,000 DNA samples in French, Americans, and Africans, they found that it did.

What are the implications of knowing that a close relative is diagnosed with LI? One should assume that it could be the result of an autosomal recessive condition. On that basis one can analyze risk to other relatives. An adult who has LI can assume he or she has two copies of the variant. Therefore, his children will be born with at least one copy. The odds of that child being affected with the common form of LI are determined by the frequency of the causative allele in the general population.

Appendicitis

Appendicitis seems pretty common. Are there genes that increase one's risk?

Appendicitis is an inflammation of the appendix, a small, worm-shaped pouch attached to the beginning of the large intestine and located in the lower right portion of the abdomen. If the inflammation (usually the result of an obstruction at the point where the appendix connects to the colon, which predisposes to bacterial infection) causes the appendix to rupture, the patient becomes very ill. A century ago, before abdominal surgery was common, the risk of death from peritonitis was high.

Appendicitis is most common in older children and young adults, with the greatest risk in adolescence. Patients typically develop severe, localized pain, nausea and vomiting, a fever, and a high white blood cell count. However, appendicitis can present in many different ways, and it is often not an easy diagnosis to make. Many surgeons have removed more than one appendix that on pathological examination appears normal. The lifetime risk for appendicitis is about 7%. Each year about 1 person in 1000 in the United States is diagnosed with this condition. It is diagnosed more often in women, with a sex ratio of 1.4 to 1. The prevalence of appendicitis varies widely around the world, and there is good evidence that in cultures which eat a high-fiber diet appendicitis is significantly less common.

Appendicitis has long been recognized to be familial, but almost nothing was known about genetic risk factors. As far back as 1937, a physician reported the detailed history of several families where the disease appeared to behave as an autosomal dominant disorder. In 1990, a research group in Belgrade reported the results of a study based on 80 consecutive cases of acute appendicitis (proven by tissue studies after surgery). They found that the comparative risk among relatives of the patients for having had appendicitis was 10 times greater than for relatives of a control group matched for age, gender, and number of siblings! The scientists extended their studies to 674 other families in which a member was diagnosed with appendicitis, matching them with control families. The larger study confirmed the smaller. Their analysis led to the conclusion that no single gene accounted for most cases, but that the total heritability for appendicitis was 56%, and that several genes contributed to risk. This model allows for the possibility that appendicitis is on rare occasions caused by a single gene.

Despite the solid evidence that risk for appendicitis aggregates in families, we still do not know the predisposing genes. There is currently little definite that can be said to families about the genetic risk for appendicitis. Because it is a common disorder, there are many thousands of families in which two or more close relatives have both had their appendixes removed. This by no means proves that a genetic factor is the cause. However, the Belgrade study strongly suggests that if a parent has had appendicitis, the risk to a child is significantly higher than the overall population risk. Practically speaking, there is little one can do about this except have a high level of concern if a child complains of abdominal pain. A high-fiber diet may have some preventive value.

Gallstones (Cholecystitis, Gallbladder Disease)

My mother and her sister both have had gallbladder operations. Am I at increased risk?

The gallbladder is a pouch located beneath the liver that stores bile, a substance made by the liver that is needed to digest fats. Bile is composed of water, cholesterol, various kinds of fats, bilirubin, and several proteins. When stimulated to do so, the gallbladder contracts, sending stored bile through the common bile duct into the intestine, where it plays an important role in digestion. Bile can sometimes precipitate to form gallstones. These are of two major types: cholesterol stones and pigment stones. Cholesterol stones (which account for about 75%) develop when there is a chronic excess of cholesterol in the bile. The cause of pigment stones (25%) is not well known, but they are found more often in people with a variety of diseases.

Gallstones are extremely common, especially after age 60, but in more than half the people who have them, they do not cause trouble. However, gallstones can move from the pouch of the gallbladder to obstruct and inflame the duct through which the bile passes. In addition to intense pain and vomiting, people in the throes of a gallbladder attack are at high risk for infection and a worsening of other problems they might have, such as coronary artery disease. Each year more than 500,000 Americans have surgery to remove an inflamed gallbladder.

Over the years, researchers have identified several risk factors for the development of gallstones. Among the most important are age, gender, obesity, diabetes, ethnicity, estrogen level, use of cholesterol-lowering drugs, rapid weight loss, and fasting. People over age 60 are more likely to have gallstones. Women between 20 and 60 are twice as likely as men of the same age to have them. More than half of Native American adults (the fraction is even higher in the Pima tribe in Arizona) have gallstones. People with diabetes tend to have high levels of triglycerides, which increase the chance for gallstones. Weight loss causes the liver to secrete extra cholesterol that predisposes to gallstone formation.

It has been known since the 19th century that gallstones "run" in families. An early German study (1937) found that gallstones were three to five times more common in the relatives of affected persons than in the relatives of a control group. In a more recent Danish study in which more than 4000 people underwent ultrasound studies, relatives of affected persons were more than twice as likely as those in a control group to have gallstones. In a 1990 study of the relatives of young affected women, the risk to relatives was threefold the background risk. Studies in Sweden, Israel, and India have made similar findings. A Swedish study of 27 children with cholesterol gallstones found that 15 mothers and 2 fathers also had them. The few twin studies suggest a concordance rate of about 40% in MZ twins, much higher than for DZ twins.

There have been only a few genetic studies of gallbladder disease (GBD). Among Mexican-Americans (a population with a generally high prevalence of gallstones), increased risk has been associated with having a variant of the cholesterol-7a-hydroxylase gene, which makes a protein involved in cholesterol metabolism. Since the biology of bile formation and secretion is well understood, there is a long list of suspect genes, but none has been indicted, let alone convicted. However, late in 2003, a lead suspect may have been identified. A research team in San Antonio reported that in Mexican-Americans with symptomatic (as opposed to silent) GBD, a locus near the tip of the short arm of chromosome 11 was unusually prevalent. If this finding is replicated in a separate study population, it will provide strong evidence for the first susceptibility gene.

Although there is good evidence that the risk for GBD runs in families, we do not yet know of any genes that are directly linked with risk of GBD. However, the connection of risk for GBD with obesity, which is significantly influenced by genetic factors, is impressive. Obese women aged between 20 and 30 have a sixfold greater risk for GBD than do comparably aged women of normal weight. This risk may be due to the fact that obese persons make much more cholesterol, from which most gallstones form. Adult-onset diabetes, which is also heavily influenced by genetic susceptibility, is a known risk factor for having gallstones.

A positive family history about doubles a woman's risk for having gallstones and somewhat increases the risk for GBD. The most helpful response to that history is probably to keep a close eye on one's weight.

ENDOCRINE DISORDERS

Adult-onset Diabetes (NIDDM, Diabetes Type II)

My father and his brother developed diabetes while in their 50s. How much are my risks increased?

In marked contrast to juvenile diabetes (which is characterized by the death of the insulin-producing cells in the pancreas), adult-onset diabetes (diabetes mellitus, non-insulin-dependent diabetes [NIDDM], diabetes type II) arises when the body becomes resistant to the insulin that is secreted by the pancreas. This impairs the ability of muscle and other cells to take up the glucose that they depend on for energy. The most obvious early sign of diabetes is an elevated blood sugar level. Unfortunately, because the onset is insidious, people may go months or years with undiagnosed diabetes. At the time the disease is diagnosed, much more damage may have occurred to a variety of organs than is readily apparent. People with diabetes, especially those in whom it is not well controlled, are at much greater risk for heart attacks, kidney failure, blindness, and amputations than are unaffected persons of the same age.

NIDDM is disturbingly common, and the number of affected individuals has been rising sharply for some time. More than 5% of adults in the population have diabetes—perhaps as many as 17 million people in the United States alone. For every person with diabetes type I, there are more than 20 with diabetes type II. The typical adult diabetic patient is diagnosed in his late 40s or 50s, is overweight, and often has affected relatives. These facts alone are sufficient to strongly indict both lifestyle and genes as causative agents.

The epidemic of diabetes type II is in large part a consequence of our overall success as a species in gaining almost unlimited access to calories. This has fostered a "thrifty genotype" hypothesis. In essence, this idea postulates that genes in early humans that favored energy storage (in the form of fat) had a survival advantage, but that today those same genes predispose to obesity and diabetes. Perhaps the most disturbing new development is that NIDDM is approaching epidemic proportions in children, a group in which it used to be rare. These children are usually significantly overweight and do not exercise enough.

Diabetes is a complex disease, and various expert medical groups regularly debate (and sometimes revise) the criteria for diagnosis. When a person presents with the classic symptoms of full-blown diabetes (increased urination, increased thirst, abnormal body chemistry, and weight loss), the diagnosis is easy. Today, far more cases are being picked up through blood sugar screening tests. The risk for diabetes, as defined by blood sugar level, is constantly being reassessed.

From 1979 to 1997, the experts defined persons as having diabetes if they had a fasting glucose above 140 mg/dl or a level above 200 when measured 2 hours after ingesting 75 mg of glucose. In 1997, the American Diabetes Association (ADA) expanded the diagnostic criteria. Today, a fasting glucose above 126 is considered highly suggestive of diabetes, and a level between 110 and 125 is considered to be an "impaired fasting glucose." Because these new numbers expand the diagnosis of diabetes to millions of persons in the United States alone, there is controversy about their use. This is in part because there is not yet medical consensus on what advice to offer the patient with the slightly elevated blood sugar levels.

Physicians have long been aware that heredity plays an important role in the risk for diabetes. One 2000-year-old Hindu text identifies two causes: "the seed" and rich diet! In family surveys, as many as half of persons with diabetes have a positive family history, whereas only 15% of age-matched non-diabetics report having an affected relative. The concordance rates for MZ twins range from 45% to 90%, three times higher than in matched DZ pairs. Furthermore, the older the MZ twins and the more careful the study, the higher are the concordance rates, sometimes nearly 100%. The prevalence of diabetes type II varies widely among ethnic groups. In the United States, the highest rate of diabetes is probably among the Pima Indians in the southwest (about 40% of the population is affected).

The fact that NIDDM is so common a disorder makes it difficult to sort out the role that genes play. It is highly likely that many different gene variants contribute to the risk. This means that in any family with several affected members, it is possible that more than one predisposing gene is involved. There are probably even different types of NIDDM. In 10 years we may recognize several clinically distinct forms of the disease that at the moment we cannot clearly delineate. For example, in studies that examine the risk of diabetes in family members of affected persons as a function of the weight of the diabetic relative, the *less* obese the patients, the higher the risk that their siblings will develop the disease!

In the mid 1990s, extensive study of more than 20 candidate genes uncovered evidence that could explain only about 1% of all cases of

Table 19. *Adult-onset diabetes: Familial risk*	
Prevalence	In Hispanic families with type 2 diabetes, about 30% of patients have affected first-degree relatives and about 15% have affected second-degree relatives.
Characteristics of high-risk families	Early age of onset (between 25 and 40). Multiple affected family members. Presence of other signs of insulin resistance including hypertension, abnormal lipids, and early CAD.
Risk	In Hispanic families, twofold risk to first-degree relatives of affected individuals. In Caucasian families, threefold risk to first-degree relatives of affected individuals.

Adapted, with permission, from Rimoin D.I., Connor J.M., Pyeritz R.E., and Korf B.R. 2002. *Emery and Rimoin's principles and practice of medical genetics,* 4th edition. Churchill Livingstone, London; © Elsevier.

NIDDM. Mutations in the gene coding for insulin may cause about 1 out of every 300 cases. In the last few years, there have been a number of genome-wide searches to find regions that may contain predisposing genes, and a number of suspicious areas have been located, including a strongly positive finding on chromosome 12 in a Finnish population. However, none of these studies has led to identification of a major genetic risk factor for type II diabetes. But, as our mapping abilities grow, so do the chances of finding predisposing genes. In the summer of 2003, a study conducted in Iceland of nearly 1000 non-obese patients with diabetes, and their relatives, localized a susceptibility gene to the long arm of chromosome 5. If this study holds up, we will have the first common predisposing gene for NIDDM.

One major success has been the discovery of genes that play a major role in an uncommon subtype of type II diabetes called maturity onset diabetes of the young (MODY), which was first recognized as a discrete disorder in 1996. In particular, a gene on chromosome 7, which codes for an enzyme called glucokinase, is responsible for many cases of MODY (which explains about 2% of all diabetes). There are at least five other genes that seem to be responsible for most of the rest of the cases of MODY, but there must be at least one other culprit gene to be discovered, as about 20% of patients with MODY do not have any abnormalities in the known causative genes.

Groups connected with the International Type II Diabetes Consortium are currently cooperating in several gene search projects. They have found many suspect regions of the genome, but there is nothing to suggest that variants in two or three genes account for most cases. There is some evidence that genes which substantially influence inflammation significantly affect the pace with which diabetes develops and the risk for its common complications (eye disease, kidney disease, and heart disease). Variations in the interleukin-1 gene may be associated with risk for heart attacks in diabetics, as well as in the development of both eye and kidney disease. The gene variants do not cause the complications, but they seem to accelerate their development.

Counseling of close blood relatives of persons diagnosed with NIDDM is based on empirical evidence. The lifetime risk to a first-degree relative of an affected individual is in the range of 20–30%, which is three to four times greater than the risk to the general population. In the case of a man whose father *and* paternal uncle both have NIDDM, the lifetime risk would be higher, perhaps 35%. Of course, such estimates are greatly influenced by the presence or absence of other risk factors, such as obesity.

There are two important actions that close relatives of persons with type II diabetes can take to reduce their risk of developing the disease. First, they should pay strict attention to maintaining a healthy diet and avoiding becoming overweight. Second, they should consult with their physicians about undergoing periodic blood sugar tests. The good news for those who are at increased genetic risk is that simple interventions can almost certainly both decrease the likelihood of developing the disease and delay by many years its onset.

Obesity

How familial is the tendency to be overweight? What do we know about the influence of genes?

Obese individuals have an abnormally high amount of fat in relation to their lean tissue mass. The standard unit of measure to determine obesity is body mass index (BMI), which is weight divided by the square of one's height. For example, a man who is 5'7" tall (1.7 meters) and weighs 185 pounds (84 kilograms) has a BMI of 29, which is the result of dividing 84 by 1.7 x 1.7. In general, persons who exceed their ideal body mass by up to 20% are considered overweight. Persons who are heavier than that are considered obese. Put another way, persons with a BMI of 25–30 are overweight. Those above 30 (essentially the 95th percentile of the idealized population curves) are obese. By these criteria, more than 50% of adult Americans are overweight! There are twice as many obese people per capita in the United States as there are in Australia or England. The prevalence of obesity has risen so dramatically over the last 50 years that some have called it a pandemic. The World Health Organization estimates that more than one billion people are overweight or obese.

Given the potential impact of obesity on one's long-term health, the word pandemic is appropriate. Mortality studies consistently show that for persons with a BMI above 30, the overall risk of death rises sharply. In adulthood, persons with a BMI of 35 have roughly twice the risk of dying at any given age as do those with a BMI of 25. Obesity has been highly correlated with hypertension, gallbladder disease, and lung problems. Extreme obesity has long been recognized as a risk factor for heart failure. In 2002, researchers who are involved in the Framingham Heart Study extended this knowledge by showing that in a study of 5881 middle-aged people, the risk for heart attack rose steadily with increase in BMI, even for mildly overweight persons. For every single unit rise above a BMI of 25, the risk of heart failure in men went up 5%; in women it was 7%. At any age, individuals with a BMI greater than 30 had double the risk for heart failure compared to those with a BMI less than 25.

There are a number of well-defined, but rare, causes of obesity, including several neurological, endocrinological, and single-gene disorders. Collectively, these account for only a tiny percentage of cases. A major research focus is to study the genes which make the hormones that, when normal, regulate the appetite centers of the brain. In addition to leptin, a hormone sent by fat cells to the brain, researchers are studying a pair of genes called MC4R and a-MSH. In 2003, scientists showed that mutations in a-MSH caused a subtype of extreme obesity associated with binge eating. Particularly important has been the finding that mutations in MC4R may account for 6% of all childhood-onset obesity (making it the most common single-gene cause of this disorder). Despite this finding, the irrefutable fact is that most obesity arises due to a subtle imbalance in the regulation of appetite and energy storage that has become much more debilitating in a modern world that is awash in calories. If a person of college age gains just 2 pounds a year, he will be obese by his mid-40s. One needs only to gain 1/10th of an ounce a day to become seriously overweight over two decades.

Americans have become progressively heavier for the last century, which certainly emphasizes the role of environmental factors. A good example is provided by data from a multi-decade study of children in Muscatine, Iowa. In 1971, 17% of the girls and boys aged 12–14 were obese; in 1992, 31% of the girls and 28% of the boys of the same age were obese. One disturbing sign of the burgeoning problem of childhood obesity is the decision by the FDA in 2003 to permit use of a weight loss drug called Xenical in children. The major environmental risk factors are gender, race, and poverty. More women than men, more blacks than whites, and more poor than rich persons are obese.

On the other hand, the fact that virtually everyone in our society has easy access to an abundance of calories, yet only some people become obese, indicates that there must be important genetic regulators of how individuals acquire and maintain excess weight.

How important are genes in obesity? As one reviewer frankly put it, "unassailable evidence now shows that genetic factors play a dominant role in determining body weight within a given environment." What do family studies tell us about the heritability of obesity? A dozen studies of the parents of obese children repeatedly show a high prevalence of obesity in at least one parent. The range in this group is from a low of 44% to a high of 85%. This makes the tendency to become obese (not merely overweight) among the most heritable of any physical traits! In these studies, the mother was twice as likely as the father to be obese. *Both* parents were *obese* in about a quarter of the families, a finding that is far in excess of the prevalence of obesity in the general population. Studies that begin by ascertaining obese couples and then studying their children report comparable results. As the mean BMI of the parents increases, so does the likelihood that their children will be obese in adulthood. Of course, such research is unable to untangle genetic from environmental factors—but adoption studies can.

They consistently report that children who are given for adoption grow up to have a BMI significantly more like that of their biological than of their adoptive parents. One of the best such studies used data from an adoption registry for Denmark. The scientists studied 400 women and 400 men who had been adopted. They found no statistical correlation of their body mass with that of their rearing parents. On the other hand, the more obese the adopted persons, the more likely that one or both of their biological parents was also obese.

Perhaps most impressive are the twin studies. In one study comparing

Table 20. *Obesity: Risk in young adulthood based on obesity in childhood and in parents.*

Age	Obese as child? yes v. no	Number of obese parents	
		1 V. O	2 V. O
1–2	1.3	3.2	13.6
3–5	4.7	3.0	15.3
6–9	8.8[a]	2.6	5.0
10–14	22.3	2.2	2.0
15–17	17.5	2.2	5.6

Adapted, with permission, from Rimoin D.I., Connor J.M., Pyeritz R.E., and Korf B.R. 2002. *Emery and Rimoin's principles and practice of medical genetics,* 4th edition. Churchill Livingstone, London; © Elsevier.

[a]For example, an obese 8-year-old child is nearly 9 times more likely to be obese in his 20s than is a child of that age who is not obese.

44 pairs of MZ twins reared together with 44 pairs of twins reared apart, the researchers found that the mean difference in weights in the twin pairs was the same regardless of their rearing, a finding that seems to speak strongly in favor of genetic factors in setting BMI. There have been several large longitudinal studies of BMI in twins. One compared the weights of 1983 MZ twins and 2104 DZ twins at about age 20 and again at about age 45. In both groups, there was a trend to be heavier, but the weights of the MZ twins were much closer to each other than those of the DZ twin pairs. Overall, the MZ concordance rate is 0.7, among the highest of any trait ever studied. Other data suggest that genetic factors are more important earlier in life and environmental factors are more influential in middle age and beyond.

Studies of obesity in extended families find somewhat lower, but still impressive, correlations. In a Norwegian study involving 75,000 persons, the heritability coefficient was 0.4. Related studies of the distribution of abdominal fat have also found a high heritability within families, about 0.5. Risk for obesity rises markedly if a first-degree relative is extremely obese (BMI> 40). In one study, relatives in 235 families in which the proband (first patient) in each family had a BMI above 40 were 25 times more likely to also be severely obese than a person randomly selected from the population!

During the last few years, there have been major advances in our understanding of the physiology of obesity. Most of the key work has been done with inbred strains of mice. In 1991, a group at Rockefeller University, working with mice known to be obese because they carried two copies of a mutant gene, successfully cloned that gene. They showed that the obese mice were deficient in the protein for which the gene codes and that if the mice were given the protein, it cured their obesity. The group named the protein leptin and designated the gene LEP. Their work gave hope that perhaps a common variant in the human version of LEP on chromosome 7 would be found to play an important role in risk for obesity. That has not turned out to be the case. The subsequent cloning of the leptin receptor gene in mice also provided important new insights into the etiology of obesity. Mutations in the human version of this gene have been found in a few extremely obese persons, but they account for only a minuscule fraction of obesity.

Since 1995, there have been many efforts to study the DNA of families with several members who met the criteria for obesity. Genome-wide hunts for genes that predispose to obesity have yielded equivocal results, mainly because the physiology is so complicated. According to the Obesity Gene Map Database, as of late 2003, at least 80 genes have been associated with obesity, many of which are involved in the formation of fat cells. Despite the genetic complexity, several major advances were made in 2002. A group led by Dr. Steven Stone at Myriad Genetics, Inc. in Salt Lake City studied a large Utah registry that collects health data from high school graduates. They invited families in which at least two members were more than 100 pounds overweight to participate in a gene hunt. They also contacted individuals identified through study of a local hospital registry of 8000 patients who had undergone gastric bypass surgery. Because obesity develops due to multiple environmental and genetic factors, the scientists used stringent criteria for selecting families for the DNA study, selecting only families in which at least three relatives had a BMI greater than 40.

They conducted the DNA search with 628 markers and analyzed the data in three ways: females only, males only, and without regard to gender. Neither the families dominated by male obesity nor the families in which obesity was studied without regard to gender yielded particularly impressive results. However, in the case of the 37 families in which there were three or more profoundly obese women, the DNA analysis offered impressive evidence that a gene predisposing to obesity was localized on the short arm of chromosome 4. The scientists then expanded their study, adding 14 large, extended families. Ultimately, more than 1000 persons were involved. The second study strongly supported the first. Their results suggest that a single gene may be frequently implicated in severe female obesity. The gene should be cloned by the time this book is in print, and we may soon have the first real genetic test for predisposition to obesity (although it will be valuable to only a small number of families). More important, we may gain new ideas about approaches to prevention and therapy.

Also in 2002, a team of scientists from China and Creighton University in Nebraska reported on their study of 53 families containing 630 persons chosen by identifying individuals in a database who have unusually low bone mass. Low bone mass is strongly associated with low BMI. Using 380 markers, this group performed a genome-wide scan for evidence of genes affecting BMI. They found that just one region on the long arm of 2 could account for more than 25% of the variation in BMI. A few months later, another group of scientists analyzed the results of eight genome-wide hunts for obesity genes involving 6849 subjects and four ethnic groups. They found strong evidence for a predisposing gene at 3q27, a region already implicated by earlier studies.

What is the bottom line? Adult weight is a highly heritable trait (heritability is estimated from a low of 0.5 to a high of 0.9). The best predictor of adult weight in otherwise healthy people is parental weight. Nearly 80 years ago, Charles Davenport, an early human geneticist, published perhaps the first study that compared the body mass of parents with that of their children. In a study of 528 parents and 1671 children, he found a strong heritability for body habitus. Basically, as the body mass of parents increased, so did the body mass of their children. Marriages between 23 pairs of two slender parents did not produce any children who became obese. Marriages between two obese parents never produced children who remained slender. Putting aside the small number of families with single-gene causes for obesity, the majority of obese individuals are so because they have a genetic predisposition to store calories as excess fat and live in a world of plenty.

Osteoporosis

My grandmother is all hunched over because of several collapsed vertebrae. I have heard that is due to osteoporosis. What is my risk?

Osteoporosis is the term used to describe a slowly progressive loss of bone mass and erosion of bone architecture that is associated with increased risk for certain fractures. Technically, bones are said to be osteoporotic when their density is more than 2.5 standard deviations below the mean for young adults aged 25 of the same gender and race (the definition used by the World Health Organization). People who have comparatively low bone mineral densities, but who do not fall below the 2.5 standard deviation threshold, are said to be osteopenic. Osteoporosis is a common condition, affecting otherwise healthy men and women, and is especially prevalent in older women. In the United States, about half of all post-menopausal white women have low bone mass, and 20% meet the WHO definition.

Although skeletal growth stops in adolescence, our bones remodel themselves throughout life. Humans have their peak bone mass in young adulthood. During middle age and beyond, peak bone mass gradually declines. This is usually because of a slight imbalance in activity of the cells involved in breaking down old bone when compared to those charged with making new bone tissue. In people with osteoporosis, the bones are thin and their centers have less of the important structural elements (called the trabeculum). The prevalence of osteoporosis varies substantially with gender, race, and age. Other common risk factors are cigarette smoking, alcohol abuse, lack of exercise, and prolonged use of certain medicines that may affect calcium metabolism. Many uncommon disorders (such as cystic fibrosis and Crohn disease) also increase the risk for osteoporosis.

The highest-risk group is postmenopausal white women. The lowest is African-American men. White women have about twice the lifetime risk of black women of having a bone fracture of any kind. The major risk associated with osteoporosis is fracture. One group has estimated that each year in the United States, 1.5 million people suffer an osteoporosis-associated fracture. It is estimated that it costs $10 billion a year to treat this disorder. In the last decade, low-cost bone densitometry methods have been developed that are fairly accurate at measuring bone mass. Bone densitometry studies confirm the epidemiological data. On average, post-menopausal white women have thinner bones than age-matched black women.

The most common associated fractures are of the wrist, collarbone, hip, and vertebra. The frequency of these fractures varies with the age and activity level of the individual. As is well known, hip fractures are most common in elderly women, and not infrequently precipitate a decline that ends in death. A woman with a hip fracture has about a 10% greater chance of dying within a year of that event than a similar woman who has not had the fracture. In one large survey of American women, there was more concern about vertebral fractures than the others, even though these usually do not cause significant clinical problems. Many women fear the cosmetic effects of one or more vertebral fractures, which often lead to a wedge-shaped deformity of the bone, a loss of height, and in severe cases, the "dowager's hump."

Much research supports a major role for genetic factors in the development and maintenance of bone mass and in the related risk of osteoporosis. Family studies indicate that bone mineral density is highly heritable (the mean correlation coefficient is about 0.6). A few studies even suggest that gene variants influence risk for particular types of fractures. How strong is the genetic contribution? Studies of twins have found that the heritability of bone density at both the femoral neck (the site of hip fractures) and the lumbar (lower) spine range from 60% to 90%, which is quite high. There is a strong correlation in bone density between mothers and daughters. Siblings of persons with osteoporotic fractures are six times more likely to have low bone mineral density. Risk for fracture is also highly correlated between mothers and daughters and between maternal grandmothers and granddaughters. That is, if one of the pair has had a fracture, the other has a greater likelihood of having had one than expected by chance.

Given that osteoporosis is usually a disorder of older age and that many genetic and environmental factors must play a role in its development, it is hardly surprising that the search for particular causative genes has been challenging. Nevertheless, over the last decade, several research teams have had some success in their search for genes that influence risk for osteoporosis.

About 20 candidate genes have been associated with bone mineral density. For example, a gene known as COL1A1, which encodes the protein called α-1-collagen that is part of the skeletal matrix, plays a role in influencing bone density and fracture risk. The presence of a polymorphism (variation) in this gene has been associated with decreased bone density. The only relevant long-term study suggests women with this polymorphism may be at increased risk for fractures in the lumbar spine. Other studies have suggested that variations in the gene (VDR) that codes for the vitamin D receptor protein, a collagen gene called COL2A1, interleukin-6 (IL-6), and a gene (TGF-β) for transforming growth factor all affect bone turnover in a way that may increase or decrease the risk for osteoporosis.

Table 21. *Osteoporosis: Familial risk*	
Prevalence	About 45% of women and 30% of men with osteoporosis have a positive family history.
Characteristics of high-risk families	No significant differences between familial and non-familial cases as to age at diagnosis, gender, fracture history, and bone mineral density scores.
Risk	Maternal history of hip fracture confers twofold risk of hip fracture in daughters. About 33% of mothers and 5% of fathers of affected women have osteoporosis.

So far, none of these genes has been shown to explain more than a small fraction of the overall risk, but others may turn out to play a bigger role.

In 2003, researchers reported strong evidence that among Icelandic people, several relatively common variants of a gene involved in bone formation called BMP2 increased the risk ratios for osteoporosis from two-to sixfold. About 30% of persons in Iceland with osteoporosis carry one of the three variants. If this were generally true for persons of northern European extraction, it could turn out that BMP2 is a major risk gene.

It has long been suspected that genes also influence the risk for the type of fracture to which a person with osteoporosis is likely to succumb. A large study in Utah recently confirmed this. The research team ascertained hundreds of persons with hip fractures and then studied their DNA to see whether variants of several genes known to predispose to osteoporosis were more or less common among them. Polymorphisms in three genes (vitamin D receptor, estrogen receptor, and osteocalcin) were associated with hip fracture in women, and variations in COL1A1 were associated with increased risk for hip fracture in both women and men.

One common, genetic predisposition to osteoporosis may be due to polymorphisms in interleukin-1 (IL-1). This gene, which plays a critically important role in generating the inflammatory response, also is important in regulating the constant turnover or remodeling of bone. Indeed, when it was first studied, it was named osteoclast-activating factor (OAF). Osteoclasts are the cells that break down old bone. One study has found that vertebral fractures are significantly more common among women who were born with a common variant (present in about 30% of white women) of the IL-1 gene than in those who were not. If further studies support that finding, it could lead to the development of a simple risk-assessment test that women could take at any age. For such a screening test to add real value, it must, in addition to identifying those truly at increased risk, connect the individual to a course of preventive action beyond standard approaches to bone wellness, such as taking calcium supplements.

Currently, a few DNA-based risk assessment tests are commercially available. However, they look at genes that only explain a small percentage of all osteoporosis. It is likely that low-cost genetic risk-assessment tests, which analyze the DNA of a large panel of known risk genes, will be commercially available in the next few years. Although they will not be diagnostic of disease, health-conscious women may use them to assess their risks (as well as that of their daughters) to reinforce healthy behaviors.

The opening question in this section is hard to answer. Let us assume that the person who is asking is a healthy 30-year-old white woman, that her 60-year-old mother is in good health, exercises regularly, and does not have osteoporosis, but that her 84-year-old mother does. Based on current knowledge, the best one can say is that it is likely that the 30-year-old woman is at slightly increased risk over background, but that there is good reason to think that health maintenance activities (calcium supplementation, exercise, avoidance of cigarettes, and weight control) will reduce that risk.

Thyroid Diseases

Do genes predispose to thyroid disorders?

The thyroid gland, situated at the base of the neck, is an iodine-concentrating gland that makes and secretes two hormones, known as T3 and T4. They play a significant role in growth and development and in setting the body's baseline metabolic rate. In normal individuals, secretion of T3 and T4 are under feedback control with a pituitary hormone called TSH (thyroid-stimulating hormone). T3 and T4 course throughout the body and are taken into cells via receptor proteins. Once inside, they down- or up-regulate cellular activity. Disorders of the thyroid gland, which are relatively common, are usually characterized by overproduction of the hormones (hyperthyroidism), underproduction (hypothyroidism), and cancers. In this section, I briefly discuss what we know about the role of genes in thyroid diseases other than cancer.

The most common form of hyperthyroidism is an autoimmune condition called Grave's disease (GD). Although in severe cases there are obvious physical signs (such as velvety skin and bulging eyes), the diagnosis is biochemical. Affected persons have high levels of thyroid hormone, low levels of TSH, and no evidence of pituitary gland disease. The vast majority of affected persons make antibodies (B cells) directed against the TSH receptors on the cell surfaces of thyroid tissue. These cells stimulate the gland to overproduce thyroid hormones.

A companion disorder, Hashimoto's thyroiditis (HT), arises when a particular type of immune cell called T cells infiltrate the gland to attack follicular cells. No one knows why this occurs, but one thought is that an infection has stimulated the T cells, which accidentally recognize the thyroid cells as foreign. Affected persons sometimes have goiters (markedly enlarged glands). For unknown reasons, this disorder is more common among Japanese persons.

These two thyroid autoimmune disorders are relatively common, each affecting about 1% of the people in the United States. Survey data indicate that women are at about fivefold greater risk for GD than are men. The lifetime risk for women is about 5%, and for men about 1%. Twin studies show a far higher concordance rate among MZ twins (30–60%) than among DZ twins (3–9%). Several large studies of the families have shown that mothers and sisters of affected persons are much more likely to be affected than are fathers and brothers. About 5–10% of sisters of affected persons also have GD, whereas only 2% of brothers and few fathers are affected.

Family studies clearly show that genes play an important, if still unclear, role in the etiology of hyperthyroidism. One persuasive bit of evidence is that risk for GD is highly associated with being born with the HLA-8/DR3 genotype. This particular combination of genes is found three times more often in patients than in the general population.

Armed with the tools of molecular biology, researchers have started to track down genes that influence risk for GD and HT. The latest study, an analysis of 102 families with multiply affected persons in which the genomes of both patients and unaffected relatives were scanned for linkage to any one of 400 DNA markers, found strong evidence to implicate that gene variants on 20q and 12q were linked with risk for GD and HT, respectively. In addition, the study supported earlier work implicating genes on 6p and 14q.

Because the major genes that predispose to GD have not yet been discovered, the most one can currently offer in genetic counseling is that there is increased familial risk, especially for women. HLA-8 women with an affected first-degree relative have a 10% chance of also developing GD. Women with the HLA-DR3 genotype and an affected relative have a 15% lifetime risk.

Hypothyroidism (due to causes other than HT), the underproduction of thyroid hormones, is relatively common, so much so that in most western nations all newborns are screened for the disorder. Worldwide, the most common cause is a diet deficient in iodine. In nations with adequate diet, the major cause is autoimmune thyroiditis. Although only 1 in 5000 babies has severe hypothyroidism, if the condition is not treated (with hormone therapy), they will be mentally retarded (a condition once called cretinism). About 1% of men develop hypothyroidism at some time in their lives. Hypothyroidism is more common in women than in men. After age 70, as many as 2 women in 100 are diagnosed with the condition. Women face nearly a 10% lifetime risk for this disorder.

Hypothyroidism clusters in families. The concordance among MZ twins is high. Genome-wide scans have found evidence for predisposing genes on chromosomes 12 and 13. As yet, there are no well-characterized genetic risk factors (including the HLA genes). The recurrence risk in future pregnancies for couples with an affected infant may be as high as 25%. The risk to sibs of adults who have been diagnosed with hypothyroidism is about 1–2%.

INFECTIOUS DISEASES

Susceptibility to Infection

Do genes influence our risk for serious infections?

Humans and the bacteria and other microbes that infect them have evolved together. Over the last million years, especially the last 5000 during which our species began to live in crowded communities that facilitated the movement of infectious agents from person to person, mutations that in some way enhance our ability to defend against infection have (because of the survival advantage) spread through the human gene pool. At the same time, mutations in bacteria, viruses, and parasites that confer an advantage in invasiveness and/or survival inside the human host have spread through their gene pools. This is the nature of the never-ending dance of host with pathogen.

For the past few thousand years, children faced a substantial risk of dying young from infectious diseases, especially diarrheal disorders and pneumonias. There is some intriguing evidence that those who survived such illnesses tended to live longer than children who were never exposed to that early winnowing process. This in turns suggests that the survivors of these epidemics were more likely to carry genes that provided them with a robust defense against infectious disease.

It is indisputable that the dramatic reduction in death from infectious disease that began in the 18th century occurred primarily because of improvements in social hygiene. The effort to improve the water quality in cities was probably the single most important intervention. Certainly, there is ample evidence that human mortality rates had been falling significantly for many decades before the routine use of vaccines and antibiotics.

During the 20th century, there was an impressive string of victories over our microbial enemies, but we have obviously not won the war. The public health literature is overflowing with reports of bacteria that have developed resistance to even our newest and most powerful antibiotics. The HIV virus and the influenza virus are famous for how rapidly they mutate. HIV is constantly evolving new subspecies that cannot be effectively contained by the drugs (called "proteases") that did so much to improve the survival of AIDS patients in the 1990s. Each year, vaccine experts play a dangerous guessing game with the influenza virus as they create a new vaccine to defend against what are predicted to be its most virulent subtypes.

Not surprisingly, the response of a large population of individuals, all of whom have been exposed to a dangerous infectious agent, takes the shape of a bell curve. At one tail will be those who do not become infected, followed by those with only mild signs and symptoms of disease. Toward the other end will be those who become severely ill, and at the tail will be those who die from the infection despite aggressive medical intervention. Assuming a population in good health that has relatively even access to medical care, what explains the range of outcomes? The answer is in large part that there is a broad range of defensive armaments built into the diversity of the human genome and that some persons are less well defended than others to handle particular invasions. Examples of this abound.

What is some of the evidence that genetic factors play a key role in susceptibility to or resistance to infections? Perhaps the most famous is the role of the sickle cell gene. Persons born with one copy of the common mutation in the β-hemoglobin gene that, when two copies are present, causes sickle cell anemia are much less likely to become infected with malaria. The sickle cell allele is present in about 1 in 10 Africans, an exceedingly high prevalence for a disease gene. The prevalence suggests that nature has traded the risk of dying from sickle cell anemia in exchange for improving the odds of surviving malaria. Similarly, persons with one copy of a mutant form of the α-hemoglobin gene are also at reduced risk of malaria.

A closely related example is that *Plasmodium vivax*, the second most common (after *Plasmodium falciparum*) cause of malaria, cannot infect a person who was born with two copies of a form of the "Duffy" blood group protein. This is because the binding-site protein on the surface of their red blood cells has an altered shape that the organism cannot use to gain entrance. On the other hand, people born with variants of a gene called TNF2 are, if they become infected with malaria, at increased risk of death from cerebral complications. Recent research in mice has shown that, in some strains, animals with a variant of a gene that makes an enzyme called pyruvate kinase are highly resistant to malaria. Whether this is also true of humans is under investigation.

There is fairly substantial evidence that the genetic background of an individual has a significant impact on his or her resistance to tuberculosis. The most gruesome evidence comes from a terrible tragedy that occurred in Germany in 1929. In that year in the city of Lubeck, 251 babies were accidentally inoculated with massive amounts of a highly virulent strain of tuberculosis. Over the next year, 72 infants died, 175 became ill but lived, and 4 showed no signs of being infected. Although the genetic risk factors for tuberculosis are of only passing interest to most readers, they illustrate the kinds of findings we will eventually make for many other infectious diseases. Several twin studies conducted about 70 years ago also suggested that host susceptibility is a major factor in determining who becomes infected with tuberculosis. About 35% of the risk for TB is a function of the particular genes in the individual. A recent genome search found evidence for susceptibility genes on chromosomes 15 and X.

In 1998, a group showed that susceptibility to TB in mice was strongly associated with a gene called NRAMP1. This gene is highly expressed in white blood cells, which are part of our defense system against invading bacteria. In a study of 410 adults with TB in Gambia, researchers found that certain variants of this gene were highly overrepresented in persons infected with TB, as opposed to a control group of unaffected persons. Variants in NRAMP1 have also been associated with risk for virulent TB in a population of Native Americans living in Canada.

The most important part of the story involves the human leukocyte antigen (HLA) genes on chromosome 6. These genes code for proteins that sit on the surface of the cell and that can bind to foreign antigens (on the surface of bacterial invaders) and "present" them to other human white cells which have the weapons to then kill them. There are more than 20 of these genes, and nearly 1000 variants of them have been found in the human genome. Immense effort has gone into unraveling the complex story of why various HLA types are associated with resistance to, or susceptibility to, infections with various microbes, but we are still at the beginning of understanding this story that has been written over millennia. It appears to be an immensely complicated, constantly changing balancing act. For example, HLA B53 has been shown to protect from malaria, but to *increase* the risk for infection with *Onchocerca volvulus*, the parasite that causes river blindness. These diseases are endemic in the same geographic regions. Various combinations of HLA genes have been shown to affect risk for more than 30 different bacteria, viruses, worms, fungi, and protozoa that together cause hundreds of millions of infections each year. In addition, they are known to affect a person's response to several different vaccines.

It is likely that genes coding for cell surface proteins also are hugely important in determining response to infection. Individuals with blood group O are at increased risk from dying if they are infected with cholera (probably because the cell surface protein that determines blood type also affects the mucosal cells which constitute the barrier that the infectious agent must penetrate to enter the host). Variants of the gene that makes the receptor for a protein called interferon-γ make the individual at increased risk for infection with *Salmonella*. Individuals with variants of the chemokine receptor 5 (CCR5) gene are resistant to HIV infection.

In 2003, an international group of researchers led by Robert Modlin at UCLA demonstrated that there are substantial, consistent differences in the gene expression profiles of patients, depending on which of the two major clinical forms of leprosy afflicts them. Leprosy is a chronic disorder caused by infection with a bacterium called *Mycobacterium leprae*. The organism, which seems to prefer tissues that are cooler than our core temperature of 98.6 degrees, attacks the skin and destroys the peripheral nerves. This causes loss of sensation and puts the patients at high risk for secondary injury. Leprosy is among the world's leading causes of hand deformities; it also creates a high risk for blindness. Although chemotherapy with dapsone and related drugs is effective, it is difficult to eradicate the bacteria.

The two clinical subtypes are tuberculoid and lepromatous leprosy. In patients with the tuberculoid pattern, the bacteria are largely contained. Patients with the lepromatous form have inadequate cell-mediated immunity (CMI), and the bacteria spread widely throughout the body. Modlin and his colleagues looked at the gene expression patterns of 12,000 human genes in biopsies taken from 11 leprosy patients (6 with the tuberculoid form, 5 with the lepromatous). They found dramatic differences in which genes were up-regulated in each group. Indeed, their findings were so persuasive that when one patient's gene pattern did not match the clinical diagnosis, they challenged it. On review, clinicians found that the patient had been misclassified. By studying the expression profiles, the scientists also developed a plausible argument concerning how alterations created the failure of CMI that permits the lepromatous form. In 2003, another group reported powerful evidence that they had identified a tiny region of chromosome 6 (6q25) where the presence of two SNPs (single-letter DNA variations) comprised a haplotype that conferred a fivefold increased susceptibility to leprosy. The finding is especially impressive because it was made in both Vietnamese and Brazilian populations.

Also in 2003, in the aftermath of the SARS virus scare, researchers at the Mackay Memorial Hospital in Taipei (Taiwan) reported that a gene known as HLA-B46 was found significantly more often among the most severely affected patients (5 out of 6) than in control groups of unaffected persons. In general, the gene was found twice as often among SARS patients, however severely affected, as among unaffected persons. HLA-B46 is found in about 15% of Asians, but is rare among Caucasians and Africans, a fact that could help explain the variations in apparent infection rates in different racial groups. The Taipei data are preliminary and will require replication in other studies. However, if they are validated, they might form the basis for a genetic risk test. For example, perhaps doctors and nurses who carry HLA-B46 should not directly care for SARS patients, given their statistically higher risk of becoming infected.

Another fascinating development has been the recent discovery that there is at least one major susceptibility locus on chromosome 22q12 that greatly increases the chance that people infected with a protozoan organism called *Leishmania donovani* will develop a particularly severe form of leishmaniasis called kala-azar. Untreated, this massive infection causes fevers and severe anemia, disrupts liver and spleen function, and is often fatal. Studies of families in villages in the eastern Sudan have shown that the chance of becoming severely (as opposed to mildly) ill from the infection (the protozoa enters the body via the bite of a sand fly) is highly correlated with DNA markers on 22. A second predisposing locus may be on chromosome 2.

We are just beginning to grasp the range of genetic factors that affect the risk that a particular individual carries for infections in general or for some special pathogen in particular. One of the more enticing recent research reports is that mosquitoes prefer attacking some people over others because of genetic differences in the potential hosts. Australian researchers surveyed 500 pairs of twins aged 12–14 about their tendency to be dined upon by mosquitoes. There was much more similarity among MZ than among DZ twins. The epidemiologists concluded that 85% of the variability in susceptibility to being bitten could be attributed to genes!

At the close of 2003, Americans were worrying whether their beef could be contaminated with mad cow disease. A similar brain disease that affects sheep is known as scrapie (affected animals rub themselves against fence posts with such force that they tear off patches of skin). Veterinarian scientists have shown that among sheep, risk for becoming infected with the scrapie virus is highly influenced by sheep genes. It is hoped that we will soon learn that there are genes that protect cows from mad cow disease.

We have much to learn about why some children are more prone to ear infections than are others, why some people live in peace with the streptococcus bacterium while others die with pneumonia from it, and why some people almost never get colds and others get several each year. In some cases it is merely luck, but in others it is surely an indirect result of one's genetic defenses. Currently, with the exception of very rare, very severe genetic disorders that cause fundamental weaknesses in the human system, physicians cannot offer much guidance about the level of risk. Someday, however, they will.

HIV/AIDS

I have heard that a few people have genetic resistance to AIDS. Is that true?

AIDS (acquired immune deficiency syndrome) is caused by a virus called HIV (human immunodeficiency virus). The now well-established worldwide epidemic that is devastating sub-Saharan Africa and knocking on the walls of all Asia can claim at least 40 million people who either have the disease, or who are infected with the virus but are not yet symptomatic. About 25 million people have died of AIDS since 1980, and the worldwide annual death rate now tops 3,000,000. About 13,000,000 children are AIDS orphans, most in the poorest parts of Africa.

The HIV virus is transmitted predominantly through direct contact with the blood or via sexual intercourse. As with many disorders, there seem to be a number of factors influencing one's risk of becoming infected, and some are genetic. During the late 1980s, as AIDS took center stage in the public health world, researchers became intrigued by two groups of people: those who seemed much less susceptible to infection despite repeated high-risk exposure to HIV and those who were known to be HIV positive, but who developed clinical signs of AIDS much more slowly than did other infected persons. Unfortunately, part of this interest grew out of failure of the medical system that is almost as gruesome as the Lubeck story. Between 1978 and 1984, about 12,000 persons with hemophilia received blood products contaminated with HIV. Although many died of AIDS, about 1 in 5 remained HIV negative, and 1 in 100 who became HIV positive did not develop AIDS.

In 1996, researchers showed that many of the persons who were at risk for becoming HIV positive, but who remained healthy despite repeated exposure to the virus, have a variant in a gene called CCR5, the gene that makes cell surface protein to which HIV attaches in order to gain entry into the cell. About 10% of Caucasians have a 32-base pair deletion in this gene that renders the protein it codes for dysfunctional. To invade human cells, HIV needs access both to a protein receptor called CD4 and to one of several other cell surface proteins called chemokine receptors. The protective mutation in CCR5 prevents the formation of the other necessary receptors on the T cell's surface. If denied access to these receptors, the HIV virus cannot successfully invade the cell. About 1% of the population is homozygous (has two copies) for the CCR5 mutation. They are highly resistant to HIV.

More recently, mutations in two other genes, CCR2 and SDF1, have been shown to be protective. The former confers resistance to HIV; the latter delays progress to AIDS. About 39% of Caucasians have at least one of these three partially protective gene variants, as do about 31% of African-Americans. These genes explain some of the variance in the risk for becoming infected and in the disease trajectory.

In 2000, a group working at the National Institutes of Health discovered that certain people who are HIV positive but who have a small variant of a gene called RANTES take about 40% longer to develop clinical signs of AIDS than do those who do not have the variant. This finding is especially fascinating because people with the RANTES variant are also at increased risk for infection if exposed to the virus. How can these two facts be reconciled? No one knows. However, it may be that people with the RANTES variant make more of the protein that is pro-inflammatory. This may make it easier for the virus to enter the body, but harder to enter each cell.

A small percentage of the population is somewhat resistant to HIV, and an even smaller percentage has a genetic profile that retards the progress of AIDS. Of course, no one, not even the few persons who have both copies of the protective CCR5 variant, should regard himself or herself as immune from this devastating disease.

RHEUMATOLOGICAL DISORDERS

Rheumatoid Arthritis

What role do genes play in rheumatoid arthritis?

Rheumatoid arthritis (RA) is a chronic autoimmune disease, the hallmark of which is inflammation of the membranes lining the joints and the slow erosion of the membranes and the bony surfaces within those joints. The destruction is due to enzymes released by the white blood cells that are somehow provoked to attack the tissues in the joints. From an evolutionary perspective, inflammation is one of nature's oldest and most basic defenses. In RA and some other disorders, some defensive cells erroneously identify tissue in their own bodies as foreign. Patients with RA are harmed by "friendly fire." As with other autoimmune disorders, no one knows exactly what causes RA. The dominant theory is that some environmental agent, perhaps exposure to a virus or a bacterium, triggers a response in people who are genetically predisposed. Epstein-Barr virus, mycobacteria, and a bacterium called *Proteus mirabilis* have all been suspects, but there has not been enough evidence to convict.

Typically, the patient with RA suffers from chronic intermittent pain, swelling, redness, and stiffness in several joint spaces. The discomfort is usually worse on awakening. RA is a systemic disorder, and some doctors really prefer to call it rheumatoid disease, rather than rheumatoid arthritis, a term that emphasizes only the involvement of the joints. Persons who are severely affected often develop anemia, respiratory problems, and heart disease. Unfortunately, in the worst cases, RA is severely crippling; people lose much of their hand function, become very weak, and often have trouble walking.

The clinical spectrum of RA is wide and, especially in mild cases, the diagnosis can be difficult. In 1987, the American Rheumatism Association developed a rigorous set of diagnostic guidelines. A person has RA if he or she has 4 of 7 criteria, each being present for at least 6 consecutive weeks. They are morning stiffness, involvement of three or more joints, arthritis of the hand joints, symmetrical arthritis, arthritic nodules, a positive blood test for rheumatoid factor, and joint changes discernible on X-ray.

RA is fairly common. Among white populations, the lifetime risk is 1%. In African populations, the disease affects only about 1 in 1000 persons. Interestingly, two studies of Native Americans, the Chippewa and the Pima, have found a prevalence of 5%, about 5 times higher than in Europe and 50 times higher than in some sub-Saharan African peoples. Overall, RA is 3 times more common in women than men aged 30 years, but there is no discernible difference in sex ratio in persons who are diagnosed after age 65.

There have been many twin studies of RA, all of which have found relatively low (15–20%) concordance rates in identical twins. In 2002, researchers in Denmark reported that in reviewing the medical records of 37,000 twins, they found only 13 MZ pairs in which one member had RA. In none of these pairs was the other twin affected. Of the 36 DZ pairs they found in which one member had RA, in only two cases were both twins affected. A large twin study in Finland involving 4137 MZ and 9162 DZ twin pairs found concordance rates of 12% and 3%—evidence that supports only a small genetic contribution to a disorder with other important predisposing factors.

Still, genetics is not unimportant. Risk in siblings of affected persons is about sixfold greater than in the sibs of unaffected persons. The level of risk varies with the severity of the disease in the first affected sib—the more severe the RA, the higher the risk to brothers and sisters. There have been many studies of possible linkage between RA and various alleles of the genes that direct our immune system. The most consistent linkage is with carrying a copy of the DR4 gene. Recent studies associate having DR4 with an earlier age of onset. Unfortunately, the predictive power of the presence of DR4 in healthy persons is weak. Those few people who have subtypes of the gene called 0401 and 0404 seem to have the highest lifetime risk for RA, perhaps 80%.

Several groups conducted genome-wide scans of families with two affected sibs in the late 1990s, but the results did not strongly implicate any particular chromosomal region. In 1997, the National Institutes of Health and the Arthritis Foundation announced the world's largest study of the role of genes in RA. Scientists at a dozen major medical centers are enrolling 1000 families in which two or more siblings between the ages of 18 and 60 have the disease. The researchers are analyzing the DNA of

Table 22. *Rheumatoid arthritis: Relative risk by inheritance of HLA genes*

Genotype	Relative risk in patients versus controls as a function of HLA genotype
DRB 04/04	25
0401/0401	15
0401/0404,8	49
0404,8/0404,8	14
DR4 04/DR1 01	16
0401/DR1 01	21
0404,8/DR1 01	9
DR 04/DRX	5
0401/DRX	6
0404,8/DRX	4
DR1 01/DR1 01	5
DR101/DRX	3
DRX/DRX	1

Adapted, with permission, from Rimoin D.I., Connor J.M., Pyeritz R.E., and Korf B.R. 2002. *Emery and Rimoin's principles and practice of medical genetics*, 4th edition. Churchill Livingstone, London; © Elsevier.

affected siblings to look for genetic regions that they share more frequently than would be expected by chance. They predict that they will find different predisposing genes in different families. The ultimate goal is to develop more refined approaches to therapy for what will probably turn out to be a group of diseases.

Perhaps the most exciting development in the field of RA in the last 5 years has been the appearance of new drugs to treat persons with severe cases. Two of these medicines, all of which were created using genetic engineering technology, target a protein called tumor necrosis factor (TNF); the other targets a protein called the interleukin-1 receptor. Both of these proteins play a key role in RA. These new drugs, which cost more than $10,000 each year, are known to be highly effective in about 60% of patients, but only mildly effective or ineffective in the rest.

There is currently much interest in developing pharmacogenetic tests to assist physicians to choose the best drug for each RA patient. Early results are encouraging. In 1999, scientists at Amgen, the maker of the IL-1 receptor antagonist called anakinra, reported that some patients responded markedly better than did others, and that the persons in whom the drug appeared to be more efficacious were much more likely to have a certain common genetic variant in the IL-1 gene. In 2001, researchers in Sweden reported on a study of 123 RA patients who had been treated with the TNF blocker, etanercept. They found that patients with either one of two polymorphisms—one in the interleukin-10 gene, the other in the TNF-α gene—were most likely to respond to therapy.

The bottom line? RA can be familial, and it is likely that there are several as-yet-undiscovered predisposing genes. At the moment, the increased risk to first-degree relatives is based on empirical studies.

Osteoarthritis

My grandmother and my father have osteoarthritis. Am I at high risk to end up this way?

Osteoarthritis (OA), also known as degenerative joint disease (DJD), is one of the most common disorders of middle and old age. It is caused by a gradual breakdown of the cartilage tissue that lines the body's joints. This causes bones to rub against each other, which in turn causes pain and swelling. OA affects mainly weight-bearing joints, especially feet, knees, and hips, but the hands also may be affected. About 80% of persons over the age of 65 show some signs of OA on X-rays. OA generates millions of visits to the doctor each year, and estimates of the annual cost to the United States economy in medical care and lost work run over $50 billion.

The hallmark of OA is a disease of the joints, ranging from mild erosion of cartilage to actual bone loss. Other features include new bone growth, an increase in the density of subchondral bone, and inflammation. A simple scale developed in 1963 to use X-rays to evaluate narrowing of joint space is still in use. OA may be primary or secondary. Primary OA means that there is no obvious cause for the process; secondary OA indicates an antecedent cause such as trauma. Known risk factors for primary OA are age, sex, occupational history, ethnicity, obesity, and positive family history. Risk rises steadily with age into one's 70s. Men are at higher risk for OA before age 50; women are at higher risk in later decades (which suggests that loss of estrogen may be a risk factor). Persons who work as manual laborers are at higher risk. OA seems to be less common in Asians than in Caucasians.

Despite the fact that it is so common a problem, OA is not an inevitable consequence of aging. Much of it derives from sports- or work-related injuries. Being chronically overweight also puts an individual at increased risk for the disorder. In addition, there is growing evidence that there are genetic risk factors. Credit for this recognition belongs to rheumatologists who were struck by the number of families they saw with many affected members.

Two large intergenerational studies have found impressive correlation for risk of serious OA between parents and children. In 1998, Dr. Alex MacGregor of St. Thomas Hospital in London reported that an X-ray study which compared the presence of signs of OA in 616 pairs of MZ and DZ twins found a much tighter correlation for three measurements among identical twin pairs than nonidentical twin pairs. He estimated that genetic risk factors are responsible for 50% of osteoarthritis of the hip.

In 2000, researchers in Nottingham, England, reported on their X-ray studies of 392 patients who had undergone hip replacement surgery and 604 of their siblings, comparing them with a control group of 1718 other patients. They found that siblings had a fivefold greater risk of developing OA of the hip when compared with the unrelated individuals. In 1999, scientists at the University of Maryland began a 3-year study that enrolled 1400 families in which there are two or more siblings with generalized primary osteoarthritis (a relatively severe form characterized by the involvement of many different joints). The study is comparing clinical records and X-rays with scans of DNA samples to look for regions of the human genome that are found more often than expected in affected persons.

One particularly interesting project is focused on a large family in The Netherlands in which OA manifests as a dominantly inherited disorder. Most of the candidate genes (those coding for collagen proteins) have been excluded as causing the disease in this family. Genome scanning with more than 300 markers has located one region that is suspected of harboring an as-yet-undiscovered OA risk gene. Other groups, especially researchers at Oxford University in England and DeCode Genetics, a company in Iceland, have launched large studies of OA families with two or more affected sibs. In 2002, the Oxford Group reported evidence of a gene predisposing to knee OA on chromosome 2 and to genes for hip OA on chromosomes 2, 6, and 11.

In 2003, scientists at DeCode Genetics reported the first discovery of a gene in which certain variants were highly associated with a form of OA limited to the joints of the hand. They conducted a genome scan that pointed out three suspicious regions, one of which overlapped with a region known to contain a gene called matrilin-3 that makes a protein important in building the cartilage in joints. Next, they sequenced that gene and found a mutation in affected persons. It accounts for only about 2% of hand arthritis, but it may offer insight into the disease and suggest new ways to treat it.

Although much work is needed to track down the genes, I have little doubt that in the next decade we will identify several genetic risks factors for OA and have risk assessment tests that can be used to warn those at special risk for the disease. These tests may be especially important to persons in the prime of life, such as college and high school athletes, because they may be motivated to take precautionary measures that they might not otherwise have followed.

The answer to the question posed at the opening of this section is "Yes." The risk cannot be quantified. The best preventive strategies are to maintain a healthy body weight and to avoid repetitive trauma to the joints.

Gout

Does gout run in families?

Gout is caused by the body's inability to control its level of uric acid (a ubiquitous substance, as it is a component of the base pairs that make up the nucleic acids in every cell). In affected individuals, chronically high levels of uric acid (hyperuricemia) eventually cause the formation of urate crystals, which become deposited in the joint space, the kidney, and elsewhere, resulting in a chronic, very painful condition. The first attack of gout is often a suddenly painful big toe, ankle, knee, or elbow. A painful big toe is so common a presentation that it has its own name, podagra.

Physicians recognized the disease centuries ago, and it has long been associated with indulgences of the good life. The classic image of the gouty patient derives from 18th-century England. Patients were typically well educated, wealthy, corpulent men who could afford a diet rich in cheese, meat, and alcohol (especially port, which in earlier times had high amounts of lead, which is known to precipitate urate). Today, it is well recognized that obesity, diabetes, and alcohol all predispose to gout. Untreated, the disease progresses slowly from an occasional arthritic flare involving one or two extremely painful joints that resolves to a severe, debilitating chronic arthritis. Fortunately, a number of drugs are effective in treating gout. These include antiinflammatory medications, colchicines, and agents that increase excretion of urate. A mainstay of treatment is a drug that inhibits the action of the enzyme that produces uric acid. All the medications have potentially serious side effects, so they must be used cautiously.

About 1 in 3000 adults in the United States is diagnosed with gout each year and, overall, about 5 in 1000 adults have the disease. It is most common in men over 40. In Europe, the highest prevalence is in older French men; worldwide, gout is most prevalent in the Maori people of New Zealand, where 1 in 25 adult men is affected.

Gout has long been recognized as a familial disease. As far back as 1823, an English physician found that 60% of his 522 patients reported that one or both parents also had gout. During the mid-20th century, more than a dozen family studies found evidence for a significant predisposition to gout. None of the research supported a single-gene disorder, but it is certainly possible that there are subtypes of gout which are caused by the action of primarily one gene. Since gout arises due to a disorder of uric acid metabolism, some researchers have studied the genetic influences on the relative physiological pathways. The evidence fits best with a model involving the separate influences of several genes. In one study of 65 adult men with gout, 42 had relatives with urate levels at or above the 95th percentile. In several large studies of adults with primary hyperuricemia, family history of gout is markedly positive. Twin studies consistently show that identical twins are much more likely to both have gout than are fraternal twins.

Persons with gout often have one or more associated disorders, including obesity, high cholesterol levels, high blood pressure, and coronary artery disease, but there is little firm evidence that any of them plays a major role in causing the primary disorder.

Since gout results from the presence of excess uric acid in the body, a gene variant that significantly influenced serum urate levels would also constitute a risk factor for gout. A number of general population studies of serum urate levels have not found evidence of a single gene predisposing to elevated urate. However, in studies of the families of persons found to have high blood levels of urate or actual gout, there are often a much larger number of relatives with elevated urate than would be expected by chance. Studies of the first-degree relatives of affected persons are most compatible with the existence of a single dominantly acting gene with late-onset, sex-dependent (gout is more common in men) expression. This is compatible with the few twin studies of gout, which show a high concordance rate (80%) among MZ twins.

Gout is often familial, and close relatives, especially sons of affected fathers, are at markedly increased risk. Female relatives are also at higher risk than women without affected relatives. Adult first-degree relatives of affected individuals might benefit from having their serum uric acid levels checked perhaps every 3–5 years. Presymptomatic evidence of hyperuricemia, which suggests that the individual may in time develop gout, should reinforce dietary restrictions. It would be especially prudent to keep trim and consume little alcohol.

Lupus

How much of the risk of lupus is genetic?

Lupus (systemic lupus erythematosus, SLE) is an autoimmune, inflammatory disorder characterized by a loss of tolerance to many "self-antigens." In affected persons, the immune system generates a wide variety of antibodies that attack normal tissue. The disease varies greatly in its symptoms and its course. So variable are its manifestations that the diagnostic criteria agreed to by the American College of Rheumatology require only that any four of eleven findings be present, together or serially, during the course of care. The eleven different criteria include involvement of the skin, mouth, joints, kidneys, brain, and blood. The most common physical feature is a red facial rash.

Historically, the most feared complication of SLE was renal failure, which was its leading cause of death. However, persons with lupus are also at high risk for early, severe heart disease (almost certainly due to inflammation of the coronary arteries). Because of solid strides in treating the renal failure, heart disease is now the major killer. For lupus patients under 40, one important study found nearly a fivefold increased risk for coronary artery disease.

Lupus is uncommon, but not rare. Its incidence and prevalence vary almost tenfold among different racial groups. Lupus is about three times more common in Asians and Native Americans than in Caucasians. It is most common among Africans and Afro-Caribbean peoples—on the order of 1 in 500. Estimates of the number of people in the United States with the disease vary widely—from over a million (probably too high) to 200,000. Epidemiological studies have documented that African-American women are at highest risk, about fivefold higher than white women. Of the several hundred thousand persons with SLE in the United States, only a few thousand are white men.

The disease has long been viewed as a multifactoral disorder with important genetic risk factors. It primarily affects women of childbearing age. A typical patient comes to the doctor complaining of fatigue, joint pains, and a facial rash. When risk by gender is stratified by age, lupus is diagnosed in postmenopausal women at about the same rate as it is in older men, suggesting an important role for sex hormones. Laboratory testing is often helpful. Most lupus patients have a positive ANA (antinuclear antibody). Some patients are found to have circulating antibodies that are seen in virtually no other diseases. In 2003, a study of stored serum samples collected by the Department of Defense in the mid-1980s showed that about 90% of persons who were later diagnosed with SLE had disease-related autoantibodies on average more than 3 years before they developed clinical signs of the illness.

The chance of finding lupus in close relatives of affected persons is comparatively high, with reports ranging from 10% to 15%. The concordance rate in MZ twins has been reported in the 30–50% range, about tenfold higher than the chance that a DZ twin of an affected person will also be diagnosed. The risk that a sibling of an affected person will develop lupus is 40 times higher than the background risk for the general population.

There have been only a few family studies of SLE. A Baltimore study of the families of 77 patients found that race (African-American) and age at diagnosis (less than 30) were the strongest predictors for finding a second affected family member. In a study in the United Kingdom of 74 patients with SLE, 10 out of 335 first-degree relatives were also affected. This indicates that having a first-degree relative with SLE confers a tenfold above-background risk on individuals. Of course, because the background risk is so low, the absolute risk for first-degree relatives of affected persons is also low. In one study of MZ twins, in 11 out of 16 pairs, both twins were affected. Combining most twin studies, the concordance rate for MZ twins is 34%, much higher than the 3% concordance in DZ twin pairs, a finding that strongly implicates genetic risk factors.

In recent years, scientists have developed several mouse models that mimic human lupus. Much of the current research focuses on studying the human genes that are homologs of the genes which, when mutated or deleted, are known to cause the disease in mice. There are currently three genetic hypotheses, all involving failure of the immune surveillance systems, for the etiology of lupus in mice.

In 1997, a study of 52 affected sib pairs found evidence for a predisposing gene on the long arm of chromosome 1. Subsequently, three larger genome scan studies also all found evidence of a predisposing gene in that location. The suspect region has been narrowed to 1q23. About ten other suspect regions for which the evidence is less impressive have also been called out. In addition, new linkage studies have suggested that there are genes on chromosome 5 and chromosome 10 that predispose lupus patients to kidney disease, a devastating complication of this disorder. Of even greater interest is the growing evidence that variations in a gene called RUNX1, which codes for a receptor protein that helps other proteins enter cells, may predispose to lupus, psoriasis, and rheumatoid arthritis, three of the most common autoimmune disorders.

In February 2003, a research team led by Timothy W. Behrens at the University of Minnesota reported an important new finding about persons with severe lupus. He and his colleagues used DNA microarrrays to ask whether there were differences in which genes were active in patients

Table 23. *Lupus: Relative risk by HLA genes*

Genes	Relative risk
DRB1*1501/DQB1*0602	
Heterozygote	1.5
Homozygote	3.5
DRB1*0301/DQB1*0201	
Heterozygote	2.3
Homozygote	2.3
DRB1*0801/DQB1*0402	
Heterozygote	1.9
Homozygote	1.0
Heterozygote for 1 of 3 above	1.3
Compound (2) haplotypes	5.2
All homozygotes	3.0

Adapted, with permission, from Graham R.R., Ortmann W.A., Langefeld C.D., Jawaheer D., Selby S.A., Rodine P.R., et al. 2002. Visualizing human leukocyte antigen class II risk haplotypes in human systemic lupus erythematosus. *American Journal of Human Genetics* **71:** 543–553; © University of Chicago.

with severe disease compared to those in healthy controls. They found that of the thousands of genes studied, 14, all of which were turned on by the activity of a protein called interferon, were more robustly expressed in the severely affected individuals. The finding suggests that therapeutic agents that block interferon pathways may offer a new approach to containing this terrible disease.

What can we say about hereditary risk for SLE today? Unfortunately, both the genetic and the environmental risk factors are poorly understood. On the basis of empirical data, we know that depending on racial group, the first-degree relatives of affected persons face a lifetime risk between 1 in 25 and 1 in 300. This is far greater than the population risk, but still fairly low. The highest risk is to first-degree female relatives of affected African-American women. Such persons may face up to a 4–5% lifetime risk. The risk to male relatives is probably less than half of that. The recent discovery that antibodies are often present in the blood before SLE becomes manifest may make it valuable to test first-degree relatives of affected persons for biochemical warning signals.

Fibromyalgia Syndrome

My mom developed fibromyalgia when she was in her mid-20s. What is the risk to me?

Fibromyalgia is a chronic disorder characterized by pain and tender points in the muscles and ligaments, especially in the neck, back, shoulders, and hips. It is far more common in women than men (8:1 ratio). Age of onset is typically in young adulthood, but it is also diagnosed regularly among children and teenagers. At least 2% of adult women have this disorder. That means that more than 2,000,000 women are affected. With each passing year, the estimates of the prevalence of this disorder increase.

Although cases in younger persons have been associated with hypermobility (excess joint flexibility), no one knows the cause of the disorder. Some studies suggest that some physical trauma (such as a whiplash injury) may trigger its development, but in most patients, the trauma that is recalled is mild. The American College of Rheumatology has developed formal diagnostic criteria for fibromyalgia. The diagnosis requires that there be widespread pain for at least 3 months and that at least 11 of 18 points located in precise anatomical sites be tender to touch at a certain pressure. Affected patients have a wide range of presentations and are often bothered by other problems, especially disordered sleep.

There are no known chemical abnormalities on standard blood tests. However, in recent years, studies of the spinal fluid of affected persons has found that a protein called Substance P is elevated about threefold over the values typically found in a control group. This finding has been crucial to the growing dominance of a theory that fibromyalgia is really a neurological disorder that arises due to a change in the threshold of how the brain perceives pain from peripheral nerves (a transmission system that relies on Substance P).

There have been few formal studies of the heritability of fibromyalgia, but there are families with many affected relatives, which certainly infers a role for genes. The first modern gene hunting efforts are now under way. A consortium of research teams that run a project called the Fibromyalgia Family Study recently reported the results of their efforts to establish genetic linkage in 80 fibromyalgia families. They found that a subset of families characterized by younger age of onset, comparatively less pain, and lack of a commonly associated symptom called inflammatory bowel disease were significantly more likely to be linked to a gene called the serotonin receptor 2A (HTR2A). In contrast, later age of onset was linked to the HLA region. Although it is hard to quantify, having a mother with fibromyalgia definitely confers some measure of increased risk. Current research is focused on understanding the neurobiology, finding drugs that suppress production of Substance P or that suppress the reuptake of serotonin and norepinephrine, both of which have been found to be depressed in affected persons, and on novel approaches to maximizing physical fitness.

SKIN DISORDERS

Atopic Dermatitis

Both my Dad and I have atopic dermatitis. My wife does not. How high is the likelihood that our kids will be affected?

Atopic dermatitis is a common skin disorder (often called eczema in children) characterized by lichenification (popular or bumpy eruptions). The skin lesions have a distribution that varies by age, but they are almost always itchy. Most researchers think that increased levels of a protein called immunoglobulin E are present in nearly all affected persons. Atopic dermatititis is part of a spectrum of disorders, including allergic rhinitis (hay fever) and asthma, that are often found in common (or sequentially) in affected persons.

Although few formal studies have been done on the heritability of atopic dermatitis, those that have been done suggest that genes contribute

Table 24. *Atopic dermatitis: Risk to children of affected persons*

	Number	Affected offspring
Proband affected, spouse unaffected	164	180/321 (56%)
Proband and spouse affected	26	48/59 (81%)
Proband affected, spouse affected with respiratory involvement	80	88/149 (59%)
Total	270	316/529 (59%)

Adapted, with permission, from Uehara M. and Kimura C. 1993. Descendant family history of atopic dermatitis. *Acta Dermato-Venereologica* **73:** 62–63.

significantly to risk. Surveys of affected patients find that on the order of 20% of first-degree relatives also are affected and that another 20% have asthma. About half of the children of affected parents are also affected, and if both parents are affected, the number rises to about 80%, a finding that suggests the presence of a few dominantly acting genes.

Psoriasis

My sister has psoriasis. What is my risk?

Psoriasis is a chronic, relapsing skin disease that affects about 1% of the white population. The hallmarks of the disease are red, scaly, oval, plaque-like lesions that are found most often on the elbows, knees, scalp, and lower back. If one removes the scales, there is a small amount of bleeding. The lesions tend to develop on areas that have been injured. The disease varies widely in severity, but about 1 out of 5 affected persons is badly affected and feels significantly compromised in his lifestyle. The disease typically has its onset in early adult life, but may develop in older persons. Whites are affected more often than are blacks. At least 10% of patients (usually those with more severe skin involvement) also develop arthritis as a feature of their disease.

Although the cause of psoriasis is not yet known, there is much evidence to support characterizing it as an autoimmune disorder. The sudden appearance of many skin lesions in a previously unaffected person is commonly associated with a drug reaction. The disease waxes and wanes, which is typical of such disorders. Certain infections, especially streptococcal bacterial infections, seem to trigger the disorder. Currently, the favored hypothesis is that some invader (a virus or bacteria) activates the body's T cells, which attack skin cells or closely related cells that in turn secrete proteins which drive the formation of the scaly plaques.

Over the years, dermatologists have described about a dozen subtypes of psoriasis, but it is not yet known whether these clinical variants are associated with distinct causes or cofactors. Psoriasis is rare in Asians, Eskimos, and Africans, and relatively common in whites. It seems to be particularly common in Denmark and Sweden, especially on the Faroe Islands.

Family studies and twin studies indicate that the risk of psoriasis is strongly tied to underlying genetic risk factors. Psoriasis is twice as common in children of an affected parent as in children without an affected parent. In one large Swedish study, about 16% of the siblings of affected persons also had psoriasis. The risk to a full sibling of an affected individual is about five times greater than the background risk. It has been nearly 30 years since scientists first recognized that certain variations in the HLA genes on chromosome 6 conferred an increased risk. Subsequently, it was shown that people with an allele called HLA-Cw6 were 20 times more likely to have psoriasis than expected by chance. No causative genes have yet been apprehended. However, linkage studies have found strong statistical evidence for predisposing genes on 6p21 and 17q24-25. These putative genes have been tentatively named PSOR1 and PSOR2. Family studies have shown that they explain about half of the genetic risk for this disorder. Early in 2003, the International Psoriasis Genetics Study reported that it had found evidence for susceptibility genes on chromosomes 10q and 16q.

In the autumn of 2003 at the annual meeting of the American Society of Human Genetics, a group at Washington University led by Dr. Ann Bowcock confirmed the presence of a risk gene on 17q24-25 and showed that persons with psoriasis were unusually likely to have a single DNA base-pair change in a nearby region known to be a binding site for an important protein called RUNX1. Variations in the RUNX1-binding site have now been associated with three genetically influenced autoimmune disorders, potentially offering a new approach to studying how these conditions arise.

Another important discovery presented at the same meeting was the finding that a variant in a gene called SLC12A8 on chromosome 3 is highly associated with psoriatic arthritis. This is the first susceptibility gene to be linked to this disorder.

What can we tell relatives of persons newly diagnosed with psoriasis? In a recent study of more than 3000 patients, the risk to children of an affected parent was about 8%. In the few families in which both parents were affected, the risk was about 35%. The lifetime risk to the brother or sister of an affected person is about 10%.

Baldness

My dad is bald. Am I going to go bald?

Although no one would call it a disease, male pattern baldness, which affects more than half of all men by age 60, is a major cosmetic concern for millions of people. Affected men spend more than $2 billion each year for cosmetic products, for medicines intended to slow the progress of the balding, and for surgical treatments. Male pattern baldness is distinctly different from a much less common form of baldness called alopecia areata (which affects about 2 million adult men), for which the cause is unknown.

The prevalence of common male baldness varies widely among racial groups. Chinese are the least affected; Caucasians are most frequently affected. In a 1968 study of 119 men with significant baldness (scoring grade IV or greater on the Hamilton scale of hair loss), 103 had a positive family history. A 1998 study of 3000 individuals found no clear pattern of inheritance. There have been no adoption studies or adequately sized twin studies of this subject. The available data best fit with the hypothesis that male pattern baldness is due to the action of a few dominantly acting genes. There is no evidence supporting the common claim that baldness is associated with high levels of testosterone.

In 1998, a research group headed by Dr. Angela M. Christiano at Columbia University reported that it had discovered the first gene for baldness in humans. They studied a rare form of baldness, called alopecia universalis (affected persons have no hair on their bodies), in a group of families in Pakistan in which there had been many cousin marriages (if there is a gene variant in a family that predisposes to a recessive condition, cousin marriage raises the odds of its manifesting).

In 2003, a consortium of research teams from Tel Aviv University, the University of Antwerp, and several others reported that they had discovered the cause of a rare autosomal dominant form of early baldness called hypotrichosis simplex. Affected individuals (of both sexes) begin to lose hair in childhood and are usually totally bald before they are 30. The disorder is caused by mutations in a gene called CDSN, which encodes a protein called corneodesmosin. This large protein is thought to function as a kind of intercellular glue that controls the adhesion of keratinocytes (the most superficial layer of the skin). By better understanding the biology of corneodesmosin, researchers may gain new insights into how to prevent other kinds of baldness.

Although it had always been thought to be benign, in 2000 a large research study concluded that male pattern baldness was a marker for risk for heart attacks. In a study of baldness and heart disease among more than 22,000 men, epidemiologists found that men with severe vertex balding were 36% more likely than those in a matched control group to have heart disease; men with moderate balding were at 32% increased risk, and men with frontal balding were at 9% increased risk. The risk was even higher if the bald men had a history of high blood pressure or high cholesterol. This does not of course suggest a causative relationship; rather, both phenotypes may share underlying causes.

Our ignorance about the genetics of most cases of male pattern baldness was succinctly stated recently by an expert who opined that one's grandmother could do just as good a job assessing risk in any particular man as could a geneticist. The only known intervention to prevent baldness is castration, which is unlikely to prove popular. Nevertheless, one can predict with some degree of confidence that in time we will identify the genes that predispose to baldness and develop effective treatments to counter their effects. In an exuberant moment, one scientist working in the field has even suggested that someday it will be possible to genetically engineer hair color in humans. One can imagine some bizarre potential outcomes.

CANCER

Breast Cancer

My mother and my grandmother both died of breast cancer. How great is my risk?

Excluding skin cancers, breast cancer is the most common form of cancer diagnosed in women in the United States and Europe. In the United States today, there are about 1,000,000 women who have been diagnosed with the disease and about 1,000,000 who have breast cancer, but do not yet know it. In 2000, more than 225,000 new cases were identified, and nearly 40,000 women died of the disease. Among all cancers, only lung cancer kills more women. In the United States a woman has about a 1 in 9 chance of being diagnosed during her lifetime. It is important, however, to remember that the risk is highly dependent on age. For example, the chance of a woman being diagnosed during her 40th year is less than 1 in 100, whereas the chance of being diagnosed in her 70th year is 1 in 10.

There are several different types of breast cancer, defined mainly by the cell of origin. Most breast cancer arises in the epithelial cells of the mammary gland. These cells include both the milk-producing lobules and the ducts through which the milk travels. The most common form (about 80% of all cases) of breast cancer is intraductal carcinoma. Infiltrating lobular carcinoma accounts for about 10%, and several rare forms account for the rest.

The risk of developing breast cancer varies widely by country. One large study conducted several decades ago showed that white women in the urban United States were diagnosed nearly six times more often than women in Osaka, Japan. The difference does not appear to be due to genes that vary among ethnic groups. Studies of Polish, Italian, and Japanese women who migrated to the United States show that the immigrants acquire the risk of the country in which they live.

Breast cancer arises due to a series of mutations (occurring over a span of years), which as they accumulate, eventually cause cell division to become disordered. There are almost certainly many factors that can cause these mutations. During the second half of the 20th century, great effort was expended to try to identify them. Among the most important are age, family history, reproductive history, diet, exposure to radiation, and history of a first breast cancer. Unfortunately, despite extraordinary efforts, we understand the risk factors that have been implicated in only the most general way.

Age is the major risk factor—the older the woman, the greater her risk. White women and black women are at higher risk than Asian women. People of high socioeconomic status (better educated, wealthier) are at 2–3 times higher risk than those in lower economic groups. Having a mother or sister with breast cancer is a risk factor, but that does not necessarily implicate genes, because close relatives tend to have similar environments. Both early menarche and late menopause increase the risk, as does nulliparity (never having been pregnant) or having a very late first pregnancy. These facts strongly implicate length of exposure to one's own hormones as a risk factor. Exposure to radiation and a past history of having had breast cancer also increase the risk. Despite many studies, scientists remain uncertain about the influence of diet, consumption of alcohol, and weight on overall risk. The use of oral contraceptives is not thought to be a risk factor for breast cancer.

Of course, the likelihood of being diagnosed with breast cancer depends in part on one's economic status and the structure of the available health care system (if, indeed, there is one). In the United States, the dramatic rise in the apparent incidence of an early form of breast cancer, called ductal carcinoma in situ (DCIS), from 1983 to 1995 reflects the dramatic rise in the use of mammography. The sharp rise in the diagnosis of breast cancer must include many cases of early cancer that would never have been diagnosed in other times or in other nations.

A number of researchers have developed tools for predicting a woman's age-specific risk of breast cancer. The best known is the Gail model (based on a large sample of women undergoing regular mammograms). It uses a formula that factors in current age, age at menarche, age at first live birth, number of affected first-degree relatives, and number of previous breast biopsies. The Gail model does not incorporate a number of genetically related risk factors (such as having a first-degree relative with ovarian cancer), and recent research confirms that it underestimates hereditary risk. The Claus model, which uses data from a longitudinal study of almost 5000 American women, focuses on family history of the disease. However, it also underestimates risk in families in which a causative gene is being transmitted through the generations. In families with unimpressive disease histories, either of these two models can be used. For example, the Claus model predicts that a 39-year-old woman with a single affected first-degree relative who was diagnosed at age 43 has a 1% chance of currently having breast cancer and a 13% chance of having it at age 79. Two other models, the Couch model and the Frank model, specifically address risk in families in which BRCA1 or BRCA2 mutations (see below) are present.

Physicians began to publish papers about families in which there was a large clustering of breast cancer more than 120 years ago, but it was only in the last 25 years that predisposing genes took center stage as important potential risk factors. During that time, epidemiological studies repeatedly showed that 10–20% of women with breast cancer have a first-degree relative (mother, sister, or daughter) or second-degree relative who is also affected. In such families, the mean age of onset tends to be a decade earlier, and there are more patients with cancer in both breasts. For example, one study showed that the sisters of women diagnosed with bilateral breast cancer before age 40 have 10 times the risk of also having breast cancer than does an age-matched control group. Among identical twins, when one twin develops breast cancer, the lifetime risk to the other is about 30–35%, more than three times greater than the risk to the general population. Among dizygotic twins, the inci-

Table 25. *Breast cancer: Familial risk*

Prevalence	About 10–20% of affected women have a positive family history. Of these, about 50% are consistent with a high familial risk.
Characteristics of high-risk families	Early onset of disease (< age 50), several affected relatives, bilateral and/or multifocal disease, and affected men.
Risk	An affected first-degree relative increases risk about 2.5-fold (higher in Ashkenazis).
	If the first-degree relative has cancer in both breasts, the increase is 3-fold.
	A family history of prostate, endometrial, or ovarian cancer also increases the risk of breast cancer to first-degree relatives.

Adapted, with permission, from Rimoin D.I., Connor J.M., Pyeritz R.E., and Korf B.R. 2002. *Emery and Rimoin's principles and practice of medical genetics,* 4th edition. Churchill Livingstone, London; © Elsevier.

dence of breast cancer in the co-twin of the first affected twin is also higher, but not dramatically so.

A series of landmark discoveries in the 1990s greatly advanced our understanding of the role of genes in breast cancer. Today there is widespread agreement that about 10% of all breast cancers arise mainly due to the effect of a mutation with which the individual was born. The simplest way to think about the role of genes that predispose women to breast cancer is to divide them into three categories. The first category is genes that so dramatically increase the lifetime risk that they can be thought of as causing an autosomal dominant disorder with incomplete penetrance (so-called because not all persons with the mutation develop the cancer). Scientists have identified two such genes, and there is good reason to think that there must be at least one or two more. The second is a group (potentially, quite large) of "low penetrance" genes that increase the risk, but not to the level that the families in which they are found stand out as "breast cancer families." The third category is a group of very rare single-gene disorders that include breast cancer as a feature. These account for only about 1% of all breast cancer (I do not discuss them here).

In the mid-1990s, a team at the University of Utah led by Dr. Mark Skolnick found the BRCA1 gene on the long arm of chromosome 17. About 2 years later, a team in England and Skolnick's group identified BRCA2 on chromosome 13. Mutations in BRCA1 and BRCA2 are unquestionably associated with a very high lifetime risk of developing breast cancer. Persons born with one of these mutations are also much more likely to develop cancer at an early age and are at higher risk for developing more than one tumor.

A woman carrying a causative BRCA1 mutation has roughly a 30% chance of developing breast cancer by age 50 and a 65% chance of developing it by age 70. The risk to age 70 for carriers of a BRCA2 mutation is about 45%. Together these two genes appear to account for 80–90% of the breast cancers in heavily burdened breast cancer families.

Today, a DNA sequencing test that examines thousands of base pairs in these two genes is commercially available through a company called Myriad Genetics that Dr. Skolnick co-founded. Using empirical studies of families in which there are many cases of breast cancer, the company has constructed a series of algorithms that can be used by physicians to estimate the likelihood that a particular person will be found to have a causative mutation in the BRCA1 gene. If at-risk persons and their physicians adhere to these algorithms, there is about a 1 in 6 chance that the person tested will be found to have a mutation, a yield that is quite high compared to most medical screening tests.

For a few years, there was some controversy about the value of this test (which costs about $2500, but which is reimbursed by insurers). The major argument against taking it has been that all women should regard themselves as at high risk for breast cancer and adopt appropriate monitoring behaviors (monthly self-exam, periodic mammograms). However, for the woman who because of family history may be at 1 in 2 risk for having inherited a mutation that vastly increases the risk of breast cancer, the possibility that the test will show that she does not carry any of the recognized BRCA1 and BRCA2 mutations may be helpful. The test is especially valuable in families in which the causative mutation has already been identified.

One gene that confers modest, rather than high, risk is called CHEK2. It controls a checkpoint in the cell cycle and thus could influence cell division. In a study of 718 families in which two or more women developed breast cancer before age 60 and who did not have BRCA1 or BRCA2 mutations, more than 4% of the women with disease had a CHEK2 mutation called 1100delC. This is about four times the number of mutations found among women without breast cancer who acted as a control group.

For women who learn that they do carry a high-risk BRCA1 or BRCA2 mutation, there are important options. Because these mutations are also associated with increased risk for ovarian cancer, many women undergo oophorectomy soon after they have completed their families. A few women decide to undergo bilateral mastectomy, but most simply engage in vigilant monitoring of their breasts. The earlier it is detected, the easier and more effective is the treatment of breast cancer.

After the BRCA1 and BRCA2 genes (which are as prevalent in men as in women) were cloned, epidemiological studies found that about 1 in 40 Ashkenazi Jews carries a mutation in one of them, a prevalence about threefold greater than in the background Caucasian population. About 1 out of 3 Ashkenazi women who are diagnosed with breast cancer before age 42 carry a BRCA1 mutation. This finding probably accounts for much of the relatively high incidence of breast cancer in Jews, an observation that historically had been attributed to dietary or other environmental factors.

A number of studies have implicated still other genes as predisposing to breast cancer, although not nearly to the same extent as BRCA1 and BRCA2. The most intriguing is a gene which, when mutated in both germ-line copies, causes a very rare disease called ataxia telangiectasia. About 1 in 100 women carries just one copy of this mutated gene. They do not have the disease, but appear to be at higher risk for breast cancer. One study estimated that mutations in the A-T gene account for 4% of all breast cancers. The evidence is controversial, and there has been no call for screening women for A-T mutations.

Some researchers have sought to implicate several other genes which have in common the fact that they code for proteins that detoxify chemicals that enter the body. The favorite targets are the cytochrome p450 genes, two N-acetyl transferase genes, and the gene that codes for glutathione S-transferase. Thus far, epidemiological results have been mixed. There is no reason at this time to think that variations of these genes are important risk factors for breast cancer. However, it is impossible to rule them out as minor risk factors in the general population or as major risk factors in a small subset thereof.

There is not yet uniform agreement among physicians about what constitutes a sufficiently high risk for breast cancer to justify an expensive DNA sequencing test of BRCA1 and BRCA2. The table lists some criteria that should stimulate a woman to seek counseling at a clinic that specializes in evaluation of high-risk families. The lifetime risk to first-degree relatives of a woman with breast cancer of also developing the disease drops over time because hereditary breast cancer presents earlier than does the more common form.

Women in families in which three or more relatives have been diagnosed with breast cancer at any age, or in which there are two women with breast cancer and one or more with ovarian cancer, or in which any woman has been diagnosed with either disease before age 40, should consider themselves at risk for having a major risk gene. As for the question that I used to open this section, for a woman who is the daughter and granddaughter of affected women, age at diagnosis is key information. If both relatives were diagnosed before age 60, her risk of being a BRCA1 or BRCA2 carrier is about 15%. Even if only one of her two relatives was diagnosed before 60, she should consult a physician about the possibility that she is at increased risk for genetic reasons.

Table 26. *Breast cancer: Guidelines for referral to a high-risk clinic*

Mother or sister diagnosed before age 40.

Mother or sister diagnosed before age 50 and a close blood relative with cancer of breast, ovary, colon, or endometrium or a sarcoma, before age 65

Mother or sister diagnosed between 50 and 65 and one other close blood relative with cancer of the breast, ovary, endometrium, or colorectum, or a sarcoma, before age 50; at least one of the tumors occurred before age 50 and the breast cancer occurred before age 65.

Dominant history of disease (four cases of breast or ovarian cancer or both, on same side of the family, at any age of onset).

History of related malignancy in mother or father (cancer of colorectum, ovary, or endometrium, or sarcoma, before age 50) and at least one close relative with breast cancer before age 50.

Two or more cancers of related types (breast, ovary, colorectum, endometrium, or a sarcoma) in close relatives on father's side, but not necessarily including father, with one diagnosed before age 50.

Adapted, with permission, from Rimoin D.I., Connor J.M., Pyeritz R.E., and Korf B.R. 2002. *Emery and Rimoin's principles and practice of medical genetics,* 4th edition. Churchill Livingstone, London; © Elsevier.

Ovarian Cancer

I have two close blood relatives with ovarian cancer. How high are my risks?

Ovarian cancer is the fifth leading cause of cancer deaths among women. The American Cancer Society has estimated that in 2001 about 23,000 women in the United States learned that they have ovarian cancer, and about 14,000 American women died of the disease. The background risk to any woman of ever developing this disease is about 1%. Unfortunately, it is an insidious disorder that rarely causes symptoms in its early stages. At the time it is diagnosed, ovarian cancer has spread beyond the ovary to the abdomen (stage III) in about 75% of patients. Only about 25% of such patients survive for 5 years.

Most ovarian cancers (80–90%) arise in the serosal tissue layer. In addition to the ovary, the cancer can also arise in the cells that line the pelvic wall (which originate from the same embryological tissue). There are three main types of ovarian cancer: epithelial-cell, germ-cell, and stromal-cell tumors. Because epithelial ovarian carcinomas (EOCs) account for most ovarian cancers, I only discuss that type here.

Little is known about the causes of ovarian cancer. Age is an obvious risk factor. The highest incidence is in women in their late 70s (about 57 cases in 100,000 women). As with breast cancer, incidence varies sharply by country; rates in Sweden are five times higher than those in Japan. Also as with breast cancer, risk in Japanese women rises if they migrate to Europe or the United States. The best evidence is that risk for ovarian cancer is increased by the amount of physiological trauma associated with ovulation itself. For example, risk for ovarian cancer is about twice as high in women who have never been pregnant as it is in women who have been pregnant several times. Several studies have shown that users of oral contraceptives have a lower lifetime risk of ovarian cancer than non-users.

In families with two close relatives with ovarian cancer, 1 of at least 3 possible genetic syndromes could be present: hereditary breast-ovarian cancer syndrome (caused by mutations in BRCA1 or 2), hereditary ovarian cancer syndrome, or hereditary nonpolyposis colon cancer (HNPCC). In most cases, however, the family will not fit any of these syndromes. If three close relatives have been diagnosed with ovarian cancer, the odds that the family is burdened with a single-gene disorder are much higher.

Between 5% and 10% of EOCs arise due to germ-line mutations, mainly mutations in the BRCA1 and BRCA2 genes that also cause breast cancer. The lifetime risk of hereditary ovarian cancer varies depending on the gene involved. For those with predisposing mutations in BRCA1, the risk of developing ovarian cancer is about 40%. For those with BRCA2 mutations the risk is about 10–20%. The lifetime risk of ovarian cancer in the general population is only about 1–2%. Thus, the cumulative lifetime risk to BRCA1 carriers may be 2000% higher than background. In the case of BRCA2 carriers, the comparative risk is at least 500% higher. In addition, if the BRCA2 carrier has a mutation in the part of the gene called exon 11, the risk of ovarian cancer is higher than if it is located in some other part of the gene.

There are a few families in which ovarian cancer clusters independently of breast cancer. It appears, however, that the majority of these ovarian cancers are still caused by mutations in BRCA1 or BRCA2. An excess of ovarian cancers has been reported in families that meet the criteria for being primarily at risk for hereditary colon cancer (HNPCC fami-

Table 27. *Ovarian cancer: Familial risk*

Prevalence	About 5% of women with ovarian cancer have a positive family history. About 20% of these familial cases are at high genetic risk.
Characteristics of high-risk families	Ovarian cancer in two or more close blood relatives strongly suggests an inherited susceptibility. High risk/hereditary ovarian cancer may be classified as site-specific ovarian cancer, breast-ovary syndrome, or hereditary nonpolyposis colon cancer, each accounting for about one-third of high-risk cases.
Risk	Relative risk of ovarian and breast cancer for first-degree relatives of women with ovarian cancer is increased to about 2.8- and 1.6-fold. Among first-degree relatives of women with breast cancer, the relative risk for ovarian cancer is 1.7. The relative risk for ovarian cancer to Jewish women with an affected first-degree relative is 8.8.

Adapted, with permission, from Rimoin D.I., Connor J.M., Pyeritz R.E., and Korf B.R. 2002. *Emery and Rimoin's principles and practice of medical genetics*, 4th edition. Churchill Livingstone, London; © Elsevier.

lies). A woman who has a mutation in one of the genes responsible for HNPCC has about a 10% risk of developing ovarian cancer by age 70. Women with a family history of ovarian cancer are at increased risk. The lifetime risk to first-degree relatives is about three times greater (about 5% by age 70) than for a woman without a positive family history. If a woman has two affected first-degree relatives, her lifetime risk of ovarian cancer is closer to 30%. The cumulative risk may be even higher among Ashkenazi Jews.

A positive family history of ovarian cancer should make a woman consider BRCA1/2 testing. Having even one first-degree relative who was diagnosed with ovarian cancer before age 50 is a significant risk factor. Unfortunately, there are not good monitoring techniques for women who undergo BRCA1/2 testing and learn that they do carry a mutation. One is to undergo annual pelvic ultrasound exams and an annual blood test for a substance known as CA-125. Neither test is particularly valuable as a screening tool for the population at large. However, some studies of high-risk groups suggest that they are useful in catching some cancers at a time when curative interventions are possible.

In 2002, researchers from a company called Correlogic, using a technique called proteomics (which compiles a profile of gene activity in tumor tissue that can be compared and contrasted with the profile of normal tissue), claimed what may be a major advance in screening for ovarian cancer. Among 113 subjects, about half of whom had ovarian cancer and half did not, its new blood test correctly identified every patient with cancer, while falsely diagnosing the disease in only three women in the control group. The test is currently still in clinical trials.

The 1995 NIH Consensus Statement on Ovarian Cancer recommends that women at known genetic risk of ovarian cancer have their ovaries removed after having their children or at age 35. Many such women are choosing to have their ovaries removed. This surgery reduces their risk for ovarian cancer by about 90%. It cannot completely eliminate the risk because a layer of tissue that arises from the ovary during embryological development also lines the pelvic peritoneal wall, and it cannot be removed. One recent study has shown that removal of the ovaries in BRCA1/2 carriers reduces the risk of both ovarian and breast cancer, a double benefit. We do not yet know if the drug Tamoxifen (an anti-estrogen which is widely prescribed to women who have been treated for breast cancer) reduces the risk of either breast or ovarian cancer in BRCA1/2 carriers.

Endometrial Cancer

I have heard that cancer of the uterus is not familial. Is there any evidence to the contrary?

Endometrial (uterine) cancer is the most common gynecological cancer and the fourth most common cancer in women. More than 39,000 American women were diagnosed with the disease in 2002, and more than 6,000 died from it. The major risk factors for endometrial cancer are obesity, nulliparity (having had no children), and use of estrogen. All three of these risk factors create a relative excess of estrogen over progesterone that, in turn, causes the atypical hyperplasia which is the forerunner of cancer. Fortunately, in about 75% of affected women the cancer has not spread beyond the uterus at the time of diagnosis. This is why the 5-year survival rate in white women is about 85%. The long-term survival rate is not as good in African-Americans, due in part to lower access to health care. By far the most common form of endometrial cancer is the endometroid form of adenocarcinoma which, thankfully, does not spread as quickly as less common forms.

Historically, endometrial cancer has not been regarded as being much influenced by genetic predisposition, but that view is fading quickly. In May of 2003, molecular geneticist Paul Goodfellow, who works at Washington University in St. Louis, showed that among a group of 30 patients whose family history suggested they were at high risk for this disorder, 7 had been born with mutations in a gene called MSH6. Especially interest-

Table 28. *Endometrial (uterine) cancer: Familial risk*

Prevalence	About 15% of women with endometrial cancer have a positive family history.
	About one-half of such families have hereditary non-polyposis colorectal cancer syndrome (HNPCC).
Characteristics of high-risk families	Two or more close relatives with endometrial cancer, often before menopause.
	Many high-risk families may have HNPCC.
Risk	Family history of endometrial cancer increases the risk threefold.

Adapted, with permission, from Rimoin D.I., Connor J.M., Pyeritz R.E., and Korf B.R. 2002. *Emery and Rimoin's principles and practice of medical genetics*, 4th edition. Churchill Livingstone, London; © Elsevier.

ing is that the women with the mutations were on average 10 years younger than the other women. This gene is known to code for a protein that corrects DNA replication errors, and mutations in it are already strongly associated with increased risk for colon cancer. Although MSH6 mutations probably directly cause only a small fraction of all endometrial cancer, Goodfellow's discovery suggests new approaches both to establishing risk and thinking about novel therapies. His research team has also shown that if the tumor tissue contains cells that show two phenomena called microsatellite instability and lack of methylation, risk for other cancers may be significantly increased.

Over the last decade, several scientific groups have focused on trying to understand the genetic profile of endometrial tumor tissue. They want to know whether there are unusual genes or combinations thereof that might play a key role in the progression of mutated cells to cancer. In 1997, researchers at the University of Maryland showed that in about 50% of all endometrial tumors, a gene called PTEN is mutated. By 1999, a group in Spain found that genes called K-ras, c-erbB2/neu, and p53 were also frequently mutated. The list continues to grow.

The new understanding of the role of MSH6 in uterine cancer should renew the appreciation for risk of endometrial cancer in women who are members of families with a strong history of colon cancer. In addition, if one has a relative who developed endometrial cancer at a comparatively young age (less than 55) and for whom the standard risk factors are not present, the index of suspicion for genetic risk should be fairly high. On the basis of current knowledge, it is safe to assume that at least 5% of all endometrial cancers arise substantially due to hereditary risk, reason enough to take seriously a positive family history.

Colon Cancer

Several of my older relatives have had colon cancer. What does that mean for me?

Colon cancer is among the most common of all non-skin cancers. About 150,000 new cases are diagnosed annually in the United States, and about 70,000 people die each year of the disease. The vast majority of colon cancers are adenocarcinomas. The disease can arise anywhere in the colon. Most colon cancers arise from small polyps that are initially not cancerous. Because surgical treatment of early cancers is often curative, physicians have long taken an aggressive stance in favor of screening. Because most of these polyps are easy to locate during colonoscopy, it is the gold standard for screening. As of 2004, advances in using MRI to scan the colon for abnormalities appear to have matured to the point where one can expect that "virtual" colonoscopy will soon be a clinical option.

The incidence of colon cancer varies widely among countries. The highest rates are in the United States and Europe (about 44 cases per 100,000 persons per year); the lowest rates are in sub-Saharan Africa, about one-fifth that of the United States. Researchers have found that populations moving from low-incidence regions to high-incidence regions acquire the risk of their new homes. In analyzing risk by country, it appears that persons who exist on high-fiber, low-fat diets are at significantly less risk than other persons. Men face a risk for colon cancer that is about 50% greater than that of women.

Thanks to the efforts of many groups, but especially the team led by Dr. Bert Vogelstein at The Johns Hopkins School of Medicine, we have learned a great deal over the last 15 years about the molecular events that convert a cell in the large intestine into a cancer. Dr. Vogelstein and his colleague, Dr. Eric Fearon, proposed that cancer arose in a multistep process. They hypothesized, and then proved, that the progression of a colon cell from normal to metastatic cancer requires the accumulation of about 5–7 distinct mutations in the daughter cells as the tissue evolves from a set of hyperproliferating cells to an early adenoma, then to late adenoma and cancer. In the early 1990s, other researchers showed that mutations in a gene called APC led to a rare form of colon cancer that behaves like a dominant disorder. In sporadic (nonhereditary) forms of the disease, mutations in the same gene seem to be the most important step in initiating the pathway to cancer.

The hereditary risk of colon cancer is best thought of in three categories: familial adenomatous polyposis (FAP), hereditary nonpolyposis colorectal cancer (HNPCC), and other familial colon cancer. FAP is a rare autosomal dominant disorder in which patients develop hundreds or even thousands of precancerous colonic polyps, often before adulthood. Unless treated by removing the colon, all FAP patients develop colon cancer. FAP accounts for less than 1% of colon cancer, so I do not further discuss it here.

Although physicians have known of colon cancer families for a century or more, it was Dr. Henry Lynch, a clinical geneticist at Creighton Med-

Table 29. *Colon cancer: Familial risk*

Prevalence	About 20–25% of affected persons have a family history of colorectal cancer. About 1% of familial cases are high-risk for polyposis syndromes. About 25–50% of familial cases are consistent with HNPCC syndrome.
Characteristics of high-risk families	Early-onset colon cancer and increased risk for multiple primary tumors. Family history of colon cancer *and* other malignancies.
Risk	About 3.5-fold increase in incidence and mortality from colorectal cancer in first-degree relatives of persons with colon cancer.

Adapted, with permission, from Rimoin D.I., Connor J.M., Pyeritz R.E., and Korf B.R. 2002. *Emery and Rimoin's principles and practice of medical genetics,* 4th edition. Churchill Livingstone, London; © Elsevier.

ical School in Nebraska, who convinced the medical establishment that at-risk families were quite common and that much could be done to identify them and reduce deaths. Known today as Lynch syndrome or hereditary nonpolyposis colon cancer (HNPCC), this familial form of the disease is defined by a set of clinical criteria agreed upon at a meeting held in Amsterdam in 1991. Somewhat simplified, the Amsterdam criteria are (1) there must be three relatives in the family who have been diagnosed with colon cancer, (2) the cases must span two generations, and (3) one case must be diagnosed before age 50.

HNPCC is characterized by a dominant pattern of inheritance with a high penetrance rate. About 70% of men and 30% of women who inherit a causative gene develop colon cancer. Age of onset is typically 40–45 years, and the patients are at risk for multiple colon cancers. In addition, they are at increased risk for cancer of the uterus, the ovary, the stomach, the kidney, and several other locations.

Today, we know there are at least five genes (MLH1, MSH2, MSH6, PMS1, and PMS2) that if mutated can cause HNPCC. Of these, MLH1, MSH2, and MSH6 account for about 90% of the cases. In one recent study of 49 HNPCC families, researchers found mutations in 45, all but 3 in the

MSH2 or MLH1 genes. Clinical testing of these genes is now available. These are called mismatch-repair genes. They make proteins that are involved in correcting errors which occur at low frequency during the doubling of DNA that precedes normal cell division. When these proteins are dysfunctional, uncorrected DNA errors result in a condition called microsatellite instability (MSI). Most colon cancer tissue has MSI. Colon cancer in classic HNPCC families probably accounts for 3% of all colon cancers.

It is clear that there are many families that do not meet the Amsterdam rules, but which are burdened with an obviously increased risk for colon cancer. A person in a known HNPCC family who has a parent with colon cancer must be considered as having a 50% chance of having inherited a causative mutation. Members of families with less impressive histories may have an a priori risk of having been born with a causative mutation of anywhere from 5% to 50%.

Anyone who has a close relative with colon cancer diagnosed before age 50, or who has a family history of two or more affected relatives of any age, should so inform his or her physician and should undergo screening. Some experts recommend that members of HNPCC families undergo annual colonoscopy starting at age 40. For members of families that do not

Table 30. *Colon cancer: Screening recommendations by family history*

One affected first-degree relative	standard screening[a] from age 40
Two such affected relatives	colonoscopy every 5 years, from 40
One such relative with colon cancer before 50	colonoscopy every 5 years, starting 10 years earlier than age of youngest case
One second-degree relative affected	standard screening from age 40
Two second-degree relatives affected	standard screening from age 40
One first-degree relative with a polyp	standard screening from age 40
Known carrier of HNPCC mutation	colonoscopy every 1–2 years from 25

Adapted, with permission, from King R.A., Rotter J.I., and Motulsky A.G., eds. 2002. *The genetic basis of common diseases,* 2nd edition. Oxford University Press, United Kingdom.
[a]Standard = Fecal occult blood test.

meet the Amsterdam criteria, but who are at increased risk on the basis of history, there are no formally recognized guidelines. However, it would be wise for such persons to undergo colonoscopy at an age that is at least 3 years lower than the earliest known manifestation of colon cancer in the family, as well as at least every 2 years after that. In addition, they should strongly consider genetic testing. Caught early, colon cancer is a completely curable disease.

Prostate Cancer

My dad was diagnosed with prostate cancer at 68 and his brother developed it at 72. What is my risk?

Prostate cancer, the second leading cause of cancer in men, is diagnosed in nearly 200,000 people annually in the United Sates. About 40,000 men die of prostate cancer each year. Age is an obvious factor, and the risk seems to rise steadily as a man grows older. About 75% of all cases are found in men over 65. The widespread use of the PSA (prostate specific antigen) screening test has greatly increased the number of cases diagnosed, especially those in which the cancer is small and localized (and clinically silent). This, in turn, has led to uncertainty, particularly in regard to patients over the age of 75, with regard to how aggressively to treat such small tumors. Autopsy studies have shown that at death many men have undiagnosed prostate cancer that was never clinically apparent.

Little is known about the cause of prostate cancer, but there is good evidence to incriminate both environmental and genetic risk factors. Studies of diet, vitamins, weight, and a variety of other factors yield inconsistent results. Black men are about twice as likely to die of prostate cancer as are white men, but this could be an effect of poverty and less good access to regular medical care. Studies of Chinese men (who while in China have a much lower incidence of prostate cancer than do whites) who have migrated to the United States show that the longer they have lived a western lifestyle, the more closely their risk approximates that of white men raised in the United States.

A positive family history is a definite risk factor. Studies of Mormon families in the 1980s indicated that heredity plays an even bigger role in prostate cancer than it does in breast or colon cancer. Current estimates suggest that 15% of all cases arise in the presence of an inherited mutation.

Table 31. *Prostate cancer: Familial risk*	
Prevalence	About 15% of prostate cancer is familial. About 30% of these familial cases are high risk.
Characteristics of high-risk families	Prostate cancer in two or more close relatives, often with early age of onset.
Risk	Men with an affected father or brother have 2-fold risk. Men with two affected first-degree relatives have a 5-fold risk. Men with three affected first-degree relatives have an 11-fold risk.

Men with two affected first-degree relatives have about five times the risk of prostate cancer as that faced by men without a positive family history. As the number of affected family members rises, so does the risk. Men with first-degree relatives who developed prostate cancer between 45 and 50 are at vastly increased risk (about 15 times greater than background) for developing the disease in the same 5-year period. Germ-line genetic factors may explain as many as half of all prostate cancers that manifest before age 55.

The first successful effort to localize a predisposing gene grew out of a study by researchers at the NIH, Johns Hopkins University, and the University of Sweden, who in the mid 1990s studied the DNA of 91 families with at least three affected members. In 2000, they reported that they had localized a causative gene to a narrow band of chromosome 1. They named it hereditary prostate cancer one (HPC1). Since then, these scientists have found five other regions of the human genome that appear to harbor a predisposing gene. Of special interest is that some patients are born with a mutation in the gene that codes for the androgen receptor protein.

In January 2002, some of the same researchers reported that they had identified a particular gene, called ribonuclease L (RNASEL) that is mutated in some persons with prostate cancer. A search for mutations in this gene in men with nonfamilial (sporadic) prostate cancer indicates that it accounts for only a few cases. However, the few mutations that were found were identified in men with a significantly earlier age of onset. Thus, a mutation in RNASEL may contribute to altering the risk threshold in men who carry it.

One of the most troublesome clinical dilemmas in caring for patients

Table 32. *Prostate cancer susceptibility genes*

Gene	Chromosome ·	Function
RNASEL	1q24-25	breaks down RNA
ELAC2	17p11	unknown
MSR1	8p22	encodes a cell surface receptor
AR	Xq11-12	encodes androgen receptor
CYP17	10q24	encodes enzyme for sex hormone biosynthesis
SRD5A2	2p23	encodes enzyme that converts testosterone to dihydrotestosterone

with prostate cancer is that many of the cancers are indolent, while others are highly aggressive. This greatly complicates the decisions that the physician and the patient must make about therapy.

Currently, the hottest research effort is in using DNA microarrays to refine our understanding of prostate tumors. This technique is used to determine how patterns of gene expression differ among different kinds of tissue. For example, it is likely that the different behavior of the most and least aggressive tumors is due to significant differences in which genes are active and inactive (turned on or off) in the tumor. This can provide insights for both prognosis and choice of therapies. A recent study showing that changes in a gene on 7q32 called PODXL are strongly associated with having an aggressive tumor hold out hope that someday soon genetic profiling will help some patients defer surgical intervention in favor of less-invasive therapies.

Prostate cancer is so common that many families include at least one man who has the disease. The diagnosis of the disease in two men about age 70 does indicate a familial genetic risk, but it does not constitute a significant risk for early-onset disease in younger relatives. The warning signs of an increased genetic risk are straightforward: two or more affected relatives or a single first-degree relative who was diagnosed before age 55. In men who are members of such families, annual PSA screening and regular physical exams should be initiated at about age 40. The yield in such a screening strategy will be low, but worthwhile. Despite the clinical dilemmas, prostate cancer is much more successfully treated when the diagnosis is made early. Although routine genetic screening for hereditary risk factors is not yet clinically available, it will be used in limited circumstances soon.

Kidney Cancer

My mother has kidney cancer. How much does that fact increase my risk?

Each year about 30,000 Americans are diagnosed with kidney cancer, and about 11,000 die of the disease. It is the eighth most common cancer in men and the tenth most common cancer in women. Usually called renal cell carcinoma (RCC) by doctors, this cancer has four major types; the subdivisions are based on the appearance of the tumor cells. They are clear-cell, granular-cell, mixed-granular and clear-cell, and spindle-cell cancers. About 85% of all adult cases of RCC are clear-cell carcinoma. There are a number of other rare forms of kidney cancer (for example, Wilms' tumor that arises in children) that I do not discuss here.

Most of the renal cancers found in adults are adenocarcinomas that arise in the proximal tubule, a part of the kidney that plays a crucial role in maintaining salt and water balance. As with many other solid tumors, the development of RCC is insidious. It is often discovered accidentally when a routine urinalysis finds red blood cells. About 25% of patients have metastatic cancer at the time they are diagnosed. This is unfortunate, because when RCC is diagnosed early while it is still confined to the kidney, it is often curable (80–90% surgical cure rate). One of the most important new therapies for patients with metastatic RCC is a drug called aldesleukin (marketed under the name Proleukin), a genetically engineered form of a protein known as interleukin-2. Although only a small number of patients respond well to the therapy, those that do sometimes enjoy long-term survival from this potentially fatal disease.

Not much is known about the environmental factors that increase the risk of developing RCC. Age is clearly a risk factor. Most kidney cancers are found in people between 50 and 70. Gender is a risk factor; RCC is almost twice as common in men as in women. A substantial history of smoking cigarettes doubles the risk for RCC, a fact that may contribute to the increased risk among older men. Some research suggests that people who use medicines that contain phenacetin for long periods are at increased risk for RCC, but this association is unproven. Substantial exposure to heavy metals, especially lead and cadmium, may also be a risk factor.

Hereditary factors account for only a small percentage of all RCC, probably about 2% of all cases. However, because the vast majority of RCC arises sporadically, any family with two cases should be evaluated for genetic risk. Furthermore, any time that a kidney cancer is diagnosed in a person under age 50, a careful family history should be undertaken.

Most hereditary RCC arises in persons who are burdened with a dominantly inherited cancer gene that causes Von Hippel-Lindau (VHL) disease. The disease is named for a German doctor who reported his findings of two affected patients in 1904 and a Swedish pathologist who studied the lesions in the 1920s. About 10,000 Americans have this condition, and about 20,000 are (because of a positive family history) at risk. The hallmark of this syndrome is being affected with tumors called hemangioblastomas which, beginning in early adulthood, can affect the retina, spinal column, and cerebellum. About 10% of patients have cancers of the adrenal gland called pheochromocytomas. In about 10% of patients, the first sign of trouble is RCC. By the time they reach age 60, more than half of the patients with VHL disease have been diagnosed with RCC. The gene that causes this rare disorder was cloned in 1994, and diagnostic testing is available in persons born with a 1 in 2 risk of having a mutation.

There are a few published reports of large families in which many members have RCC, but no other problems suggesting VHL disease. Thus, there must be at least one other rare autosomal dominant gene that causes hereditary RCC. A variety of evidence suggests that this disease is caused by a gene on chromosome 3.

In the vast majority of cases, a renal-cell carcinoma is a sporadic event that does not confer increased risk to other family members. The exceptions to this are if the RCC is found in a person who has been diagnosed with VHL disease, if there is a positive family history of RCC over two generations, or if the first individual (index case) develops the cancer before age 50.

Bladder Cancer

I know that bladder cancer is less common than it used to be. Does that mean that it is mostly caused by environmental factors?

Although its incidence (new cases each year) is now relatively low in the United States and Europe, bladder cancer is more common than most people realize. It is the fourth most commonly diagnosed cancer in men and the ninth most commonly diagnosed cancer in women in the United Kingdom. Because many patients live a fair number of years with the disease, bladder cancer is overall the second most prevalent cancer in that nation. There is a high (95%) survival rate for the stage at which the cancer is usually found. More than 55,000 new cases are diagnosed in the United States each year, and about 12,000 people die annually of the disease.

About 90% of all bladder cancers (and the only ones I consider here) are transitional-cell carcinomas. They are unusual in that once a person has presented with his or her first tumor, it is highly likely (unless he or she is near death from metastatic disease) that he or she will, as the years pass, be afflicted with several more cancers arising at different spots on the bladder wall. The patient is also at increased risk for new cancers elsewhere in the urogenital organs. Bladder cancer demands a very high level of vigilance after it is first treated.

Bladder cancer is found three times more often in men than in women. Incidence rates vary across nations and time. For example, the incidence has tripled in Scotland since the 1960s. Epidemiological research strongly suggests that cigarette smoking and chronic exposure to certain chemicals, especially aniline dyes, are important risk factors. The genetic changes in bladder tumor cells have been studied intensively. The most consistent finding is that, during the course of their development, most bladder cancer cells lose a part of chromosome 9. A number of researchers have unearthed evidence that a gene that suppresses bladder cancer is located on chromosome 9, and a candidate gene has been proposed. If it indeed is the culprit, a new avenue for therapeutic research could open. Mutations in the p53 tumor suppressor gene are also very common in bladder tumors.

Although a few families have been reported in which there are clusters of affected patients, in general there is little evidence that hereditary predisposition to bladder cancer accounts for more than a tiny fraction of all cases. The two exceptions are for individuals in families with more than two documented cases (and who have not had suspicious occupational exposures) and families known to segregate one of the genes for hereditary nonpolyposis colon cancer (HNPCC). Persons who inherit one of these mutations are at increased risk for bladder (and several other) cancers.

At the moment, there is little evidence that germ-line mutations account for even a small fraction of bladder cancer. Nevertheless, in families with more than one case or with even one case of early onset (before 50), first-degree relatives should think of themselves as at increased risk and make sure that their doctors know of the family history.

Stomach Cancer

I have heard there is much more stomach cancer in China than in the United States. Is that partly due to genetic factors?

Although there are several rare forms of stomach cancer (gastric lymphoma and sarcoma), about 90% are adenocarcinomas. They arise from a particular cell type, the epithelial mucous cell. The most fascinating aspect of stomach cancer is the dramatic change in the number of cases diagnosed each year over the last century. In 1930 in the United States, gastric cancer was the most common cancer diagnosed in men, and it remained the leading cause of cancer death in men until 1947. Since then, the rate of gastric cancer has dropped by 75% in men and nearly 85% in women. Today in the United States, it ranks only twelfth among all cancers, with about 20,000 new cases diagnosed in the United States each year. A similar trend has been noted in most other countries, especially Japan, which once had extremely high incidence rates.

Even though the incidence of stomach cancer has fallen markedly in the developed nations, it is still the third most commonly diagnosed cancer in the world. It is highly prevalent in Asia, especially China. Both the sharp decline in incidence and the more than tenfold range in incidence rates across different countries suggest that environmental factors play a major role in the disease. The speculation that is most often made is that the decline in gastric cancer in the United States is due to better food preservation, which has, in turn, greatly reduced the amount of bacteria in the stomach. Another possibility is that certain methods of food preservation (pickling, salting) that are much less common today in the West, but that are still common in China, may predispose to the disease.

The risk for gastric cancer has been associated with a variety of stomach ailments, especially atrophic gastritis. Recently, one research group suggested that this association has genetic roots. A bacterium called *Helicobacter pylori* is commonly found in the human stomach. It is established that infection with *H. pylori* is more common in families of persons who have gastric cancer. It also appears that this risk is even higher in individuals who are also born with a variation in the interleukin-1 gene that is important in shaping the body's inflammatory response to both acute and chronic injury. People with the gene variant that creates the most robust response are more able to destroy *H. pylori*; but the inflammation that comes with killing sharply reduces the amount of chloride ions in the gut,

sometimes leading to a condition called achlorhydria, which in turn causes atrophic gastritis and increased risk for cancer.

For many decades, physicians have occasionally reported on gastric
cancer families. The oldest and best-known example of a genetic finding
that modestly increases risk is the more than 50 studies showing that persons with Blood Group Type A are on average 20% more likely than others to develop gastric cancer.

Recent research lends support to two theses about the role of genes in
stomach cancer. First, there is now solid evidence that a small fraction
(10%) of all stomach cancer is due primarily to the action of one or more
inherited genes (much like the story in breast cancer). Second, there is also
evidence to think that other, less influential, genes can contribute to risk.
One enticing finding that stimulated interest in searching for a causative
gene in gastric cancer comes from the tiny country of San Marino (a 23-
square-mile country situated within Italy) where stomach cancer causes
nearly 10% of all deaths!

A study in northern Italy in the late 1980s of the families of 154 persons diagnosed with gastric cancer found a large excess of stomach cancer
in their siblings compared to the siblings of an age-matched control group.
About the same time, a Finnish study also found that the risk for gastric
cancer was higher in relatives of affected persons than in relatives of a control group. In 1992, a very large case control study of cancer patients in
northern Italy found that first-degree relatives of 628 gastric cancer
patients had a relative risk of 2.6 of also having the disease.

In 1998, a research team in New Zealand discovered that germ-line
mutations in a gene called E-cadherin caused diffuse (this term refers to
the form of the cancer that spreads along the stomach wall) gastric cancer
in a large gastric cancer-prone family. E-cadherin is an adhesion molecule
found in epithelial cells that play an important role in controlling tissue
growth. The researchers quickly looked for mutations in other similar
families and found them. Today it is established that mutations in E-cadherin are an important risk factor for gastric cancer. For persons who
inherit such a mutation, the lifetime risk of gastric cancer may be as high
as 60–80%. However, the E-cadherin mutations have been found in only
about 30% of the diffuse gastric cancer-prone families that have been studied, so there must be one or more other important predisposing genes.

In 2003, researchers in Colombia, where stomach cancer causes the
most cancer deaths, showed that a relatively common deletion in a gene

that makes an enzyme called glutathione S-transferase is highly associated with increased risk for stomach cancer. Since this enzyme plays a key role in detoxifying environmental carcinogens, it is plausible that when it is defective, risk of certain cancers would rise.

What are the important facts in assessing risk for gastric cancer? Because virtually all gastric cancer families have the diffuse form of the cancer, it is important to know about the tumor type in the family. Next, it is crucial to remember that most gastric cancer is not familial. One is categorized as being a member of a hereditary diffuse gastric cancer (HDGC) family only if one of two criteria is satisfied: (1) there have been two or more documented cases of gastric cancer in first- or second-degree relatives of whom one is under age 50 or (2) regardless of age, there are three first- or second-degree relatives with the illness. It is also important to make sure that the gastric cancer is not a manifestation of some rare familial cancer syndrome that is due to a single gene.

Unfortunately, persons who find that they meet the criteria for being in a gastric cancer family do not have an easy path to follow. E-cadherin testing is not yet available outside the research setting. Furthermore, even if an at-risk person can gain access to the test in a research setting, a negative result is only really helpful if the causative mutation has been identified in the affected relative. Otherwise, a negative test cannot rule out a mutation that has not yet been associated with the disease. The toughest part is that there is no easy way to monitor people who are at high risk for early signs of gastric cancer. Current recommendations are for endoscopy every 6–12 months. Furthermore, treatment options are bleak. Gastric cancer is frequently treated by removing much of the stomach. Because the median age of being diagnosed with gastric cancer in these families is 38, a typical patient will face the problems associated with having the stomach removed for decades. Of course, most people who have a relative with gastric cancer are not part of an HDGC family. Unless the affected relative is unusually young, most physicians do not recommend routine use of endoscopy.

Cancer of the Pancreas

My brother died of pancreatic cancer at 59. What are my risks?

Pancreatic cancer is diagnosed in about 30,000 Americans each year. It is the second most common gastrointestinal cancer and the fifth leading cause of cancer death. It affects slightly more men than women and, on average, it is diagnosed somewhat earlier (median age 65) in men than in women (median age 70). Pancreatic cancer is insidious. It typically presents with unexplained weight loss, abdominal pain, and/or jaundice. It is usually diagnosed when it is too advanced to hold out much hope for cure. Far fewer than half of the newly diagnosed patients live for one year.

We know little about the causes of pancreatic cancer. Cigarette smoking is widely agreed to be a risk factor. One large study comparing those who smoked in college to those who did not found that smokers have a 2.6-fold increased risk. Some studies have shown that a high-fat diet increases the risk, but the evidence is mixed. We do know that the incidence of pancreatic cancer is increasing, which suggests there are important environmental risk factors that have not yet been detected.

All cancers arise and progress because of serial changes (called somatic mutations) in the DNA. Over the last decade, scientists have shown that the majority of pancreatic cancer tissues have mutations in a family of tumor suppressor genes called the RAS proto-oncogenes. These mutations are thought to contribute more to starting the cancer than to helping it spread. In addition, pancreatic cancers also usually have mutations in the p53 and/or p16 gene (the numbers refer to the molecular weight in kilodaltons of the protein for which the gene codes), both of which are also commonly mutated in other forms of cancer. The presence of the p16 mutation in particular is associated with metastatic disease and a poor prognosis.

Physicians have long known that there are families in which pancreatic cancer seems to cluster. Family survey studies have shown that persons with a positive family history have a lifetime risk of pancreatic cancer that is about three times greater than that in the general population. A few studies have reported substantially higher risks. On the other hand, the largest twin study of pancreatic cancer, a study of thousands of pairs of twins in Scandinavia, found only modest concordance rates. Currently, the best guess is that about 10% of all cases of pancreatic cancer arise in large part due to a hereditary predisposition. Most of these are associated with dominantly inherited cancer syndromes (associated with the BRCA2, HNPCC, and Li-Fraumeni syndromes). However, there is a small number of families with what is called site-specific pancreatic cancer. In these families, the disease appears to arise due to the influence of a single dominant gene that is highly (but not completely) penetrant. The best-known of the families burdened with such a gene (or genes) is that of President Jimmy

Table 33. *Genes associated with hereditary pancreatic cancer*

Gene name	Chromosome	Syndromes
PRSS1	7	hereditary pancreatitis
P16 syndrome	9	familial atypical mole–malignant melanoma
BRCA2	13	familial breast/ovarian cancer
STK11	19	Peutz-Jeghers syndrome
ATM	11	ataxia telangiectasia
MEN1	11	multiple endocrine neoplasia syndrome

Carter. Several of his close relatives, including his brother, Billy, died of pancreatic cancer.

Since 1988, the National Institutes of Health has maintained a National Familial Pancreas Tumor Registry. In an effort to better understand familial risk, the NFPTR recently reviewed the cancer history of 5199 persons in more than 1000 families in the registry. It found a markedly increased risk for pancreatic cancer among relatives. The risk was highest for those in families with three affected persons, but still very high in families with two affected members, and moderately elevated if a person had even one affected relative.

In the hope that finding the gene or genes which cause hereditary pancreatic cancer will help in the development of new therapies, several scientific teams are currently hunting for them. The first major success came in April 2002, when researchers, led by University of Washington Professor Leonid Kruglyak (whose cousin died of the disease) reported the results of a painstaking genome scan of a very large family in which the disease behaved as though it were caused by an autosomal dominant gene. In this family, whose affected members usually develop the disease in their early 40s, the team found strong statistical evidence that a causative gene was located in a region on the long arm of chromosome 4 (4q32-34). When that gene is cloned, a new therapeutic approach to the disease may become possible. Because the genes with germ-line mutations that cause cancer are sometimes the same genes that environmental factors damage, identification of them can be crucial to improvements in treatment.

The fact that a person has a single first-degree relative who died of pancreatic cancer elevates his or her risk, but only modestly. The vast majority of cases of pancreatic cancers are, to the best of our knowledge, sporadic. However, a positive family history should be enough to encourage an individual to take seriously any signs that could be associated with the disease.

Leukemia

My aunt has chronic myeloid leukemia. Does this mean my dad (her brother) is at higher risk?

In this section I briefly discuss the two most common forms of adult leukemia: chronic myeloid leukemia and chronic lymphocytic leukemia. Leukemia accounts for 2.5% of all new cancers each year in the United States; it causes about 3.5% of all cancer deaths. Chronic myeloid leukemia (CML) is famous among geneticists because it is the first cancer in which a scientist found that the cancer cells had a distinctive chromosomal abnormality. In more than 90% of patients, the chromosomes in the cancer cells have a translocation involving numbers 9 and 22. There are no really efficacious treatments for CML, but in 2003, a new drug, called Velcade, which has a unique mechanism of action (attacking a part of the cell called the proteasome) was approved for use by the FDA. This may lead to improved survival with the disease.

Although there are families with multiple relatives afflicted with CML, this is quite rare. In answer to the opening question, barring the discovery that a person is part of a cancer family syndrome, there is no solid evidence to support increased risk based on family history.

Chronic lymphocytic leukemia (CLL) is the most common form of leukemia, accounting for about one-third of all leukemias diagnosed in Europe and North America. About 1 in every 2000 whites over 70 has CLL. In essence, the disorder arises because the body makes too many lymphocytes, white cells that are involved in defending against infection. The disease usually runs a long slow course over many years. It is staged according to the impact that excess lymphocytes have on the liver and the spleen and as to whether or not the bone marrow cells that produce red blood cells are being harmed.

CLL is rare in children and young adults but becomes steadily more common in older people. It is much more common in whites than in blacks or Asians, a pattern that does not change with immigration, suggesting a genetic predisposition in Caucasians. In families in which both a parent and a child are affected, the age at diagnosis in the child is often 10–20 years younger than that of the parent. This phenomenon, which geneticists call anticipation, also suggests a genetic predisposition. About half of all CLL patients have a deletion or translocation involving a section of the long arm of chromosome 13, a finding which strongly suggests that a gene in that area is highly associated with risk for the disease.

The long-held suspicion that relatives of patients with CLL are at increased risk for CLL and related cancers has been validated by a large study in Sweden and Denmark. It showed that first-degree relatives of CLL patients were at much greater risk (a hazard ratio greater than 7) than the general population for developing CLL and at modestly greater risk for developing both Hodgkin's lymphoma and other lymphomas. Of course, because these disorders are uncommon, the absolute risk to each first-degree relative is low. It is important not to overreact to such findings. For families with a single affected relative over age 60, there is no particular reason to be concerned about recurrence risk. If there are two affected relatives or one who was affected before age 50, those facts should be brought to the attention of a physician. However, there is no agreement about preventive actions to take based on such a family history.

DNA studies of CLL have shown that the tumor cells of some patients have mutations in the immunoglobulin genes. Those persons who do have the mutations are much more likely to have a slow, almost benign, clinical course. In microarray comparison of the two subtypes, researchers found about 160 genes that were expressly differently. One in particular, ZAP-70, could be used to distinguish the two subtypes with 93% accuracy. A test for this gene could be introduced as a prognostic tool in the near future.

One of the most important advances in our genetic knowledge of CLL is that certain changes which occur in the chromosomes of the *tumor* cells are of prognostic value. For example, tumors in which there is an extra chromosome 12 tend to be aggressive, and certain deletions in the short arm of chromosome 17 have been associated with resistance to chemotherapy and poor survival.

The most important genetic advance in the struggle against leukemias has been that DNA microarrays may someday be used to guide choice of therapy. It has been shown that patients with leukemias that overexpress a gene called HOX11 have a more favorable clinical course than do those whose cells do not.

Lymphoma

My grandfather was diagnosed with lymphoma at age 52. Does that increase my risk?

Lymphoma is a single name given to many different forms of cancer—by some counts more than 20—that are primarily categorized by the appearance of cells called lymphocytes under the microscope. For decades, lymphoma has been subdivided into two major categories: Hodgkin's disease and the non-Hodgkin's lymphomas (NHL). Together they constitute the fifth most common type of cancer in the United States, accounting for about 60,000 newly diagnosed cancers each year. Perhaps the most disturbing fact about this group of cancers is that the incidence of NHL has increased by 50% in just 20 years, a finding that strongly implicates environmental risk factors.

Hodgkin's Disease

Each year in the United States, about 7500 people are diagnosed with Hodgkin's disease. The disease has two peaks: young adulthood and old age. The median age of diagnosis in the younger group is just 28 years. The disease seems to express itself differently in different parts of the world. In poor countries, for example, Hodgkin's disease is more common in children than in adults.

The diagnosis of Hodgkin's disease is made by careful study of a biopsy of the tumor tissue. Unlike most cancers, in Hodgkin's disease most of the cells are not cancerous. Rather, the vast majority are inflammatory cells. However, in all cases of Hodgkin's disease, pathologists are able to find odd-shaped cells called Reed-Sternberg cells that recall the image of an owl's face. They are named after the two men who first described them. In general, the greater the number of those cells in the tumor, the poorer the prognosis.

No one knows the cause of Hodgkin's disease, but there is some reason to suspect that certain infections predispose individuals to develop the cancer. Patients newly diagnosed often complain of fevers, night sweats, and enlarged lymph nodes. The strongest evidence implicates the Epstein-Barr virus (EBV) and the more recently discovered human herpesvirus-6. EBV is one of the viruses that cause infectious mononucleosis. Persons who have had this infectious disorder are at increased relative risk for Hodgkin's disease for the ensuing 5 years. Their absolute risk is quite low.

It has long been thought that genetic risk factors play an important role in a subset of Hodgkin's disease, for about 5% of the cases are familial. A study done in the Boston area in the 1970s found five pairs of siblings with Hodgkin's disease, a concordance that was much higher than would be expected by chance. One fascinating aspect of the few familial studies is that affected siblings tend to be of the same sex. In 1986, a research team reported that in families in which two siblings were affected, about 60% of the risk could be explained by the sharing of certain HLA genes. The scientists argued that some cases of familial Hodgkin's disease could be due to a rare recessive gene.

In 2003, a study by Swedish and Danish scientists of the first-degree relatives of 52,000 patients with one of several cancers, including Hodgkin's lymphoma, showed that first-degree relatives are at increased risk for also developing Hodgkin's lymphoma. The risk was highest among males, siblings, and, especially, the relatives of persons whose disease manifested before 40. Despite these strong epidemiological data, the absolute risk to relatives is low. Unfortunately, these findings do not suggest a preventive action plan. They do suggest that first-degree relatives should be especially conscious of any warning signs in their health.

Currently, perhaps the most interesting genetic research in this area has been the successful effort to study gene expression in isolated Reed-Sternberg cells. Scientists have identified 2,666 genes that are turned on in this cancer cell, a first step to developing new therapies.

Non-Hodgkin's Lymphoma

About 53,000 Americans are diagnosed with non-Hodgkin's lymphoma each year. In almost every population in which the question has been asked (the only exception—for unknown reasons—is Koreans), lymphoma affects men more often than it does women. In the United States in persons over 70 there are twice as many men as women with the disease. The incidence of lymphoma rises steadily with age. Lymphoma is more common in whites than in blacks or Asians.

Lymphoma usually presents insidiously, often just as a small painless lump that when excised and studied under the microscope turns out to be a cancerous lymph node. The lymphomas are complicated disorders that can behave or misbehave in many different ways, and there are many different approaches to treatment (a topic beyond the scope of this book). In about 85% of cases, the disease arises in an immune cell called the B cell; in 14% it arises in a T cell. Rarely, lymphoma arises from some other type of immune cell.

Despite much research, scientists still know little about the causes of lymphoma. There is fairly good evidence that certain viral infections increase the risk for this disorder, but no one knows for what percentage they are responsible. Recently, scientists working with a mouse model showed that mutations in a single gene greatly enhanced the risk that a particular strain of animal (e.g., with a particular genetic background) faced of developing lymphoma.

About 40% of persons with a subtype called diffuse large B-cell lymphoma respond well to current therapy. Scientists have studied differences in gene expression in responders and nonresponders. Patients with a genetic signature indicating that the tumor arose in an area called a germinal center have a higher rate of survival 5 years after chemotherapy than do patients with other genetic profiles.

In a subtype of disease called mantle cell lymphoma, survival with cancer has been shown to be highly dependent on pattern of gene expression. People with the highest quartile of expression of genes (known as a "proliferation signature") have a median survival of more than 6 years, whereas those in the lowest quartile for that signature have a median survival of less than 1 year.

Currently, absent a highly suggestive family history (two or more affected members), there is no reason to think that having a close relative affected with lymphoma significantly alters an individual's risk for the disease.

Melanoma

My sister has melanoma. What does that mean for me?

Melanoma is the deadliest form of skin cancer. It arises from the melanin-producing cells in the basal layer of the epidermis. The vast majority of small round brown spots (moles or nevi) on the skin are harmless. Melanoma tumors tend to present as irregularly shaped, multi-shaded spots of variegated color that are usually larger than moles. Once a melanoma has metastasized, it is difficult to treat. The major known cause of melanoma is sun exposure (ultraviolet radiation). In wealthy western nations, where both occupational and recreational exposure to UV light is high and a youth-oriented culture puts a premium on tanning, melanoma is becoming more common. Indeed, the incidence seems to be doubling about every 10 years. Among white women, melanoma is second only to lung cancer in regard to the annual rate of increase of new cases. The disease is much more common in equatorial areas than in the temperate zones. Melanoma is 10 times more common in United States whites than in blacks or Asians. About 45,000 cases will be diagnosed in the United States this year.

Unlike other forms of skin cancer, risk for melanoma seems to be increased less by cumulative exposure to sunlight than by periodic, intense exposures. A history of two or more severe sunburns doubles the lifetime risk for melanoma. Other known risk factors include a positive family history, light skin, freckling, large numbers of benign nevi (moles), a single large, irregular mole, and a childhood spent in a sunny climate. Skin doctors recognize four categories of melanoma based on the appearance of the skin lesion, but little is yet known about the degree to which they can be subdivided according to underlying changes in the DNA.

The universal precaution to reduce the risk of melanoma is avoidance of sun exposure. This mainly consists of the use of broad-brimmed hats, light, long-sleeved clothing, and new kinds of beach wear, and the liberal use of UV-blocking creams on sun-exposed areas. In Australia, where melanoma is all too common, many children now routinely frolic at the beach in full-length bathing suits.

About 10% of individuals diagnosed with melanoma have at least one first-degree relative with the disease, and first-degree relatives of affected persons have a two- to fourfold increased risk. However, less than 2% of new cases arise in families with multiple affected members. In families with two or more affected persons, people tend to develop the disease about 20 years younger than do those who develop the more common, sporadic form. In both groups, one of the four recognized forms, a type known as superficial spreading melanoma, is the most common.

More than 15 years ago, researchers studied the chromosomes in tissue biopsies taken from patients and found that chromosome 9 was frequently missing, a condition known as loss of heterozygosity (or LOH). In 1992, an important study of a young woman with multiple melanomas and germ-line changes involving chromosome 9 again cast suspicion that it harbored a predisposing gene. During the 1990s, several studies led ultimately to the discovery that in about 20–25% of melanoma families, affected persons have a mutation in a gene called CDKN2A (also called p16). This gene has been intensively studied and is now recognized as a tumor suppressor gene, which when dysfunctional, predisposes to melanoma, as well as many other kinds of cancers including pancreas, bone, blood, and bladder.

Of course, since CDKN2A mutations only explain a quarter of the germ-line risk, there must be other predisposing genes. Recently, genome scanning has identified two other chromosomal regions where predisposing genes may reside. An important breakthrough came in August of 2003 when an international team that conducted the first genome-wide scan for linkage to melanoma susceptibility announced that in a study of 49 Australian families with three or more affected persons (and 82 families overall), it found strong evidence for a novel predisposing gene on chromosome 1p22. In these families, the linkage was strongest among those in which the melanoma developed at an especially early age. Because there are about 60 known genes within this region, the researchers will now focus on determining the most likely candidate genes (those known to have functions that are compatible with creating a susceptibility if a mutation is present) among them.

In 2002, an international team of melanoma researchers reported on their extensive analysis of the genetic changes inside melanoma cells. Their crucial finding was that in about *two-thirds* of all people with melanoma, the cancer cells have a mutation in a gene called BRAF that essentially leaves the gene stuck in the "on" position. This gene is part of the cell's machinery for responding to growth signals, so it is plausible that its failure to shut down when it is supposed to could cause cancer. The fact that a somatic mutation in this gene is so common in melanoma opens up important new ideas for treatment. Several research teams are currently trying to find ways to turn BRAF off.

A test for germ-line CDKN2A mutations is commercially available (under the trade name Melaris) for those families with the hereditary form of melanoma. Currently, the Melanoma Genetics Consortium does not support its use as a basis for clinical decision making. It asserts that the low likelihood of finding mutations, uncertainties about the penetrance of certain mutations, and the lack of a special intervention to help carriers render the test of little value. I disagree. In families where the causative mutation is known, at-risk persons have a 50% chance of getting good news—that they did not inherit the mutation. Individuals who learn that they were born with the mutation can redouble their efforts to minimize sun exposure. In addition, carriers of the p16 mutations are also at increased risk for pancreatic cancer; a scary fact, but one that may be helpful to know.

Everyone should be mindful of the risks of melanoma. They should avoid ever getting a sunburn. They should become familiar with moles on their skin and periodically check them for suspicious changes. Any person with a first-degree relative diagnosed with melanoma should consider himself or herself at increased risk. Such persons should consult a physician for further advice about monitoring.

Lung Cancer

Is there any genetic predisposition to lung cancer or is it all due to smoking?

Lung cancer is commonly divided into two categories: small-cell lung cancer (SCLC) and non-small-cell lung cancer (NSCLC). The latter is the more common (70%), and most cases are of three cell types: squamous cell cancers, adenocarcinomas, and large-cell cancers. Squamous cell carcinomas are the most tightly linked to a history of smoking. Adenocarcinomas are the only ones linked to a positive family history. Lung cancer is the leading cause of cancer deaths in the United States for both men and women. In 2000, more than 150,000 people died of lung cancer and nearly 200,000 were newly diagnosed.

As is well known, the number one risk factor associated with lung cancer is smoking. Smokers of both sexes are at more than tenfold greater risk for lung cancer than are nonsmokers. Other important causes are exposure to asbestos (which seems to act synergistically with exposure to tobacco smoke), exposure to radon, and chronic exposure to second-hand smoke. Together these three only account for a small percentage of lung cancer.

The role of smoking in lung cancer is so substantial that there may seem to be little reason to discuss genetic factors. Yet, the role of genes is important for at least three reasons. There are families in which lung cancer clusters, strongly suggesting the existence of genes that confer risk. All lung cancers arise because of the accumulation of somatic mutations in the DNA in lung cells. Because not all people who smoke heavily develop lung cancer, there may be protective genes, the study of which could help in the development of new medicines.

Despite the overwhelming evidence that the vast majority of lung cancer is caused by cigarette smoking, there are studies that demonstrate the influence of genetic risk factors. A study done some years ago in Louisiana found a two- to threefold excess of lung cancer in the close relatives of affected persons even when the researchers controlled for alcohol and cigarette use. Another study found a sevenfold increased risk for lung cancer among nonsmoking relatives of persons with lung cancer who were in the 40–59 age group. Most recently, researchers in Shreveport have found an intriguing association between lung cancer and carriage of a certain form of the prothrombin gene, which is also thought to increase the risk of blood clots.

Because adenocarcinoma of the lung is less associated with smoking, one might posit a stronger role for genetic factors in its etiology. In one study of 336 affected women, researchers found that even accounting for smoking history, the patients were four times more likely to have a positive family history than were a control group of healthy neighbors.

The most persuasive evidence that genes influence who develops lung cancer comes from a large study recently conducted in Iceland. Researchers identified 2756 persons who were diagnosed with lung cancer between 1955 and 2002 and linked them to an extensive national genealogical database. Their analysis showed that there was an increased familial risk for lung cancer which could not be explained merely by smoking history. The relative risk was impressive among first-degree relatives and was discernible among second-degree relatives.

The Medical College of Ohio is also spearheading a major study of genetic risk factors in lung cancer. It is conducting genome scans in families with more than one patient, families with members who developed cancer at an early age, families with relatives who have lung cancer but never smoked, and families with members who have been diagnosed with lung cancer and one other cancer.

For anyone concerned about the risk of lung cancer there is very simple advice: Do not smoke. Those very few people who are nonsmokers and have a positive family history of lung cancer in nonsmoking families should obtain genetic counseling.

BRAIN DISORDERS

Stroke

Both of my grandfathers died of a stroke. Are my risks elevated?

Stroke is a broad term used to describe a sudden, often severe, injury caused by blockage or rupture of any of the blood vessels in the brain. There are two major types of injury: (1) ischemic strokes (about 75–80%), in which the cells of the brain dependent on the blood flow from a particular vessel that has become blocked are either badly injured or die, and (2) hemorrhagic strokes (about 10–15%) in which a vessel bursts and the bleeding devastates the local tissue. A third type, subarachnoid bleeding, is the cause of about 10% of strokes. Ischemic strokes occur because the inside of one of the major brain vessels has become too narrow or because a plaque breaks off from the wall and moves downstream to block blood flow. The most important injuries, such as partial paralysis and loss of speech or understanding of language, vary greatly from patient to patient depending on the exact location of cell death. Indeed, it has often been said that medical students learn about the brain "stroke by stroke." Masterful neurologists can map the brain injury quite precisely based on a detailed examination of the patient's deficits.

Thanks largely to dramatic advances in our ability to treat hypertension and high cholesterol, there has been a significant drop in the number of strokes since the 1950s and 1960s. More recently, the decline has slowed. This, however, is partly due to our ability (using CT and MRI scans) to diagnose quite small brain injuries that would not have been recognized in earlier decades. Stroke is still the third leading cause of death in the United States. About 500,000 people will have a stroke this year, and about 175,000 will die from it. Stroke is more common in black persons than in white persons, due partly to environmental factors such as less consistent access to good health care to control high blood pressure.

The risk factors for the two common forms of stroke are the same as for heart attacks. They include high blood pressure, high cholesterol, abnormal heart rhythm (which can cause an embolus to dislodge and block a vessel), and diabetes (which predisposes to arterial disease). Each of these risks is in turn determined by various combinations of environmental and genetic factors.

There are many single-gene disorders that include among their features a high risk for stroke. However, each is rare, and together they account for only a small percentage of all cases. For the vast majority of families who learn that a relative has had a stroke, there will not be an obvious explanation, and questions about their genetic risk will be hard to answer, but there are some things we do know.

Strong, albeit indirect, evidence for the existence of genes that predispose to stroke comes from comparing stroke rates among pairs of identical and nonidentical twins. Researchers have shown that risk for stroke in the twin of an affected MZ twin is more than four times greater than it is for the sib of an affected DZ twin. About 18% of the twins of affected MZ twins eventually have strokes, whereas only about 3–4% of the twins of affected DZ twins do. Large family studies also indicate a genetic predisposition to stroke. In one study of more than 14,000 men and women, the fact that either parent had had a stroke was associated with a nearly twofold greater risk for the children. The genetic effects were even stronger when the members of the second generation had their strokes before age 50.

Many geneticists are searching for genes that contribute to the risk for stroke. In general, they do this by conducting "association studies," investigations that ask whether one or more genetic markers are found more commonly in the affected group than in the general population. Another approach is to examine variations in "candidate genes," genes that because of their function could reasonably be assumed, if faulty, to affect the risk for stroke.

Results of the first genome-wide screen of persons with the common form of stroke were reported in 2002 by researchers at DeCode Genetics, a genomics company based in Iceland that has been given access by the government to the nation's health database. Dr. Kari Stefansson, the founder, knew that his homeland was a great place to hunt for disease genes. The small population (275,000) is almost completely composed of descendants of about 1000 individuals of Norse and Celtic background who immigrated to the island about 900 years ago. For this reason, a gene variant that is associated with an increased risk for a particular disorder in one Icelander is likely also to be the same variant that predisposes a fellow citizen to the same disorder. To this, add the facts that the nation has superb geneaological records and extensive, well-maintained health records, and you have a recipe for successful gene hunting research.

The DeCode team began by identifying 2000 patients who had suffered either ischemic or hemorrhagic (subarachnoid hemorrhages were excluded) strokes during the years 1993–1997. They then studied family records in the national genealogical database, which enabled them to group the stroke patients according to how closely they were related. This in turn permitted them to select a group of families including at least one person with stroke who also had at least one relative, no farther removed than a second cousin, who also had had a stroke. The end result was a study population of 476 patients in 179 families. The scientists used 1000 DNA markers to perform a genome-wide screen on the patients and 438 of their relatives. They found a marker on the long arm of chromosome 5 that was present far more often than expected by chance in patients. This impressive study suggests that a gene in that region has one or more variants that constitute a major risk factor for the third most common cause of death in the western world.

In September 2003, the scientists at DeCode reported that by building on the 2002 study, they had found the first gene that predisposed to stroke. Among Icelanders, those with quite subtle variations in the gene, which codes for an enzyme called phosphodiesterase 4D, have a three- to fivefold increase in stroke risk. In addition to identifying a new risk factor, the team has also uncovered a potential new approach to prevention or therapy. Roche, the large Swiss pharmaceutical company that funded part of DeCode's work, is already studying the potential therapeutic uses of this new knowledge.

Given the common European heritage of both Icelandic persons and whites in the United States, this research could turn out to be important. To return to the opening question, for the vast majority of families who might be concerned about genetic risk factors because two grandparents have had a stroke, there is little one can yet say about genetic risk other than it is probably about twice the background risk. The most important preventive actions to avoid stroke are to maintain overall good health, avoid smoking, and obtain treatment for even mildly high blood pressure. It is also important to note that irregular heart rhythms increase the risk.

Although only about 10% of strokes are caused by subarachnoid hemorrhage (SAH), a term used to denote bleeding into a potential space created by a thin mesh of cells bound rather loosely to the base of the brain, they account for 25% of all stroke-related deaths. Most subarachnoid bleeds are caused by a rupture of a vessel at the base of the brain in an area called the Circle of Willis. These bleeds occur when an outpouching called a "berry aneurysm," which can grow slowly over the years to reach a diameter of a centimeter or more, bursts. Such ruptures are often devastating events which leave those that survive terribly compromised.

Genetic factors may have an important role in risk for SAH. Several research studies have shown that between 7% and 20% of relatives of persons with SAH also have intracranial aneurysms. On the other hand, autopsy studies have shown that berry aneurysms are not rare and that many people who die of other causes have aneurysms that never ruptured. Because at least 1% of all people have aneurysms, there will be families in which more than one person is affected just by chance.

If an individual has a family history that includes two or more close relatives (for example, a parent and a grandparent on the same side) who have been diagnosed with ruptured cerebral aneurysms, he or she should seek expert advice. Brain imaging techniques are very helpful in identifying aneurysms, and there are medications that may help reduce the risk of rupture. Furthermore, for aneurysms of worrisome size, it is sometimes possible to provide a surgical repair.

Table 34. *Stroke: Familial risk*	
Prevalence	About 40% of stroke patients have an affected first-degree relative.
	About 50–75% have a first-degree relative with CAD.
Chararcteristics of high-risk families	Age of onset before 60.
Risk	Twofold increase if first-degree relative has stroke.

Alzheimer's Disease

My mom, who is in a nursing home, developed Alzheimer's disease at age 74. How high is my risk?

Over the last century, as the average human life span has dramatically increased, declining mental function in old age has become an immense medical and societal problem. From 1907 when Dr. Alois Alzheimer described the autopsy study of the brain of a woman for whom he had cared over several years, until about 1960, there was relatively little attention paid to dementia in the elderly. In just 40 years, Alzheimer's disease (AD), once considered as a relatively unimportant consequence of aging, has emerged as the most serious medical problem among older patients.

The major feature of AD is a gradual (and, eventually, dramatic) loss of memory, especially for recent events. Over time, speech also declines and vocabulary shrinks. The individual tends to repeat questions asked of him or her, loses the ability to follow simple directions, and becomes easily lost in all but the best-known surroundings. Even the personality changes; the patient loses social skills and may become paranoid. Eventually, he or she has trouble walking. A person suffering from AD inhabits a world that grows smaller each day. In the end, patients are bedridden and require total care. They often die of pneumonia.

Especially in the early stages of the disease, the diagnosis is difficult to make with certainty. There is no blood test or X-ray study with which to confirm the clinical suspicion. Even today, AD is a diagnosis of exclusion, meaning that the physician will make it only after he has excluded all other possible causes. An experienced diagnostician will correctly diagnose the disease more than 90% of the time, but only a postmortem study of the brain provides absolute proof.

AD is uncommon before the age of 60 and is diagnosed in only about 1% of persons who are 65. On the other hand, AD is relatively common among people over the age of 75, and its incidence rises steadily with age. Some studies indicate that almost one-half of those over the age of 85 have signs and symptoms compatible with AD. Although there are many causes of dementia, most are thought to be due to AD. Estimates of the number of affected Americans now hover around the 4,000,000 mark. The disease seems as common in one nation as another. Many neurologists believe that the longer one lives, the more likely he or she will develop AD.

No one knows what causes AD. Over the years, many credible theories have been proposed, but none has been proven and many have been refuted. For example, at one time some scientists believed that the disease arose due to a toxic accumulation of trace amounts of aluminum. Today, the dominant theory is that AD is caused by an unusual precipitation of a brain protein called β-amyloid, but an important minority of researchers in the field continue to explore other possibilities. One, Dr. John Nash of Massachusetts General Hospital, has begun to convince people that excess copper and zinc may play an important role. He believes that the amyloid protein acts as a sponge to soak up the heavy metals which are the true culprits. A small clinical trial in which patients with AD were treated with a drug that acts to limit accumulation of these metals showed that it slows disease progression.

Physicians have long known that AD sometimes runs in families and that there are a few families in which many people develop a severe form of the disorder in their 40s or 50s. Armed with the new tools of DNA analysis, during the late 1980s and 1990s, scientists made a series of exciting discoveries concerning the role of genes in AD. Today we know of several genes, which, when mutated, confer grave risk for a very early onset form of the disease. In addition, scientists have found other regions of the human genome that appear to include genes which predispose to the far more common late-onset form of AD.

The first report of a predisposing gene for early-onset AD grew out of the observation that essentially all persons born with Down syndrome (which is caused by the presence of an extra chromosome 21) develop AD if they live into their 50s.

Amyloid, the protein that is found in excess in the brains of persons with AD, is coded for by a gene on chromosome 21 called APP (amyloid precursor protein). Examining rare families with early-onset AD, scientists eventually found a handful worldwide where the disease was clearly caused by mutations in APP.

Studying other highly unusual families, other researchers were able to find mutations in genes on chromosomes 1 and 14 that explained their early-onset disease. The gene on chromosome 14 is called the PS1 (presenilin 1) gene and that on chromosome 1 is called the PS2 gene. PS1 accounts for about half of the early-onset cases, and more than 50 different "familial" mutations have been found. Mutations in PS2 explain the early onset of AD in a cluster of families of Volga-German background. The discovery of mutations that explain only a tiny fraction of all cases still greatly helps in the effort to understand how the disease arises. Of course, the real goal is to untangle the genetic contribution to the late-onset form of AD that burdens tens of millions of people around the world. At the center of that effort is a gene called APOE on chromosome 19.

In 1991, a study showed that in families with more than one person with AD, affected individuals were more likely to have the same version of a certain part of chromosome 19 than would be expected by chance. By 1993, a team at Duke University showed that the gene in question was APOE, already well studied because it coded for a cholesterol transport protein. Large family studies soon showed that of the three common forms of the gene (E2, E3, and E4, which are found on 7%, 78%, and 15% of chromosomes among Caucasians), E4 was associated with risk for AD.

The most important discovery was that the 2–3% (a number arrived at by multiplying 15% by 15% because the chance of inheriting a copy from one parent is independent of the chance of inheriting a copy from another parent) of persons born with two copies of APOE4 were far more likely to have AD than were age-matched controls who did not have two copies. Other studies showed that E2 seemed to protect against AD. Persons with two copies of E2 were less likely to have the disease, and if they did have it, were more likely to develop symptoms at an older age.

Although APOE status is currently the most important known risk factor for AD, it alone is not predictive enough to constitute a screening test. This is because many people who develop AD do not have an E4 allele, and many who do not develop AD do carry an E4 allele. Current estimates are that APOE status explains about 50% of the genetic effect on risk for

---

Table 35. *Alzheimer's disease: Familial risk*

Three dominant genes cause three extremely rare forms of AD with early age of onset.

APOE4 allele accounts for about 55% of the overall risk for the common form of AD.

In persons born with two copies of the APOE4 allele (about 3% of northern Europeans) who do develop AD, the age of onset is more than a decade earlier than among those affected persons who do not have these alleles.

APOE4 testing is not a good predictor of risk. Many people with these alleles do not develop the disease.

late-onset disease. This raises the possibility that the discovery of one or two other relatively common genetic factors could lead to the creation of a fairly accurate risk test. Preliminary research by workers at the University of Arkansas suggests that common variants of a gene called IL-1 (which codes for a protein that plays a central role in the body's inflammatory response) may be another important risk factor.

In 2002, the National Institute on Aging launched the most ambitious effort yet to track down other genes that predispose to AD. Under the coordination of neurologist Richard Mayeux at Columbia University, researchers are recruiting 1000 families in which AD is common. Given the vast number of subjects and our ever more impressive gene-finding tools, it is likely that they will discover several new predisposing genes.

Should people with a family history of late-onset AD be tested for APOE4? Most physicians discourage such inquiries. However, there are some situations in which testing is valuable. It is most helpful in clinical situations in which a physician strongly suspects the diagnosis. If the patient has two copies of E4, that finding strongly supports the suspicion. Another context in which testing for APOE status may be helpful is if an affected parent is known to carry two copies of the E4 allele. It may be reassuring to the children to find that they carry only one copy.

To confront the question with which I opened this section, having a parent who developed AD after age 70 is so common, and the etiology is so complex, that one can say little more than that it probably suggests a somewhat greater risk to the children than if were was no family history. Currently, APOE4 testing would be of little benefit to those children. However, the risk for, and age at onset of, AD are both definitely influenced by genetic factors. It is likely that a risk assessment test with reasonable predictive value could appear in the next 5 years. Since the disease is incurable, if such a test is developed, it will be engulfed in ethical debate. Likely, the choice to use it will be driven less by clinical than by life-planning considerations.

Migraine Headaches

In my family, many people seem to get migraine headaches. Is this genetic?

Migraine headaches are typically throbbing, one-sided, severe headaches that are sometimes associated with nausea and vomiting. They vary tremendously in severity. In the more severe episodes, in addition to taking various medications, patients often seek relief by lying quietly in a darkened room. Migraine headaches are often relieved by sleep.

There are two major kinds of migraine: common migraine (also known as migraine without aura or MO) and migraine with aura (MA). In MA, the patient experiences warning symptoms, usually odd visual disturbances, such as seeing wavy lines in part of the visual field. Such auras typically last from 5 minutes to an hour. About 70% of all migraines include auras. Migraine headaches are common; about 4% of men and about 8% of women experience them. The highest prevalence is women in their reproductive years; as many as 15% of this group are affected. Migraines are much more common among whites than blacks or Asians. The cause of migraine is not clear, but the dominant thesis is that it is caused by spasm followed by dilatation of small arteries that are responsible for providing the blood supply to certain nerves. No one understands what brings on any particular attack.

Migraine headaches are a feature of several rare single-gene disorders such as familial hemiplegic migraine and episodic ataxia type 2, but these account for so few cases among the total that I will not mention them further.

Classic MA has long been known to be familial, and many neurologists have opined that it must be a genetically driven disease. At least five twin studies have found concordance rates in the range of 30–60%. Given the variations in age of onset, diagnostic uncertainties, and other factors, the precise genetic factors have been elusive. Recently, however, a study in Finland uncovered solid evidence for a causative gene on chromosome 1. The relative homogeneity of the Finnish population, combined with the nation's excellent clinical and genealogical records, have made it a popular nation in which to undertake such studies.

The research team studied 50 families among which classic migraine across two or more generations was documented in 45. To enter into the study, the families had to have at least three members with the disorder. By requiring that aura be part of the syndrome, the researchers reduced the chance of an erroneous diagnosis. They used 350 DNA markers to screen the genomes of 430 family members. They found that one marker that maps to a location on the long arm of chromosome 4 was present far more often than expected by chance in family members with migraine. This means it is highly likely that there is a nearby (linked) gene playing an important role in the disease. Elucidation of the gene could lead to a new DNA-based risk assessment test, to new insights into what causes the disorder, and ultimately to new therapies.

Migraine headaches almost certainly have a genetic component, but at the moment we cannot use that information to help in the treatment of affected persons.

Multiple Sclerosis

My 37-year-old sister has just been diagnosed with MS. What is my risk?

Multiple sclerosis (MS) is a brain disease caused by damage to the myelin sheaths, the material that wraps around and insulates the nerves. As myelin is destroyed, nerve function fails. The name is appropriate: The disease affects many different spots in the brain and the damage leads to a kind of scar (sclerotic) formation around nerve sheaths. About 400,000 people in the United States have MS, and about 10,000 new cases are diagnosed each year.

Although it can begin in many different ways, the disease typically presents with a sudden, specific loss of function such as weakness in an arm, sudden loss of vision in one eye, or dizziness. Although it can affect men and women and people of all races, the most common MS patient is a white woman in midlife. The first attack almost always resolves. The disease then takes any one of several courses, ranging from a rapid, severe progression (which is rare) to the most common, which is a waxing and waning pattern that causes gradually more handicaps over 20 or more years. This form, known as relapsing–remitting MS, accounts for about 80% of all cases. According to one recent review article, half of all MS patients require assistance in walking within 15 years of being diagnosed.

Despite a century of research, the cause of MS remains a mystery. One of the most intriguing aspects of MS is that the background risk of developing the disorder ranges from as low as 5 in 100,000 to more than 30 per 100,000, depending on the population. Even more fascinating is the fact that the risk appears to rise the farther the study population is from the equator. Some MS researchers think this fact supports the hypothesis that MS is secondary to a viral infection in childhood that elicits an autoimmune response in some people. MS is most common among northern

Europeans. It is rare among Africans. The best evidence in favor of predisposing environmental factors comes from the extremely high incidence for several decades of MS among those who live on the tiny Faroe Islands (which lie far north of the equator).

There is ample evidence that genetic predisposition is an important aspect of MS. If one member of a pair of monozygotic twins develops MS, the risk to the unaffected twin is about 30%, about 200 times greater than the risk to the general population. If one has a parent or a sibling with MS, one's lifetime risk is 3–5%, about 15–25 times greater than the risk in the general population.

Because family members usually share environments, it is very likely that unknown environmental exposures (such as viruses) also contribute to or (in some cases, perhaps) independently cause the disease. One perennial candidate is canine distemper virus, and there is modest evidence that people in homes with dogs are at slightly increased risk. Studies of the adopted siblings of affected persons have not found them to be at increased risk. This diminishes the argument for environmental factors.

What might be the culprit genes? We don't know, but there are some good suspects. MS has long been viewed as an autoimmune disorder; in essence, a problem caused by friendly fire. For 30 years, scientists have known that a certain gene variant called HLA-DW2 is found more often than expected in persons with MS. Over the last 5 years, armed with new tools for DNA analysis, scientists have repeatedly scanned the genomes of hundreds of persons for MS, but only recently have they had even mild success.

In 2002, the Multiple Sclerosis Genetics Group, following up on earlier studies which had suggested that common variants of the gene called

Table 36. *Multiple sclerosis: Evidence of familial risk*

The lifetime risk to a co-twin of an affected identical twin is more than 200-fold greater than the general population risk.

Risk to first-degree relatives of patients overall is 15-fold greater than the general population risk.

The age-adjusted MS rate among full sibs of affected persons is more than double the rate among half-sibs.

APOE on chromosome 19 were associated with the rapidity with which the disease progressed, reported on their analysis of DNA variants in that region among members of 398 families with affected individuals. They identified several SNPs (single-nucleotide polymorphisms) that were found much more often than expected by chance among people with MS. In addition, they found moderately impressive evidence that in patients who were also carriers of APOE4, the disease was severe, whereas affected persons who carried APOE2 had mild disease. Curiously, this is the same gene that has been deeply implicated as a risk factor for Alzheimer's disease. No one understands the role of APOE in MS.

What can genetic counselors say to relatives of affected persons? The data show that risk of MS to a sibling of a newly affected person is mainly a function of two factors: the age at which the disease appears and whether a parent has the disorder. The younger the age at which the proband became affected, the higher the risk to siblings. If a parent is not affected, the risk to a sibling of an affected person is low. For example, a brother of a newly affected sister in her mid-20s faces a lifetime risk of about 1–2%. A sister of a newly affected brother of about the same age has a risk of about 3–4%. The older the unaffected siblings of the affected person, the less likely they will develop the disorder. Returning to the question at the top of this section, if the person who asked is a 35-year-old brother, his lifetime risk is probably less than 1%.

One of the toughest aspects of MS is that it usually follows an unpredictable course. In 2003, scientists reported that by using a special form of brain imaging called MR spectroscopy, they could measure the decline in a certain brain chemical called N-acetylaspartate (NAA), which appears to predict disease severity.

Almost certainly, there are several genes with variants that sharply increase risk for MS. With time, we will find them, and that success will open up new lines of therapeutic research and new tests to assess risk in relatives of affected persons.

Parkinson's Disease

My father has Parkinson's disease. What is my risk?

Parkinson's disease (PD) is a late-onset brain disorder first described by Dr. James Parkinson in 1817. It is the second most common neurodegenerative disorder, after Alzheimer's disease. People with advanced PD are slow to move and have an obvious resting tremor, an expressionless face, and a stooped posture. Although the disease can arise throughout adulthood, the median age of diagnosis is about 60. There are between 300,000 and 500,000 individuals in the United States who have PD. The lifetime risk of being diagnosed with PD is about 2%.

PD is caused by the death of most of the cells in a small area of the brain called the substantia nigra. This in turn leads to loss of a key brain chemical called dopamine. Autopsy studies show that everybody loses a significant fraction of the cells in the substantia nigra as they age. Persons with PD lose them faster. Because persons with PD always have fewer cells than age-matched controls, it can be thought of as a premature aging disorder. Nearly half of persons over 80 years of age have mild symptoms (most not requiring treatment) consistent with PD. Although there is no cure, treatment with a drug called L-dopa is beneficial, because it makes up for diminished production in the brain and usually slows the advance of the disease.

Although we do not know what causes the death of brain cells, decades of investigation have uncovered some tantalizing findings. For example, shortly after World War I, an epidemic of viral encephalitis swept through Europe and the United States and left thousands of people with a disease that was indistinguishable from PD. This strongly suggested that certain viral illnesses were major risk factors. Yet, since then, PD has only rarely been associated with viral encephalitis. Perhaps the most surprising finding is that some studies have shown that cigarette smoking reduces the risk of developing PD!

Until recently, there has not been much evidence that genes play an important role in determining risk for PD. Early studies often found families with two or more affected relatives, but the disease is sufficiently common that this does not constitute strong proof of genetic predisposition. The first twin studies did not find a strong concordance for PD. Somewhat later, a study of MZ twins with early-onset (before age 50) PD found an impressive concordance rate, much higher than the rate among DZ twins. Recent studies have found that the concordance rate among MZ twins for PD is quite high if certain brain imaging techniques are used to look for early signs of the disease. Studies comparing PD among siblings of index cases to the prevalence of PD in siblings of their spouses have found rates of nearly 4% in the blood relatives of the persons with PD compared to about 2.5% to blood relatives of the spouses, a moderately increased risk.

Table 37. *Parkinson's disease: Known predisposing genes*

Locus	Gene	Location	Inheritance
PARK1	α-Synuclein	4q21	dominant
PARK2	Parkin	6q25-7	recessive
PARK3	unknown	2p13	dominant
PARK4	unknown	4p15	dominant
PARK5	ubiquitin C-terminal hydrolase	4p14	dominant (?)
PARK6	unknown	1p35	recessive
PARK7	DJ-1	1p36	recessive
PARK8	unknown	12p11.2-q13.1	dominant
PARK9	unknown	1p36	recessive
PARK10	unknown	1p32	susceptibility gene
NA	NR4A2	2q22-23	susceptibility gene
NA	Syphilin1	5q23.1-23.3	susceptibility gene
NA	tau	17q21	susceptibility gene

Adapted, with permission, from Dawson T.M. and Dawson V.L. 2003. Molecular pathways of neurodegeneration in Parkinson's disease. *Science* **302:** 819–822; © AAAS.

The major recent advance has been the discovery of a few families with rare, early-onset forms of PD. In the late 1980s, researchers described two large Italian families in which PD behaved as a dominant, one in which children of affected parents have a 1 in 2 chance of also developing the disease. In these families, the median age of onset was early (46) and the median time to death, 10 years, was much shorter than usual. A string of genetic discoveries followed.

In the 1990s, scientists proved that mutations in two genes, α-synuclein on the long arm of chromosome 4 (now called PARK1) and ubiquitin carboxy-terminal hydrolase on the short arm of chromosome 4 (now called PARK5), cause rare autosomal dominant forms of the disorder. In 1998, another group showed that a gene on the long arm of chromosome 6 (called PARK2) causes an early-onset recessive form of PD.

All these genes make proteins that are especially active in brain cells. PARK1 makes a protein that under certain biochemical conditions will clump up. PARK5 makes a protein that has a role in clearing debris from cells. In each case, it is easy to imagine how a mutant form could be very harmful.

In the late 1990s, several groups undertook linkage studies of PD. They identified at least four different chromosomal regions that appeared to harbor a PD gene. These putative genes are called PARK 3, 4, 6, and 7. As of 2003, there is also good evidence that a predisposing gene, tentatively called PARK8, causes a dominant form of PD in certain Japanese families. With the exception of PARK8, which has been found in several different countries, each predisposing gene has been found in specific ethnic groups. As these genes are cloned and studied, they may offer leads to important new therapies for this common, debilitating disorder.

Mutations in yet another gene, CYP2D6, which makes a protein that is important in clearing certain chemicals from the body, are also found more commonly than expected in people with PD. This suggests that some cases of PD arise because the individuals are genetically less able to clear environmental chemicals that with chronic exposure can cause PD.

Results of the most recent linkage study were reported in 2002 by a team of researchers led by Dr. Anita DeStefano at Boston University. They studied 103 families that included at least two persons with PD (usually siblings), with a special focus on age of onset. Her team found statistical evidence for four locations in the human genome which could harbor genes that influence age of onset. The most tantalizing, located on the short arm of chromosome 2, has also been implicated in similar studies.

Currently, there is much interest in determining the role that mutations in mitochondrial DNA play in risk for PD. All of us carry in the cytoplasm of each of our cells hundreds of copies of tiny circles of DNA (which has about a hundred-thousandth of the information found in nuclear DNA). Mitochondrial DNA makes proteins that play a key role in cellular metabolism, so a mutation can be quite harmful. Such mutations have been shown to cause PD in a few families, but they do not seem likely to emerge as a major cause.

What advice about risk can we offer today to first-degree relatives, such as the sons, of persons diagnosed with PD? In those very rare families in which PD is an autosomal dominant disorder, the risk is 50% for a person with an affected parent. All other risk estimates derive from empirical studies. The lifetime risk to the child of a person with the common form of PD is about 3–4%. The lifetime risk to a sibling of an affected person with late-onset, garden-variety PD is about 5%. That risk goes up significantly if the age of onset is below 45, if two or more first-degree relatives are affected, or if severe dementia is a prominent feature. For more distant relatives, the risk is not measurably different from that of the general population. However, as we continue to find genes that influence risk for PD, we will almost certainly determine that a significant fraction of all patients have the disease in part because of risk factors embedded in just a few genes.

Amyotrophic Lateral Sclerosis (Lou Gehrig's Disease)

My mom has ALS. Am I at risk?

Although it is less prevalent than MS and PD, amyotrophic lateral sclerosis (ALS) is almost as well known. There are two reasons. First, a whole generation of Americans followed the struggle of Lou Gehrig, the great Yankee first baseman, nicknamed the "iron man," as the disease took his career, then his life, and, finally, his name. Anyone who has seen the footage of his farewell address in Yankee Stadium remembers its poignancy. Second, there is a bizarre form of ALS that is unusually common in the western Pacific islands, especially Guam and Western New Guinea, and which defied understanding for a long time. Since physicians in the armed forces first noted just after World War II that many young adults on the islands were dying of what looked like ALS, scientists have posited many different causes. A leading contender has been that the starvation common in this region during the war led many people to consume unusual plants, one of which contained a highly toxic material.

ALS is a "motor neuron disease." Degeneration of the upper motor neurons in the brain leads to a hyperactive muscle tone (spasticity). Degeneration of the lower motor neuron causes weakness, profound muscle atrophy, and fasciculation (twitches). In addition to the muscles in the arms and legs, the diaphragm and the muscles in the tongue and pharynx also fail. Many patients die of respiratory failure.

In the United States, the lifetime risk of developing ALS is about 1 in 1000. For every two women who are diagnosed, three men are affected. About 90% of ALS is sporadic; a newly diagnosed individual is usually the first and only case in the family. The other 10% of cases are familial, and it has long been suspected that they are in each case caused by mutations in a single gene.

In the last decade, we have learned much about the genetics in the familial cases. The most common familial form in now known to be a dominant disorder, with each child of an affected parent at 1 in 2 risk.

About half the at-risk individuals develop the disease by age 45, and by age 70 about 90% of those at risk are ill. About 20% of patients with a dominant form of ALS have a mutation in a gene found on chromosome 21 called SOD1 that codes for an enzyme called superoxide dismutase. There is also an exceedingly rare autosomal recessive form that has been found in just a few ethnic groups in which cousin marriage is common. This devastating subtype of ALS typically begins by age 12.

Researchers have found more than 75 mutations in the SOD1 gene among persons with ALS. One relatively common mutation, which changes just one amino acid in the protein from an alanine to a valine, is associated with a rapid course and death within 2 years. In general, affected persons have about a 50% chance of living 5 years; about 20% of patients live 7–10 years.

One curious finding is that about 1 in 40 people who live in the Tornadelan Valley in Sweden carries a mutation in the SOD1 gene that does *not* seem to cause ALS. However, if they have inherited two copies, one from each parent, they have about a 40% lifetime risk of developing the disorder. This mutation apparently does not render the protein completely inoperable.

How does SOD1 cause ALS? Nobody knows, but there are several hypotheses. Some think that SOD1 mutants may cause a gain of function—that is, result in an altered protein that affects the size of molecules that can enter the cell. Others have observed that cells with SOD1 mutations seem programmed to die earlier than expected. Yet another theory is that cells with SOD1 mutations have too many copper ions in them, which may harm their function.

In 2001, scientists studying an early-onset form of ALS in several Arabian families discovered that it is caused by mutations in a gene on the long arm of chromosome 2. In these families, the ALS is inherited as a recessive disorder (the parents are unaffected even though they carry one copy of the mutation, but children who inherit a copy from each parent are affected), and scientists have been able to show that the severity of the disease correlates with which mutation is present in the family. In general, geneticists have a somewhat easier time studying recessive disorders. This is in part because a model of it can often be made in mice by knocking out the mouse version of the gene. Although it is exceedingly rare, molecular research involving patients with juvenile ALS may greatly aid in understanding the more common adult forms.

The summer of 2003 witnessed some important advances in understanding ALS. Focusing on families with genetic forms of ALS that could not be attributed to mutations in SOD1, two teams found strong evidence for a predisposing gene on chromosomes 16 and 20. Even more exciting was the report from a team led by Peter Carmeliet in Belgium that persons with certain variants in the promoter region of a gene called VEGF (vascular endothelial growth factor) faced twice as much risk for ALS as did those who did not carry the variants. Because the study involved nearly 1000 persons with ALS and as many controls, the results are highly statistically significant. In addition, the findings are supported by studies of mice. Mice engineered to lack the VEGF gene develop a syndrome like ALS.

ALS is such a devastating disease that scientists are working frantically to develop therapies even though there is still much to learn about the causes of the disorder. Currently, much work is being done with a mouse that has been genetically engineered to carry multiple copies of the human SOD gene and to overexpress the protein. Scientists are treating these mice (which develop symptoms that mimic ALS) with a variety of compounds that they hope will slow progression of the disease.

To return to the risk question with which I opened this section, assuming that the family history includes only one person with ALS, and that it is not one of the obvious, rare early-onset forms, the risk that a child of the affected person will also develop the disease later in life is very small.

EYE DISORDERS

Glaucoma

My mom has glaucoma. How much of the risk for glaucoma is genetic?

Glaucoma is the second most common cause of blindness in the United States. About 1,500,000 people have the disease, and about 10% of them are legally blind (their corrected vision is less than 20/200). Glaucoma is a general term used to describe a group of disorders in which the loss of vision is caused by the death of retinal nerve cells, the cells that send information to the visual cortex of the brain where it is integrated as an image that we see. There are several different causes of glaucoma, but all damage the optic nerve and, in time, cause loss of vision, usually more dramatic in some visual quadrants than others.

Glaucoma is closely associated with elevated intraocular pressures (IOP). However, many people with raised pressure never develop glaucoma, and some people with glaucoma have normal IOP. Although measurement of IOP is used as a screening test to detect those at risk for glaucoma, pressure readings are not completely reassuring if they are normal, nor powerful indicators of risk if they are mildly elevated. In those in whom the disease is diagnosed, usually through detection of visual field defects, treatment does focus on lowering IOP. Although that has been the major therapeutic approach for decades, only in 1998 did a large study definitively demonstrate that lowering IOP measurably slows progression of the disease. Currently, a form of laser therapy that destroys a part of the eye called the trabecular meshwork and that seems to enhance the drainage of fluids from the eye is a preferred therapy.

The cause of glaucoma is a mystery, but the known risk factors are compatible with the existence of predisposing genes. Recognized risk factors are: older age, black race, increasing IOP, nearsightedness, a large ratio of the measurement of the optic cup to that of the optic disc, and a positive family history. Some studies have found an association with hypertension and diabetes, but the evidence is mixed.

There is a relatively uncommon, dominantly inherited, form of glaucoma called juvenile open angle glaucoma (JOAG) for which mutations in a gene called myocilin have been shown to explain 10–20% of cases. In 2003, a team at Vanderbilt studying families with a form of JOAG that does not arise due to mutations in the myocilin gene found regions on chromosome 9q22 and 20p12 that seem to harbor other predisposing genes.

The most common form of adult glaucoma is primary open angle glaucoma (POAG). It is likely that this generic term covers several different pathological processes which share a common clinical endpoint. Twin and family studies of individuals with POAG provide moderate support for the action of as-yet-undiscovered genetic factors. For example, researchers have shown that the sibling of a person with high IOP is more likely to also have elevated IOP. The pronounced difference in lifetime risk for glaucoma between blacks and whites also permits an inference that there are predisposing genes. In whites, the lifetime risk is 1–2%, whereas in blacks, various studies suggest a risk ranging from 3% to 12%. When told they have glaucoma, blacks are much more likely than whites to identify a relative who is also affected. Interestingly, blacks tend to have larger optic cups, which some studies have suggested creates a higher risk for glaucoma. In other racial groups, the disease is quite uncommon. Among Japanese it is less than 1%, and in one survey of Eskimos, scientists found only 1 case among nearly 2000 people.

There have been several genome-wide screens of large numbers of sibling pairs with glaucoma which have identified chromosomal regions that appear to include a susceptibility gene. In 2003, a consortium that studied the DNA in three patient groups found persuasive support for predisposing genes somewhere within regions 14q11 and 15q. Since the data permit a claim that these two genes represent a significant fraction of the genetic liability for POAG, efforts are now under way to find candidate genes.

There is moderately good evidence that closed angle glaucoma, a less common form of the disease that is associated with structural abnormalities of the eye, is also influenced by genetic predisposition. Closed angle glaucoma varies widely among ethic groups, and it appears that Chinese are at higher risk than other groups. Regardless of race, within families with an affected member, relatives are at significantly higher risk than background, although the absolute risk is still low.

One promising avenue is studying animal models of glaucoma. An autosomal recessive form has been described in Welsh terriers. Whereas animals with only one copy of the disease gene have normal vision, animals with two copies start losing vision at about age 5. A strain of mice known as D2 is afflicted with a disorder called pigmentary glaucoma. This disorder arises because cells in the iris called melanosomes break and leak pigments into the intraocular space. The resulting cellular debris clogs the channels responsible for fluid drainage and causes high IOP and rapid progression to glaucoma. In addition, the pigments themselves are toxic. Using high-resolution genetic mapping, scientists have found genes in which mutations cause this instability of the melanosomes. It is likely that the human form of the disease arises from mutations in the comparable genes. The same scientists have shown that mice which have the mutations but which produce only low levels of pigments do not develop glaucoma. This suggests that agents which suppress production of the pigments could constitute a new therapeutic approach to the disease.

The observation that African-Americans are more likely to develop glaucoma led researchers at Duke to launch a research project in Ghana. The Duke team knew that there was so much familial glaucoma in Ghana that DNA studies conducted there held a much higher chance of finding a disease gene than would similar studies in the United States. Currently, the other large gene-mapping effort is in Australia, a project known as the Glaucoma Inheritance Study in Tasmania. More than 2000 persons in 400 affected families have donated DNA for research. The scientists have already shown that mutations in the gene for myocilin account for 5% of all POAG. Their work has also identified at least five other locations on the genome that may harbor a predisposing allele.

Having a parent with POAG almost certainly increases one's risk for also developing the disorder, but (with the rare exception of families in which it is a dominant disorder) only mildly so. The use of tonometry to screen for elevated IOP, although imperfect, is well worth the minor inconvenience. It is especially important for any person with a positive family history to be screened annually starting at age 40. This is of the most benefit to African-Americans with an affected parent. Their lifetime risk for POAG approaches 10%.

Macular Degeneration

My grandfather is nearly blind with macular degeneration. Am I going to get it?

The macula is composed of millions of cells at the center of the retina which, when struck by light, send nerve impulses coursing to the vision center at the back of the brain. The light images processed by the macula are the source of one's central vision. Macular degeneration (MD) is the most common cause of legal blindness in persons over age 55 in the United States. Individuals who are burdened with an advanced form of this progressive disease typically retain peripheral vision and color recognition, but wherever they focus, the image is so blurry that they are functionally blind.

MD occurs in two forms: dry and wet. The dry form, which is far more common and can affect one eye earlier and more severely than the other, develops as cells in the center of the retina break down and die. The wet form, which accounts for about 10% of all cases, is characterized by the growth of new blood vessels behind the retina. These vessels are unusually fragile. They leak fluids that are toxic to the macular cells.

The risk for MD rises sharply with age—from 2% for people in their 50s to more than 20% for people over the age of 75. In the United States, roughly 8 million people have some loss of vision due to MD; of them, about 1.3 million will experience severe visual compromise over the next

5 years. The cause is poorly understood, but women are at somewhat greater risk than men. Smoking definitely increases the risk, as may high blood levels of cholesterol. A study completed late in 2003 showed that among patients with MD, those who ate a diet rich in fatty foods (especially vegetable fats) were at higher risk for significant visual decline than those who ate a lean, fish-rich diet.

There is no effective treatment for dry MD, but, fortunately, it usually develops quite slowly over many years and is often less severe in one eye than the other. Some recent research suggests that a diet high in zinc and antioxidants may reduce the risk of developing MD by about 25%. Eye surgeons are sometimes able to treat wet MD with laser surgery to control the proliferation of the blood vessels.

Late in 2003, researchers working with Eyetech Pharmaceuticals of New York reported that in a clinical trial involving more than 1000 individuals with MD, a new drug, called Macugen, substantially slowed decline in vision. About 900 patients had Macugen injected directly into the eye every 6 weeks, while 300 had a sham procedure. At the end of a year, 45% of the control group had suffered a vision loss of at least three lines on the eye chart. Among the treated group, only 30% had suffered such a decline.

There are a variety of rare genetic diseases in which affected persons develop early-onset MD, but they represent a minuscule fraction of all cases and do not provide much insight as to the very common age-related forms of MD.

MD does run in a few families, and over the years, many eye doctors have reported on families with multiple affected members. One paper described a large family in which 6 of 13 children had MD. Two of the affected sibs were identical twins. A few twin studies also suggest a significant genetic component to MD, but specific genes have not yet been indicted. In 1998, a team led by Dr. Michael Klein studied a number of extended families with MD and found persuasive evidence for a candidate locus on the long arm of chromosome 1 (region 1q25-31), a discovery that was replicated in 2001 by another group.

In 2003, a large research team of which Klein was a member reported important new findings based on a study of 70 extended MD families. In comparing the DNA of 344 affected persons to that from 217 healthy relatives, they found solid statistical evidence to support the existence of genes predisposing to MD at five loci, three of which were novel. Also in 2003, a Boston-based group of researchers reported on their linkage study of 158 families with two or more individuals with MD. They found strong linkage to a region on chromosome 6. Of even greater importance, their work also suggested that a predisposing gene lurks on the long arm of chromosome 1, making this the third major study to reach such a conclusion. In the autumn of 2003, a consortium of researchers, completing its third genome-wide scan for susceptibility to MD, found yet more evidence to indict region 1q31. In addition, it found solid evidence for another predisposing gene on 17q25. Scientists at the University of Michigan and Harvard, performing similar studies, have found several other suspicious regions. The scientists are now using microarray technologies to identify genes that are especially active in macular cells. They have identified 92 proteins that are highly expressed in the macula.

Tracking down a gene that elevates risk for a disease of old age is particularly difficult. Older affected people usually die before their children are diagnosed, so it is hard to find families with several living affected persons, families that are likely to carry predisposing genes. Still, the search seems to be narrowing. In 2003, a Michigan team discovered that in one family with a rare form of autosomal dominant MD, the disease is associated with having a mutation in a gene called RDS. Although this does not necessarily mean that RDS mutations predispose to common forms of MD, it is possible that other mutations in the RDS gene will turn out to be risk factors in families that do not have the dominant form of the disorder.

Unfortunately, as yet we know too little about the genetics of the vast majority of MD cases to counsel persons about risk. However, we do know that risk for MD presents yet another argument against smoking and in favor of a low-fat diet.

MENTAL ILLNESS

Schizophrenia

My older sister has schizophrenia. I am 45 and healthy. What are the risks to my kids?

Schizophrenia is a frightening disease. Insidious in onset, often striking during adolescence, it robs the mind of its ability to think rationally, to feel emotions normally, and to draw boundaries to separate the real from the imagined. Until a few decades ago, when the development of antipsychotic drugs somewhat eased their plight, most severely affected individuals were incarcerated for life in chronic-disease hospitals, few of which offered more than custodial care. Untreated, severe schizophrenia destroys the patient and devastates his or her family.

Schizophrenia is an all too common disorder. The lifetime risk is roughly 1 in 100. To be diagnosed, an individual must suffer from delusions (such as believing that he can broadcast his thoughts to others or that he is under the control of aliens), or prominent hallucinations (such as persistently hearing a voice commenting on his daily life). These symptoms must persist off and on for 6 months, and an organic cause (such as certain kinds of drug abuse) must be ruled out.

Although no one knows the cause, there is ample evidence that genetic factors play an important role. The most prominent thesis is that the presence of certain gene variants sets a general threshold of risk that may or may not be breached, depending on the environmental stressors to which a particular individual is exposed.

During the 20th century, there were many family studies of schizophrenia, collectively involving more than 40,000 relatives of affected persons. These empirical studies clearly established that schizophrenia runs in families. Early research showed that about 5–6% of the parents of persons diagnosed with schizophrenia are also affected. This relatively low figure is in part due to the fact that in the past most persons with the disorder did not marry. Brothers and sisters of schizophrenics have about a 10% lifetime risk for the disease, which is about 10 times greater than the risk to the general population. The risk to children of one schizophrenic parent is 10–15%. In the few studies of couples in which both husband and wife were schizophrenics, the risk to their children approached 50%. If a parent and one child are both affected, the lifetime risk to the other siblings is about 15–20%.

Twin studies support the role of genetic factors, but also acknowledge environmental factors. In six studies comparing MZ to DZ twins, the concordance rate for identical twins was 60–65%, whereas for nonidentical twins it was about 10–15% (the same risk attributed to other siblings). The high concordance rate for MZ twins is the same regardless of whether the twins were reared together or apart.

The many studies of schizophrenics who grew up with adoptive parents consistently show a much stronger correlation of disease with the biological parents than with rearing parents. One study compared children of

Table 38. *Schizophrenia: Concordance in MZ versus DZ twins*

Country	MZ		DZ	
	number	concordance	number	concordance
Finland	17	.35	20	.13
Norway	55	.45	90	.15
Denmark	21	.56	41	.27
United Kingdom	22	.58	33	.15
United States	164	.31	277	.06

Adapted, with permission of Worth Publishers, from Gottesman I. 1991. *Schizophrenia genesis: The origins of madness.* W.H. Freeman, New York.

schizophrenic mothers who were separated by day 3 of life with a control group of children separated from healthy mothers. None of the children in the later group was diagnosed with schizophrenia, while 17% of the former were schizophrenic, and many more had other psychiatric problems.

Table 39. *Schizophrenia: Risks for relatives of persons with schizophrenia*

Relationship	Total relatives	Schizophrenics	Risk (%)
First-degree			
parents	8020	477	5.6
siblings			
overall	9921	1002	10.1
neither parent SZ	7264	698	9.6
one parent SZ	624	104	16.7
children	1578	202	12.8
children of two SZ parents	134	62	46.3
Second-degree			
uncles, aunts	2421	57	2.4
nephews, nieces	3966	120	3.0
grandchildren	740	27	3.7
Third-degree			
first cousins	1600	39	2.4
Spouses	399	9	2.3

Adapted, with permission, from Gottesman I. and Shields J. 1982. *Schizophrenia: The epigenetic puzzle.* Cambridge University Press, New York.

Almost as soon as molecular biologists acquired the tools for gene hunting, the search for genes that predispose to schizophrenia began in earnest. Over the last decade or so, there have been several gene hunts using DNA from families in which two children have been diagnosed with the disease, as well as a variety of other efforts to identify culprit genes. There have been several false starts, and at least one claim of linkage (statistical evidence that a disease-causing gene is in a certain region of a chromosome) has been withdrawn. This experience is typical of genetic studies of complex disorders. Because it is so hard to define the phenotype, and because there is so much uncertainty about how many different paths can lead to the disease, data suggesting that a disease gene has been found are often difficult to replicate.

In August of 2002, a large whole-genome scanning study reported strong statistical evidence that a gene on the short arm of chromosome 6 (6p22.3) predisposes to schizophrenia. The findings were based on a study of the DNA of 1425 persons in 270 families in which all the patients met the official diagnostic criteria for the disorder. The data are exciting because this region of chromosome 6 is known to include the location for the gene that codes for a protein called dysbindin. Mouse studies have shown that dysbindin plays an important role in organizing brain cells and in establishing their lines of communication. In January of 2003, many of the same scientists published a study of 203 other affected families that replicated the evidence against dysbindin.

Recently, scientists at DeCode Genetics have shown that at least some cases of schizophrenia may to be due to mutations in a gene named neuroregulin1. Affected persons were twice as likely to carry certain variants of that gene as were unaffected individuals. The work is especially noteworthy because the findings have been replicated in a Scottish population. In further support, mice with mutations in neuroregulin1 have a disorder that mimics human schizophrenia. Late in 2003, scientists from the United Kingdom, Sweden, and the United States reported that in a genome-wide linkage study involving 353 pairs of sibs with schizophrenia, they found strong evidence of predisposing genes on chromosomes 10q, 17p, and 22q. These findings replicate earlier studies, and they strongly support a search for candidate genes in those regions.

It now appears highly likely that in the near future scientists will identify several gene variants that confer elevated risk for schizophrenia. This knowledge may well lead to efficacious new therapies. However, far sooner it will permit us to develop genetic predisposition tests, the use of which will pose many ethical problems.

How does one counsel the relatives of persons diagnosed with schizophrenia? First, one must be absolutely sure that the patient in question actually satisfies the diagnostic criteria for the disorder. After obtaining a thorough family history, it is possible to use empirical data to support general statements about risk. The risk estimates must be tempered, however, for they are dependent on the age of the person who is worried about risk. Few at-risk people develop schizophrenia after age 40 and almost none after 50.

To answer the question posed at the beginning of this section, the risk to nephews and nieces of persons with schizophrenia is about 2%, about double the lifetime risk of the general population.

Affective Disorder (Major Depression, Bipolar Illness)

My dad's brother was diagnosed with manic depression in his 20s. I think his father, who is now dead, also had the illness. What are my risks?

Depression is a term used to classify persons suffering from a prolonged mood disorder. The dimensions of the disorder vary widely, and it should not be thought of as a single disease. The standard diagnostic criteria are set forth in the *Diagnostic and Statistical Manual IV* (DSM IV), a reference work recognized by most psychiatrists as containing the most current and widely held rules for making a diagnosis. The disorder is divided into two major categories: unipolar depression (UPD) and bipolar depression (BPD). The classic distinguishing feature of the latter is wide mood swings that include episodic manic behavior.

To meet the diagnostic standards of the DSM IV for UPD, the patient must report that he or she has experienced at least five of nine symptoms (such as feelings of worthlessness, fatigue, sleep disturbance, unintended weight loss, recurrent thoughts of death, anhedonia, and depression) over a period of 2 weeks. The symptoms cannot be due to bereavement, there must not be an underlying physiological explanation such as thyroid disease, and the symptoms must impair important areas of the patient's life.

To satisfy the DSM IV standard for episodic manic behavior associated with bipolar depression, the patient must experience a period of elevated, expansive, or irritable mood for at least 1 week. During the episode, the patient must have experienced at least three of seven symptoms: a sense of grandiosity, a reduced need for sleep, a marked increase in talka-tiveness, a sense that his thoughts are racing, easy distractability, a high increase in goal-oriented activity, or an unusual involvement in pleasure-seeking activities. These symptoms must impair his or her normal routine and they must not be due to an underlying physiological cause (such as use of illicit drugs). Patients with bipolar disease (manic-depression) do not usually experience a mixed state of lows and highs; they tend to cycle from one end of the spectrum to the other.

There are no biochemical tests to clinch the diagnosis of either UPD (also sometimes called MDD for major depressive disorder) or BPD. However, recent research suggests that a region of the brain called the amygdala (which can be accurately measured with MRI scans) is dis-cernibly smaller in affected individuals with BPD. Since this observation has been made in both adult and teenage patients who have recently become ill, a smaller amygdala may precede onset of the illness. If so, it would be the first tangible sign of risk for a major psychiatric illness. This is by no means settled.

Many family studies of depression have repeatedly confirmed that UPD cannot be separated from BPD. Most families burdened with bipolar disorder include some individuals diagnosed only with UPD and others who clearly have the manic form of the disorder. In families in which the proband has been diagnosed with depression, it is also more likely than would be expected by chance to find relatives suffering from chronic alco-holism. In these families one also finds more young women suffering from an eating disorder (discussed later). Thus far, there is no clear explanation for these observations.

UPD is a disturbingly common disorder with a lifetime risk of between 5% and 15%. BPD, which has a lifetime risk of about 1%, is by no means rare. Some health economists have estimated that by 2020, depres-sion will rank second only to heart disease in its economic impact on soci-ety. One of the most puzzling aspects of depression is that risk varies by gender. Throughout the western world, the risk is about 2–3 times higher in women than in men. This ratio could be skewed by the fact that women are more likely to seek help for this illness, but studies that have considered this question do not find much evidence to support it. In virtually all cul-tures, there are many more cases of UPD than there are of BPD.

A large number of family studies demonstrate that the first-degree rel-atives of persons with depression have a risk for also being diagnosed that is about 3–5 times greater than the risk to relatives of a control group of individuals who do not have the disease. Adoption studies strongly support a major genetic influence on risk for depression. One large study found that 30% of the biological parents of children who had been given for adoption at birth and who were later diagnosed with bipolar disorder had either UPD or BPD. Twin studies have repeatedly found that the concordance rate for both these disorders is much higher among MZ twins than it is among DZ twins. Across several studies, the concordance rate for MZ twins is about 60%, whereas for DZ twins it is about 20%.

In the late 1980s (the early days of gene hunting), two different research groups reported that in high-risk families (those chosen because depression was so common among relatives) they had linked the disease with DNA markers. One suspect region was on the short arm of chromosome 11; the other was on the X. Both claims were later retracted. How could this happen? In these family studies, if the diagnosis of even a single individual turns out to be erroneous, the statistical basis for the linkage claim can collapse. Ever more detailed genome scans continue to uncover regions of suspicion. Currently, a locus on chromosome 12 and another on chromosome 18 are tantalizing, but no one has yet cloned a gene for either UPD or BPD.

Despite much effort, there is still much to learn about how genes increase the risk for UPD and BPD. Current evidence suggests that there may be a relatively small number with large effects. In some studies, heavily affected families exhibit the phenomenon of anticipation. In essence, this means that as the generations pass, the onset of symptoms in those who become ill occurs at an earlier age. There is a well-studied group of neurological disorders (including Huntington disease) characterized by mutations that enlarge with each generation in which this phenomenon has been documented. No one has yet found such a mutation in persons with depression. A few studies have also reported that age of onset of the disease

Table 40. *Depression: Risk of either UPD or BPD among first-degree relatives of persons with UPD (summarizing many studies)*		
Diagnosis in first-degree relative	**Range of risk (%)**	**Average (%)**
Unipolar depression	6–28	14.0
Bipolar depression	0–5	1.4[a]

[a]The risk of BPD in first-degree relatives of persons with UPD is not much greater than the general population risk.

Table 41. *Depression: Risk of either UPD or BPD among first-degree relatives of persons with BPD (summary of 10 studies)*

Diagnosis in first-degree relative	Range of risk (%)	Average (%)
Unipolar depression	6–23	13
Bipolar depression	2–16	6[a]

[a]The risk of BPD in first-degree relatives of persons with BPD is markedly increased.

in the offspring of affected persons was younger if the father had the illness than if the mother was affected.

In 2002, the search for genes that predispose to BPD yielded some enticing results. Researchers who studied a group of families in a region of Costa Rica where BPD is especially common found that DNA markers in three chromosomal regions were present in affected persons much more often than would be expected by chance. The most powerful signal was localized to the short arm of chromosome 8. Several thousand miles north, a team at the University of Toronto, using a different strategy, came up with another set of positive results. Reasoning that a gene which makes a protein called brain-derived neurotrophic factor (BDNF) could be responsible for an illness like BPD, the scientists looked for mutations in affected persons. Among the affected members in 283 families, risk for disease was highly correlated with having certain variants of that gene.

In 2003, an international team of researchers reported on their investigation of whether genetic variation influenced the likelihood that stressful life events lead to clinical depression. Working with a cohort of over 1000 individuals whom they had been following since birth, they found that among persons who had similar severe life stressors, the risk of subsequent depression was significantly greater in those who carried at least one copy of a certain DNA variant in the promoter region of the serotonin transporter gene called 5-HTT. Also in 2003, a team from McGill University showed that a variant in the same region of the comparable gene in vervet monkeys was highly associated with a phenotype of "extreme anxiety." Together, these studies suggest that the serotonin transporter protein is key to mediating stress reactions.

In December of 2003, a team of scientists from Myriad Genetics in Salt Lake City published impressive evidence that they were closing in on a gene that strongly influenced risk for major depression disorder (MDD,

UPD). In a study of more than 400 large families in Utah, they identified 110 that contained at least four affected individuals. They then used a panel of more than 600 genetic markers to study the DNA of 1890 members of those large families. Because of the well-established difference in risk for the disorder by gender, they analyzed the data from that perspective. Among the samples taken from the women, they did not find evidence to link any particular genetic region to risk for depression. However, they did find a region on the long arm of chromosome 12 (a region that several earlier studies had found suspect) that has an especially important effect on risk for depression in men. From a statistical perspective, this evidence is the most powerful to date concerning efforts to untangle the role of genes in depression.

One potential near-term benefit to patients being treated for either form of depression may derive from pharmacogenetic research. Many drugs are available for the treatment of depression. In general, each works well in some patients and poorly in others. Furthermore, each has side effects that range from very mild to severe, depending on the patient. If careful pharmacogenetic studies were done, it should be possible to pick the best possible drug for each patient based in part on his or her genetic profile. Such studies are beginning, and the results should be forthcoming within the next 2–3 years. The potential clinical and economic benefits from pharmacogenetic profiling are huge.

What risks do close relatives of a person diagnosed with major depression have of developing either UPD or BPD in their lifetime? In one large, relatively recent study of the offspring of more than 600 persons with one of the two forms of depression (mostly bipolar), the lifetime risk to the children for *either* illness was about 20%. In a couple in which one parent was diagnosed with depression, the lifetime risk to the son for major depression was 8%. In a daughter, the risk was about 15%. The lifetime risk to the children (regardless of their gender) of developing bipolar disorder was 7–14%. Within that group, the risk was higher for a child who was of the same sex as the affected parent.

If both parents have been diagnosed with major depression, but there are no other affected individuals in the family, the lifetime risk of major depression for a son is about 15% and for a daughter about 25%. The risk to children rises with the number of affected first-degree relatives. In many studies, the highest calculated risk is for children born into families in which both parents and sibs are affected. These children have a lifetime risk of bipolar disorder that approaches 50%, and a risk for major depression in the 30–40% range. The risk falls off quickly as one moves out of the nuclear family. The risk to a nephew of a person with bipolar disorder of developing the same disorder is in the range of 2%, higher than the background risk, but not greatly so.

Panic Disorder

> *My 16-year-old daughter has been diagnosed with panic disorder. What risks do my other daughters face?*

Panic disorder is a common, chronic, debilitating illness that typically begins in late adolescence or early adulthood. It is characterized by several problems, especially extensive anxiety over life's relatively routine challenges and discomfort in social settings. The hallmark of the disorder is the sudden onset of extreme distress without clear provocation. The patient feels a sense of foreboding, even doom. A typical panic attack may include heart palpitations, air hunger, chest pain, dizziness, weakness, a sense of impending doom, and many other disturbing sensations. The patient may cry out, "I am dying" or "I cannot breathe" or " I am having a heart attack." The crisis peaks over about 30 minutes and recedes rather quickly. About half of the people who suffer from panic disorder also have agoraphobia. They fear crowds, traveling to new places, and public speaking.

Psychiatrists have long been familiar with this constellation of problems. Shortly after the Civil War, army doctors described this disorder as "neurocirculatory asthenia" or "soldier's heart" because so many young men mentioned symptoms referable to the heart or lungs. In 1895, Sigmund Freud used the term "anxiety neurosis" to describe what these patients were experiencing.

Age of onset is uncommon before 16 or after 35. In about 85% of cases, the severity diminishes slowly over time. Several large surveys suggest that in the United States the lifetime risk for panic disorder is about 1–2%. The same surveys indicate that about 5% of Americans experience some significant degree of agoraphobia. Multiple studies confirm that women are twice as likely as men to be diagnosed with panic disorder and are three times as likely to report feelings of agoraphobia.

Panic disorder has long been recognized as a highly familial disease. A few twin studies have found a much higher concordance rate among MZ twins than DZ twins for both anxiety disorders generally and panic disor-

Table 42. *Panic disorder: Familial risk*

Co-twins of affected MZ twins are about 5 times more likely to develop panic disorder than are the co-twins of affected DZ twins.

Risk to first-degree relatives of affected persons is about 15–25%.

The risk for panic attacks appears even higher in families in which individuals only occasionally experience the attacks.

der in particular. The studies are too small to provide reliable numbers, but they certainly support a significant genetic load. The results of about a dozen studies over the last few decades suggest that the first-degree relatives of persons diagnosed with panic disorder have about a 25% lifetime risk for this disorder. Put another way, their risk is about 10–20 times greater than that expected to be found in relatives of an unaffected control group. The risk to second-degree relatives (aunts and uncles, nieces and nephews) is about 10%, about 5–10 times greater than the background risk.

In 1951, a research team that studied the families of 139 patients and those of 80 control subjects provided strong scientific confirmation of earlier, anecdotal reports of familial clustering. In families with unaffected parents but one affected child, they found that 27% of the other siblings were also affected. If there was one affected parent, 38% of offspring were affected. If both parents were affected, panic disorder was present in 62% of the children. In 1987, a similar study of the families of 117 patients reached similar results. The presence of a single affected parent or sibling increased the risk for the disorder in other siblings to five times greater than the population risk—about 10% for men and about 25% for women. The relative risk rose sharply if there was more than one affected family member.

In 2001, a team from Spain that studied seven large pedigrees in which many individuals had panic disorder, agoraphobia, social phobias, and/or joint laxity reported the discovery that a relatively common duplication of a segment of the long arm of chromosome 15 (found in 7% of randomly selected people) was present far more often in persons with panic disorder. The team replicated their findings in a second population and is now searching for a causative gene among the 60 or so that lie along the duplicated region. The joint laxity is probably unrelated, merely reflecting the presence of a nearby gene that predisposes to that condition and is co-inherited.

Although the gene or genes have not yet been identified, the evidence that panic disorder is strongly influenced by genes is impressive. One can with some confidence tell people with affected relatives that the lifetime risk to a young sister of an affected person is about 25% (the correct answer to the question posed at the beginning of this section). The risk falls sharply with age, and rarely manifests after age 40. The severity of the disease varies widely within families, so the fact that one person is severely affected cannot be used to infer degree of severity for a sibling. Fortunately, panic disorder usually responds well to drug and behavioral therapy. Much can be done to help persons with this disorder.

Obsessive Compulsive Disorder

My wife has been diagnosed with obsessive compulsive disorder. Her symptoms remind me of some of her mother's behaviors. What is the risk to our son?

Obsessive compulsive disorder (OCD) is the name given to a spectrum of behaviors that usually manifest in adolescence or early adulthood. People with OCD have obsessions or compulsions or both. Obsessions are not merely worries. They are recurrent, episodically persistent thoughts that are intrusive and which cause the individual great stress. These unwanted thoughts or images often overwhelm the individual, even though he or she knows they are irrational. The signs and symptoms of OCD may range from mild to severely incapacitating.

Classic examples of obsessions include fear of dirt (leading to wildly excessive hand washing), repeated doubts (for example, about whether one who has left home for the day has remembered to put the dog out), an overwhelming need for order (causing the patient to spend hours each day reorganizing the contents of her closet), fear of hurting someone, and disturbing sexual imagery. Obsessions generate compulsions, the mind's attempt to counter or control them. Typical compulsions include washing, counting, checking, and arranging.

OCD is one of a group of related disorders that includes multiple tic disorders, the most famous of which is Tourette syndrome (TS). One, fortunately quite rare, manifestation is an obsession with hair-pulling so severe that it results in complete baldness. TS is a well-characterized tic syndrome that by definition has its onset in childhood. Affected children have multiple motor and vocal tics (which in about 10% of patients include an uncontrollable urge to swear or use vile language). The nature and severity of the tics change with time. Many children with TS have symptoms compatible with OCD.

OCD affects people in all ethnic groups. It affects men and women about equally. Originally thought to be relatively rare, OCD is now known to affect at least 1% of the population of the United States. TS constitutes a small subset of the total. It occurs in about 1 in 3000 boys and is quite rare in girls, who account for only about 10% of cases. As with the other major psychiatric disorders, both twin and family studies offer strong support for a large genetic contribution to risk for OCD and TS. Modeling efforts suggest that most TS is due to the action of a single dominantly acting gene. The best guess about OCD is that several genes are involved.

In the last few years, there has been major progress in understanding the molecular biology of OCD. In 1997, a group at Rockefeller University in New York City reported evidence that mutations in the gene coding for catechol-O-methyltransferase (COMT), which is normally responsible for quenching the action of two neurotransmitters, were more frequently found in men with OCD than expected. They found that men with two copies of the variant that coded for low levels of COMT were eight times more likely to have the disorder than were men with two copies of the version that resulted in high levels of COMT. In 2000, a group at the University of Toronto found that a variant in a gene coding for a serotonin receptor (a protein on the surface of nerve cells to which the important brain transmitter, serotonin, attaches) was found far more often than expected by chance in patients with OCD. This linkage study is tantalizing because the best medical treatment of OCD is drugs that inhibit the re-uptake of serotonin.

In 2003, a group at Rockefeller University reported that in a study of the families of 164 patients who met rigorous clinical diagnostic criteria for OCD, certain haplotypes in a gene called BDNF (which makes a protein that supports the growth of brain cells and is called brain-derived neurotrophic factor) were highly correlated with having the disease. The scientists also found a single amino acid change in the protein that appeared to be causative. If the results of this candidate gene study are replicated, it will mean we have identified the first known cause of this unusual illness.

What is the bottom line for families worried about their children? OCD is a behavioral disorder, the liability for which is highly influenced by genes. Risks to children of an affected parent are approximately 20%, as is the risk for any first-degree relative of an affected person. There is some evidence that the earlier the age of onset, the greater the risk that the illness will be severe. Fortunately, as with panic disorder, much can be done to help affected individuals.

Anorexia Nervosa

My niece is very ill with anorexia nervosa. Is my daughter at elevated risk?

Anorexia nervosa (AN) is a psychiatric disorder almost exclusively diagnosed in young women, the hallmark of which is obsessive fear of weight gain and refusal to eat. It is seen most frequently among white women of middle or upper socioeconomic class. AN is rarely diagnosed in Asian or black women. Less than 5% of cases occur in men. Psychiatrists recognize two other eating disorders: bulimia, which is also found almost exclusively in young women and is characterized by binge eating; and self-induced vomiting or purging. Bulimic behaviors may occur episodically in women who otherwise follow the clinical course typical of patients with AN. For this reason, there are two clinical forms of AN: anorexia nervosa in which patients do not engage in bulimic behavior (RAN) and anorexia nervosa in which they do (BPAN).

The onset of AN usually occurs shortly after puberty, sometimes in association with a precipitating traumatic event such as parental divorce or going off to college. The patient essentially stops eating, and no amount of cajoling, threats, or pleading will alter her behavior. Patients with AN become profoundly emaciated and are at risk for dying from infection. In some studies, the death rate ranges from 5% to 10%, making this a lethal psychiatric disease. Patients are usually treated with a combination of behavioral modification techniques and antidepressant drugs. In the most serious cases, management includes long-term hospitalization and forced feedings.

Neurologists have categorized these diseases as hypothalamic disorders because the region of the brain known as the anterior hypothalamus is known to control the sense of hunger and the sense of fullness. The cause of AN remains a mystery, but over the last 30 years, ever more emphasis has been placed on the possibility of a genetic predisposition. Family studies have shown that the relatives of patients with AN are much more likely than the relatives of a control group to also have eating disorders. Limited information based on twin studies shows a higher concordance rate for AN among MZ twins than among DZ twins.

In 2002, researchers at the University of Pennsylvania reported that they had found evidence of a gene that predisposes to AN. The scientists recruited 192 families, each of which had two or more siblings with an eating disorder. Each family was recruited through a patient who met the clinical definition for AN. A genome-wide scan of all the families did not yield data that strongly implicated a particular region of any chromosome. However, when the scientists studied only the 37 families in which both siblings carried the diagnosis of RAN (AN without bulimia), analysis of the data strongly implicated a region on the short arm of chromosome 1. Several teams are currently trying to track down the culprit gene, but there is much still to be done.

In 2003, the results of a study of more than 1000 patients in eight different European countries with AN or bulimia found that a variant in the gene that makes a protein called BDNF (brain-derived neurotrophic factor) was highly associated with risk for all three clinical subtypes of AN and with bulimia. The study is especially encouraging because it involves so many different populations.

What about risk to close relatives of affected persons? Because the disease is exceedingly rare in boys and young men, one can advise that the risk to the brothers and nephews of affected young women is exceedingly low. There are not many data on risk to sisters of affected persons, but it is rare to find families with more than one affected member. The best that can be said for now is that their risk is higher than the risk in the general population, but still low. Signs of an eating disorder should stimulate family members to seek help. Early intervention improves the prospects for successful treatment.

HUMAN BEHAVIOR

Alcoholism

Both my dad and his brother were alcoholics. I am afraid to drink at all.
If I did start using alcohol, would I be at increased risk?

Alcoholism is a complex disease that is both difficult to define and hard to study. The difficulty in definition and diagnosis relates indirectly to the fact that consumption of alcohol has been widespread in human culture for more than 5000 years. In a society in which most adults consume some alcohol, the diagnosis of alcoholism cannot be based on a metric as simple as the amount of alcohol one consumes over a certain period of time. What constitutes heavy drinking in one country may not even match the median level of consumption in another. In developing diagnostic criteria to define alcoholism, experts have been forced to rely on measurements of the impact of consumption on the individual's ability to maintain his or her normal activities. For five decades, the core concept of alcoholism as a disease has been that an alcoholic is a person who is physiologically dependent on alcohol and cannot function without having nearly constant access to it.

Proceeding from the idea that dependency is a core feature of the disorder, national survey data reveal that a strikingly high number of persons meet the definition of being alcoholic. In Sweden, nearly 5% of men are alcoholics, whereas only about 1% of women meet the criteria. Similar studies in the United States suggest that the lifetime risk of being diagnosed with alcoholism is 5–7% in men, but only 0.5–1% in women. These figures vary widely when studies focus on subgroups such as members of certain religions or cultures, a finding that reinforces the importance of environmental factors.

The fact that alcoholism may run in families has been recognized for more than a century. A voluminous literature consistently supports the facts that children have a higher than background risk for becoming alcoholic if either parent is an alcoholic, that brothers and sisters of alcoholics are more likely to be alcoholic than are brothers and sisters of persons who are not affected, that the incidence of alcoholism is higher in close blood relatives of alcoholics than it is in distant relatives, and that the offspring of alcoholic parents tend to become alcoholic earlier in life and to have more severe problems than do alcoholics without a positive family history.

Many studies comparing the rate of alcoholism in MZ versus DZ twins have found that among MZ twins the co-twin of an alcoholic is twice as likely to also become an alcoholic as is the co-twin of an affected nonidentical twin. In a Swedish study of identical twins reared apart from birth, of the six individuals found to have alcoholism, five of the co-twins (all of whom were unknown to them) also were alcoholic. Epidemiological studies in Sweden and the United States support the notion that there is a subtype of alcoholism characterized by markedly early age at diagnosis, far larger numbers of female alcoholics, and more severe clinical course that is driven by the action of a highly penetrant single gene or a small number of genes. This may ultimately explain about 10% of all cases of alcoholism.

Many scientists have used adoption studies to try to get a handle on the role of genes in alcoholism. These studies seek to compare rates of alcoholism in the biological (non-rearing) parents to those of the social (rearing) parents. In general, these studies found about a two- to threefold excess in alcoholism in the biological versus the social parents. Taken together, family, twin, and adoption studies suggest that the risk for alcoholism is heavily influenced by genes (the heritability coefficient is 0.5 to 0.6).

Some years ago, one of the leading researchers in the study of the heritability of alcohol abuse, C. R. Cloninger of Washington University, posited that the disorder has two major subtypes. Type I, a relatively late-onset disorder, is characterized by a personality profile of low novelty seeking, high harm avoidance, and high reward dependence. Type II individuals have an early age of onset and are more likely to be diagnosed with antisocial personality disorder. Whereas both men and women may become Type I alcoholics, virtually all Type II alcoholics are men. Although the formal psychiatric diagnostic manual (DSM IV Revised) does not recognize Cloninger's subtypes, many researchers do.

For more than a decade, a large consortium of scientists have pursued the Collaborative Study of the Genetics of Alcoholism without much success. More recently, armed with the new tools of molecular biology, scientists have tried repeatedly to map genes that predispose to alcoholism. Although no one has captured a gene, the picture that is beginning to emerge is that liability to the more common form of alcoholism is influenced by several genes, each one having a relatively small effect on altering the risk. For example, a 1998 study of a Finnish group of severe alcoholics (166 alcoholics with criminal records arising out of antisocial behavior while they were inebriated, 261 unaffected relatives, and 213 controls) found evidence linking a variant in the serotonin receptor gene (HTR1B) to risk for disease.

The answer to the question posed at the top of this section is "Yes." When compared to the general population, the children of alcoholics and the siblings of alcoholics have a three- to fivefold greater risk for the disease. For those with a strong family history of alcohol problems, the best approach is the simplest. Abstinence is a perfect prevention of alcoholism. Discussing her extended family's severe problems with alcohol, Mariel

Hemingway, the actress and granddaughter of the great writer, said in a *New York Times* interview that she does not touch alcohol. In her words, "I know that genetically I walk a fine Hemingway line" which if crossed can lead to disaster.

Drug Addiction

Is there evidence that people who become drug addicts are genetically driven to do so?

Lay people and scientists alike have long speculated about the role of genes in the greater prevalence of abuse of illicit drugs in some families than in others. As far back as the 1870s, long before the rediscovery of Mendel's laws of inheritance, Richard Dugdale, a prison inspector, impressed by the fact that certain families were so overrepresented in the jails of upstate New York, suggested that hereditary predisposition to opium abuse may have sealed their fates. Over the last three decades, some researchers have built a convincing argument that about 10% of alcoholics suffer their disorder because they were born with gene variants which increased their risk of dependency on that drug.

There have been far fewer studies of the possible role of genes in altering risk for drug addiction than for alcoholism. Furthermore, there is much evidence that socioeconomic factors and other cultural forces have a huge impact on risk for drug abuse. For example, about one of every four American adults smokes cigarettes regularly, despite widespread knowledge of the danger to health and a gargantuan antismoking public health campaign. Each day in the United States, 3000 teenagers start smoking. The percentage of adult smokers in some other nations, notably China, is much higher. Clearly, environmental influences must be very important. Still, there is a growing body of evidence suggesting that genes affect the threshold of risk and the likelihood of remaining hooked.

Genetic studies of nicotine addiction typically look at the age at which the individual started smoking, because it is well established that the earlier one starts, the less likely he or she will ever stop smoking. In 1999, two groups reported that a common variant of the dopamine transporter gene (SLC6A3-9) strongly influenced risk for smoking. Dopamine is a neurotransmitter, the action of which is thought to influence the personality traits of extraversion and novelty-seeking behavior. The researchers were prompted to do the study because they speculated that early smokers were more likely to have the genetic profile that predisposed to novelty seeking. In their study of more than 200 young smokers and a control group, the scientists found that persons with SLC6A3-9 started smoking later, made more efforts to quit, and succeeded more often at quitting. A second research group extended their research by looking at the distribution of the gene variant among more than 1100 nonsmokers, current smokers, and former smokers. Smokers who carry the SLC6A3-9 allele were 50% more likely to quit than smokers who did not.

In 2000, researchers at St. Louis University found that among 3356 pairs of twins, genetic factors (61%) were a stronger influence on smoking than were environmental factors (39%). A similar study conducted at the Medical College of Virginia on 949 twin pairs attributed 78% of the risk of becoming a smoker to genetic factors. In 2002, a group led by Carlyn Lerman showed that women and men who inherit a particular form of the gene involved in synthesizing serotonin (a neurotransmitter) tended to start smoking at a significantly younger age, a finding compatible with the suggestion that the decision to smoke or use other drugs may be closely related to impulse control.

What is certain is that once they have become addicted to nicotine, smokers find it extraordinarily difficult to stop. In one recent study of 557 smokers who said they wanted to quit, researchers attempted to use the fear of cancer to motivate them. They divided the subjects into two groups. Both were given nicotine patches to ease withdrawal. In addition, members of one group were tested for GSTM1, a gene that helps the body to cleanse itself of the poisons in cigarette smoke. The subjects who were told that they have a version of the gene that would not protect them were no more likely to quit than anyone else.

In June 2002, Jack Sipe and his team at the Scripps Research Institute in California published the results of the first large-scale search for gene variants that are connected with drug abuse. They scanned the DNA of a large number of admitted street drug abusers and compared the results to the same DNA scan of samples taken from a control group of Caucasians who did not use these substances. They made the remarkable finding that a homozygous (two copies) variant of a single gene was four times more common in the drug-abusing population than in the control group. The chance that this finding was merely the result of random sampling was calculated at less than 1 in 1000. Even more enticing is the finding that the variant does not appear to be more common in persons who abuse only alcohol or only nicotine.

The gene in which they made their discovery is responsible for producing a protein that metabolizes certain drugs. The gene, known as FAAH, codes for a protein called fatty acid amide hydrolase, which is responsible for breaking down certain cannabinoids, the chemicals in marijuana. The gene variant affects the stability of the protein, making it more susceptible to degradation. A disproportionate number of drug abusers may have enzymes that function differently from the normal version.

People who use drugs or become regular smokers do so under the influence of myriad environmental and genetic factors. There clearly are genetic factors affecting risk for starting and likelihood of quitting, but they are enmeshed in a host of other factors that are exceedingly difficult to untangle.

Homosexuality

My uncle is gay. Are gay genes transferred through the mother?

Homosexuality is defined as a preferential erotic attraction during adulthood to members of the same sex. Depending on the particular study, about 1–5% of American men are exclusively homosexual. Homosexuality in women—lesbianism—is about half as common as it is in men. The prevalence of homosexuality is roughly the same across all racial and ethnic groups.

Over the last century, there have been many studies of the heritability of homosexuality. Twin, family, and adoption studies all provide evidence that a genetic factor or factors play an important role in the development of homosexuality. Taken together, five twin studies in men have shown that 57% of identical twins of gay men are also gay. The prevalence among other brothers is 13%—much lower, but still about threefold greater than the prevalence in the general population. On the other hand, the twin and family studies also make clear that there must be important environmental factors at work in the emergence of homosexuality.

Despite many efforts, no one has ever identified a biochemical cause of homosexuality in humans. However, several studies of certain anatomical aspects of the brain have found discernible differences in the brains of gay men when compared with the brains of heterosexual men. One, in 1992, found that the shape and size of the anterior hypothalamus in gay men was the same as in women, and distinctly different from that in straight men. Another reported that in gay men the area known as the suprachiasmatic nucleus was larger than in heterosexual men. It is impossible to draw firm conclusions from these studies. First, they have not been replicated. Second, it is impossible to differentiate cause from effect.

In 1993, Dr. Dean Hamer, a researcher at the NIH, and his team reported on the results of a detailed genetic study they had performed on the DNA of gay men. By advertising in gay-oriented newspapers, they recruited 40 pairs of homosexual brothers. They then performed what by today's standards was a relatively modest linkage study, seeking to see whether the pairs of gay brothers shared any DNA segments much more frequently than would be expected by chance. Hamer reported that there was a region on the long arm of the X chromosome that was the same in 33 of the 40 brothers, a dramatic deviation from the expected number of 20. He calculated the odds of this occurring by random chance as 1 in 10,000 and argued that a candidate gene for homosexuality was located in that region. Hamer and his team conducted a similar study of 32 other pairs of gay brothers in 1995 and reported results that, although less robust, supported his thesis. In 1999, however, when a research group led by Dr. George Rice replicated the study, they found no evidence at all to support the notion that there was a gay gene on the X chromosome.

Despite the molecular genetic studies, today we still have only empirical data to rely on. There is evidence that the sons of mothers who have gay brothers are more likely to be homosexual than are the sons of mothers without gay brothers, a finding that does support an X-linked predisposing gene. If one has a gay brother, the risk of being gay is about 10%, about 2–3 times the background risk. However, one cannot easily claim that increase to be due to genetic causes, as brothers usually share environments. There may well be genes that increase the chance one will become homosexual, but there is little direct evidence that they play a major role.

Conclusion

Having completed a survey of the role that genes play in the majority of conditions, disorders, and diseases that preoccupy us as we move through the life cycle, what is the bottom line? Although we are still in the earliest days of our effort to understand the role that common gene variants play in altering the threshold of risk for disease, evidence that they are important is accumulating rapidly. All too often, however, the suggestion that one's risk for an important ailment is for genetic reasons greater than that of other individuals is not accompanied by a prescription that provides a course of action to ameliorate that risk. For the moment, for many of the conditions discussed in this book, genetic risk information will mainly serve to reinforce well-established norms for healthy behavior. Some will react cynically to such an admission, opining that the information is not worth having. Others will see the acquisition of such information as a positive step forward because it will reinforce optimal health practices as they are currently understood. Of course, we have much to learn. However, we have the tools to learn and to apply that knowledge to create a new era of health.

Genetic medicine is still in its infancy, but as infants do, it will grow rapidly. How will genetic knowledge have changed the practice of medicine 20 years from now? How much better will we be at predicting the risk of disease based on family history and genetic tests? These questions are impossible to answer with certainty, but it is beyond dispute that long before 2024 we will have much better answers to many of the questions that I audaciously took on in this book. One way to support that assertion is to look back 20 years and note the gains in medical genetics during that time.

Even the most astute geneticist could not have predicted the time course and shape of the genetic revolution that took place in the 1990s. In

1984, the polymerase chain reaction (PCR), a technology that permits researchers to make limitless copies of any segment of DNA of interest to them (and a technology without which the Human Genome Project would never have been contemplated), had not yet been invented. Molecular biologists were just beginning to scale-up DNA sequencing technologies. Clinical geneticists were not equipped with the tools to establish the genotype–phenotype correlations that created the knowledge upon which much of this book is based. All but a few physicians thought of genetic disorders as rare conditions affecting children which arose because of a mutation in a single gene. No one had yet grasped the implications of the natural variability of the DNA sequence. DNA diagnostics was just beginning. Gene therapy was considered science fiction. Cloning mammals was not even the stuff of dreams.

In 1984, no one predicted that in the year 2000 the President of the United States, surrounded by scientists, would hold a press conference to declare that the human genome had been sequenced. Indeed, when the Human Genome Project was first contemplated in the mid 1980s, there were many skeptics. The doubters had good reasons. They knew that to learn the consensus sequence of the human genome in 15 years, the scientific teams would have to reduce significantly the cost of identifying each nucleotide while increasing the speed of doing so severalfold. They did.

The history of human genetics, especially since the 1970s, has been one of accelerating discovery and rapid transfer of new knowledge into medical practice. During the next 20 years, there will doubtless be many discoveries of major clinical importance that I cannot possibly anticipate. Knowing the futility of hazarding guesses about the nature of genetic medicine in 20 years, are there, nevertheless, predictions that one can make with some reasonable certainty? I think so.

In 2004, DNA-based susceptibility testing will be a standard part of routine preventive medicine. At each child's birth, genetic screening programs will routinely analyze a DNA sample to look for hundreds of genetic variants that predict risk for various disorders. Starting in childhood, lifestyle and wellness programs will be keyed in part to each individual's genetic profile. At first, physicians will mainly focus on the few variants with strong risk profiles; gradually they will incorporate more subtle risk information into prevention programs.

It will be possible to sequence and analyze a person's entire genome (about 26,000 genes) in less than one hour for about the cost charged today for sequencing just two genes (BRCA1 and BRCA2) in order to determine whether any cancer-predisposing mutations are present. Inexpensive sequencing machines that easily fit on a small table will be available in all hospitals and at many other locations. When surgeons operate on a person for cancer, they will send tumor tissue to a lab for genetic profiling. The genetic signature of the tumor will determine what drugs the doctor chooses to prevent recurrence of the disease. A person's sequence will be routinely compared to massive databases that correlate genotype with risk for disease.

Clinicians will routinely draw upon a wide array of biomarkers, one or more chemicals easily assayed in blood and other tissues, to help them identify people who are developing, but who have not yet shown any of the standard signs or symptoms of, particular diseases. Examples of this are already emerging, such as the discovery that biochemical signs of lupus are present as much as three years before any physical signs of ill health. Biomarkers will also be widely used to screen for occult disease. This will be especially helpful in catching and curing insidious and incurable diseases such as ovarian and pancreatic cancer. These will be sophisticated versions of tests like those used to screen for prostate cancer today.

Pharmacogenetics will be a central feature of drug discovery and choice of therapy. Today, the pharmaceutical industry develops, the FDA reviews and sometimes approves, and physicians prescribe, drugs that all know will benefit usually at most no more than 70% of the patients who take them. Long before 2024, all filings for the approval of new drugs made by the pharmaceutical companies before the FDA will be required to include pharmacogenetic data—information about how the efficacy of the particular compound varies with particular (common) genetic variants in the human subjects in whom the drug was tested. New drugs will be labeled to indicate that their use is indicated or contraindicated in people with certain genotypes.

Nutritional genetics will be a central feature of wellness programs. Motivated individuals will adhere to diets and consume particular nutraceuticals based on compatibility with their genetic profile. The rapidly growing nutrition business will be based on far more credible scientific evidence than it is today. Nutritional counseling will be replete with genetic analysis. Much of the focus will be on using a combination of genetic information, dietary choice, and fitness regimes to pursue a robust wellness into the ninth decade. Current ideas about extending the human life span will lead to the creation of products that really do increase the chances of becoming a centenarian.

Somatic cell gene therapy will be a central part of medical care. New treatments for cancer (based on proteins that block the actions of renegade cancer cells), heart disease (gene therapy to re-vascularize coronary arteries), and Alzheimer's disease (recombinant proteins to clean up the toxins that destroy brain cells) will be in use. Neurological diseases that we today think of as incurable, such as Parkinson's disease, amyotrophic lateral sclerosis, and Huntington disease, will be successfully treated by delivering genetically engineered cells that contain "normal" versions of disease genes directly to the involved areas of the brain where the faulty tissue is degenerating. Early warning signs of adult-onset diabetes will evoke a preemptive intervention that will ensure the ability of the pancreas to supply adequate insulin in a timely fashion.

Significant efforts will be under way to use genetic knowledge to treat language and learning disorders. For example, it has recently been shown that a gene called FOXP2 is essential to the development of language in humans. In one English family, mutations in that gene render people unable to articulate sounds or write properly. Germ-line gene therapy to treat single-gene disorders, to modify important genetic risk factors, and even to enhance certain aspects of phenotype such as height will be available.

Despite the controversies that will occasionally engulf it, there will be immense progress in behavioral genetics. We will identify gene variants that strongly predispose individuals to such disorders as schizophrenia and bipolar depression, as well as to more murky conditions such as addiction and violent behavior. Such findings will have huge implications for social policies affecting activities as diverse as adoption, funding of special education programs, managing behavioral issues in the classrooms, the practice of psychiatry, instructing juries on determination of guilt and innocence, and sentencing and parole decisions.

Knowledge of one's genetic profile will be crucial to a long and vigorous life. The concept of a medicine will be broadened, and the line between drugs and nutritional substances will be almost completely erased. In the economically powerful nations, most of medicine will be aimed at maximizing the chances of living vigorously until 100. Individuals who have the resources and the good sense to incorporate genetic risk information into their lives, much as do people today who are committed to healthy diets and logical exercise regimens, will be far more likely to reach that goal.

For Further Information

INTRODUCTION: GENETIC MEDICINE

King R.A., Rotter J.I., and Motulsky A.G., eds. 2002. *The genetic basis of common diseases*, 2nd edition, Oxford University Press, Oxford. This single-volume work (1076 pages) is probably the most accessible single reference for the practicing physician who wants to learn more about the role of genes in common diseases.

Molecular advances in genetic disease. 1992. *Science* **256:** 766–813. A series of articles exploring how new molecular knowledge has refined our understanding of causation in genetic disorders.

Online Mendelian Inheritance in Man (OMIM). For decades, every clinical geneticist has had a copy of Victor McKusick's monumental atlas (published by John Hopkins Press) on his desk. Now OMIM is easily accessible on-line at www. ncbi.nlm.nih/gov/omim/.

Rimoin D.L., Connor J.M., Pyeritz R.E., and Korf B.R. 2002. *Emery and Rimoin's principles and practice of medical genetics,* 4th edition. Churchill Livingstone, London. This three-volume, 4250-page tome is the bible of clinical genetics.

The puzzle of complex diseases. 2002. *Science* **296:** 685–704. A series of articles exploring the interaction of genes with environmental factors in the development of late-onset disorders.

Vogel F. and Motulsky A.G. 1986. *Human genetics: Problems and approaches,* 2nd edition. Springer Verlag, Berlin. This 807-page work, authored by two of the most influential teachers of human genetics, provides succinct material on areas of basic science ranging from evolution and population genetics to gene action and the role of mutation in disease.

www.genetests.org is a comprehensive site concerning clinical genetics that includes 225 short articles by experts providing overviews of mostly single-gene disorders and an extensive list of available genetic tests and laboratories that offer them. It is a federally funded site run as a not-for-profit operation by staff at the University of Washington, Seattle.

GENES AND MUTATIONS

Balmain A., Gray J., and Ponder B. 2003. The genetics and genomics of cancer. *Nature Genetics* (suppl.) **33:** 238–244.

245

Cold Spring Harbor Laboratory maintains the Dolan DNA Learning Center: http://www.dnalc.org.
Cooperative Human Linkage Center: (CHLC), http://www.chlc.org.
Diagnostic Interview for Genetic Studies: http://zork.wustl.edu.nimh.digs/newpage11.htm.
Guttmacher A.E. and Collins F.S. 2002. Genomic medicine—A primer. *New England Journal of Medicine* **347**: 1512–1521.
Marshfield Center for Medical Genetics: http://www.marshfieldclinic.org/research/genetics.
The National Library of Medicine has a website (http://ghr.nlm.nih.gov/Omim/ that is designed to teach both interested lay persons and physicians about the basics of genetics and the role of genes in disease.
UK Human Genome Mapping Project Resource Center: http://www.hgmp.mrc.ac.uk
Whitehead Institute: http://www-genome.wi.mit.edu.

PREGNANCY

Infertility

American College of Medical Genetics. 2001. Consensus statement on factor V Leiden mutation testing. *Genetics in Medicine* **3**: 139–148.
De Braekeleer M. and Dao T.N. 1991. Cytogenetic studies in male infertility: A review. *Human Reproduction* **6**: 245–250.
Layman L.C. 2003. Genetic causes of infertility. *Endocrinological and Metabolic Clinics of North America* **32**: 549–572.
Magli M., Granaroli L., Munne S., and Ferraretti F. 1998. Incidence of chromosomal abnormalities from a morphologically normal cohort of embryos in poor prognosis patients. *Journal of Assisted Reproduction and Genetics* **15**: 297–301.
Olesen C., Hanson C., Bendsen E., Byskov A.G., Schwinger E., Lopez-Pajaous I., et al. 2001. Identification of human candidate genes for male infertility by digital differential display. *Molecular Human Reproduction* **7**: 11–20.
Seminara S.B. and Crowley W.F. 2002. Genetic approaches to unraveling reproductive disorders: Examples of bedside to bench research in the genomic era. *Endocrine Reviews* **23**: 382–392.
Urbanek M., Legro R.S., Driscoll D.A., Azziz R., Ehrmann D.A., Norman R.J. et al. 1999. Thirty-seven candidate genes for polycystic ovary syndrome: Strongest evidence for linkage is with follistatin. *Proceedings of the National Academy of Sciences* **96**: 8573–8578.
Van Assche E., Bondvelle M., and Toumaye H. 1996. Cytogenetics of infertile men. *Human Reproduction* (suppl. 4) **11**: 1–24.

Endometriosis

Bischoff F.Z. and Simpson J.L. 2000. Heritability and molecular genetic studies of endometriosis. *Human Reproduction Update* **6**: 37–44.

Simpson J.L., Elias S., Malinak L.R., and Buttram V.C., Jr. 1980. Heritable aspects of endometriosis. I. Genetic studies. *American Journal of Obstetrics and Gynecology* **137**: 327–331.

Simpson J.L., Malinak L.R., Elias S., Carson S.A., and Radvany R.A. 1984. HLA association in endometriosis. *American Journal of Obstetrics and Gynecology* **148**: 395–397.

Stefansson H., Geirsson R.T., Steinthorsdottir V., Jonsson H., Manolescu A., Kong A. et al. 2002. Genetic factors contribute to the risk of developing endometriosis. *Human Reproduction* **17**: 555–559.

Treloar S., Hadfield R., Montgomery G., Lambert A., Wicks J., Barlow O.H. et al. 2002. The international endogene study: A collection of families for genetic research in endometriosis. *Fertility and Sterility* **78**: 679–685.

Uterine Fibroids

Center for Uterine Fibroids, Brigham and Women's Hospital, Boston, Massachusetts. www.fibroids.net/html/welcome.htm.

Treloar S.A,. Marin N.G., Dennerstein L., Raphael B., and Heath A.C. 1992. Pathways to hysterectomy: Insights from longitudinal twin research. *American Journal of Obstetrics and Gynecology* **167**: 82–88.

Vikhlhaeva E.M., Khodzhaeva Z.S., and Fantschenko N.D. 1995. Familial predisposition to uterine leiomyomas. *International Journal of Gynaecology and Obstetrics* **51**: 127–131.

Weremovicisz S., Somberger K., Dah Cin P., Vanni P., and Morton C.C. 1998. Characterization of HMGIC gene rearrangements in uterine leiomyomas by fluorescence in situ hybridization (FISH). *American Journal of Human Genetics* **499**: A91.

Consanguinity

Fraser G.R. and Mayo O. 1974. Genetic load in man. *Human Genetics* **23**: 83–110.

Freire-Maia N. 1989. Genetic effects in Brazilian populations due to consanguineous marriages. *American Journal of Medical Genetics* **35**: 115–117.

Morton N., Crow J.F., and Muller H.J. 1956. An estimate of the mutational damage in man from data on consanguineous marriages. *Proceedings of the National Academy of Sciences* **42**: 855–863.

Stoll C., Alembik Y., Roth M.P., and Dott B. 1999. Parental consanguinity as a cause of increased incidence of birth defects in a study of 238,942 consecutive births. *Annals of Genetics* **42**: 133–139.

Race and Ethnicity

Cao A., Pintus L., Lecca V., Olla G., Cossu P., Rosatelli C. et al. 1984. Control of homozygous beta-thalassemia by carrier screening and antenatal diagnosis in Sardinia. *Clinical Genetics* **26**: 12–22.

Kittles R.A. and Weiss K.M. 2003. Race, ancestry, and genes: Implications for defining disease risk. *Annual Review of Genomics and Human Genetics* 4: 33–68.

Merz B. 1987. Matchmaking scheme solves Tay-Sachs problem. *Journal of the American Medical Association* 258: 2636–2637.

Risch N., de Leon D., Ozelius L., Kramer P., Almasy L., Singer B. et al. 1995. Genetic analysis of idiopathic torsion dystonia in Ashkenazi Jews and their recent descent from a small founder population. *Nature Genetics* 9: 152–159.

Rutkow I.M. and Lipton J.M. 1974. Some negative aspects of the state health department's policies related to screening for sickle cell anemia. *American Journal of Public Health* 64: 217–222.

Recurrent Pregnancy Loss

Bricker L. and Farquharson R.G. 2002. Types of pregnancy loss in recurrent miscarriage: Implications for research and clinical practice. *Human Reproduction* 17: 1345–1350.

Brigham S.A., Conlon C., and Farquharson R.G. 1999. A longitudinal study of pregnancy outcome following idiopathic recurrent miscarriage. *Human Reproduction* 14: 2868–2871.

Li T.C., Makris M., Tomsu M., Tuckerman E., and Laird S. 2002. Recurrent miscarriage: Aetiology, management and prognosis. *Human Reproduction Update* 8: 463–481.

Stephenson M.D., Awartani K.A., and Robinson W.P. 2002. Cytogenetic analysis of miscarriages from couples with recurrent miscarriage: A case-control study. *Human Reproduction* 17: 446–451.

Preeclampsia

Arngrimsson R., Bjornsson S., Geirsson R.T., Bjornsson H., Walker J.J., Snadeal G. et al. 1990. Genetic and familial predisposition to eclampsia and pre-eclampsia in a defined population. *British Journal of Obstetrics and Gynaecology* 97: 762–769.

Arngrimsson R., Sigurardottir S., Frigge M.L., Bjarnadottir R.I., Jonsson T., Stefannsson H. et al. 1999. A genome-wide scan reveals a maternal susceptibility locus for pre-eclampsia on chromosome 2p13. *Human Molecular Genetics* 8: 1799–1805.

Laivuori H., Lahermo P., Ollikainen V., Widen E., Haiva-Maallinen L., Sundstrom H. et al. 2003. Susceptibility loci for preeclampsia on chromosomes 2p25 and 9p13 in Finnish families. *American Journal of Human Genetics* 72: 168–177.

Twinning

Bulmer M.G. 1970. *The biology of twinning in man.* Clarendon Press, Oxford.

Hall J.G. 2003. Twinning. *Lancet* 362: 735–743.

Meulemans W.J., Lewis C.M., Boomsma D.I., Derom C.A., Van den Berghe H., Orbbele J.F. et al. 1996. Genetic modeling of dizygotic twinning in pedigrees of spontaneous dizygotic twins. *American Journal of Medical Genetics* 61: 258–263.

White C. and Wyshak G. 1964. Inheritance of human dizygotic twinning. *New England Journal of Medicine* **271:** 1003–1005.

Premature Births

Chan E.C., Fraser S., Yeo Y.S., Kwek K., Fairclough R.J., and Smith R. 2002. Human myometrial genes are differentially expressed in labor: A suppression subtractive hybridization study. *Journal of Clinical Endocrinology and Metabolism* **87:** 2435–2441.

Dizon-Townson D.S. 2001. Preterm labour and delivery: A genetic predisposition. *Paediatric and Perinatal Epidemiolgy* (suppl.) **2:** 57–62.

NIH Guide: Program Annnouncement: Reproductive Genetics http://grants2.nih.gov/grants/guide/pa-files/PA-01-005.html.

Romero R., Kuivaniemi H., and Tromp G. 2002. Functional genomics and proteomics in term and preterm parturition. *Journal of Clinical Endocrinology & Metabolism* **87:** 2431–2434.

Wang X., Zuckerman B., Kaufman G., Wise P., Hill M., Niu T. et al. 2001. Molecular epidemiology of preterm delivery: Methodology and challenges. *Paediatric and Perinatal Epidemiology* **15:** 62–77.

INFANCY

Congenital Malformations (Birth Defects)

Aylsworth A.S. 1992. Genetic counseling for patients with birth defects. *Pediatric Clinics of North America* **39:** 229–253.

Boughman J.A., Ferencz C., and Neill C.A. 1989. Genetic advances in pediatric cardiology. *Current Opinion in Cardiology* **4:** 53–59.

Carter C.O. 1983. Congenital pyloric stenosis. In *Principles and practice in medical genetics* (ed. A.H. Emery and D.L. Rimoin), pp. 879–883. Churchill Livingstone, Edinburgh.

Christiansen B., Arbour L., and Tran P. 1999. Genetic polymorphisms in methylenetetrahydrofolate reductase and methionine synthase, folate levels in red blood cells, and risk of neural tube defects. *American Journal of Medical Genetics* **84:** 151–157.

Hook E.B. 1992. Chromosome abnormalities: Prevalence, risks, and recurrence. In *Prenatal diagnosis and screening* (ed. D.H. Brock et al.), pp. 351–367. Churchill Livingstone, Philadelphia.

Palmer R.M., Conneally .PN., and Yu P.L. 1974. Studies of the inheritance of idiopathic talipes equinovarus. *Orthopedic Clinics of North America* **5:** 99–110.

Rietburg C.C. and Lindhout D. 1993. Adult patients with spina bifida cystica: Genetic counseling, pregnancy and delivery. *European Journal of Obstetrics, Gynecology and Reproductive Biology* **52:** 63–70.

Wyszynski D.F., ed. 2002. Cleft Lip and Palate: From Origin to Treatment, Oxford University Press, United Kingdom.

Newborn Genetic Screening

Chace D.H., Kalas T., and Naylor E.W. 2002. The application of tandem mass spectrometry to neonatal screening for inherited disorders of intermediary metabolism. *Annual Review of Genomics and Human Genetics* **3:** 17–46.

Dussault J.H., Coulombe P., and LaBerge C. 1975. Preliminary report on a mass screening program for neonatal hypothyroidism. *Journal of Pediatrics* **86:** 670–674.

Pollitt R.J. 2001. Newborn mass screening versus selective investigation: Benefits and costs. *Journal of Inherited Metabolic Disorders* **24:** 299–302.

Waisbren S., Albers S., Amato A., Ampola M., Brewster T.G., Demmer L.R. et al. 2003. Effect of expanded newborn screening for biochemical genetic disorders on child outcomes and parental stress. *Journal of the American Medical Association* **290:** 2564–2572.

Wilcken B., Wiley V., Hammond J., and Carpenter K. 2003. Screening newborns for inborn errors of metabolism by tandem mass spectrometry. *New England Journal of Medicine* **348:** 2304–2312.

Deafness

Connexin-Deafness Homepage:http://www.crg.es/deafness/.

Cryns K., Orzan E., Murgia A., Huygen P.L.M., Moreno F., and del Castillo I. 2003. A genotype-phenotype correlation for gjb2 (connexin 26) deafness. *American Journal of Human Genetics* (suppl. to Volume 73, Abstract 2337).

Fraser G.R. 1976. *The causes of profound deafness in childhood.* Johns Hopkins University Press, Baltimore.

Friedman T.B. and Griffith A.J. 2003. Human nonsyndromic sensorineural deafness. *Annual Reviews of Genomics and Human Genetics* **4:** 341–402.

Hereditary Hearing Loss Homepage: http://www.uia.ac.be/dnalab/hhh/.

Petit C., Levilliers J., and Hardelin J.-P. 2001. Molecular genetics of hearing loss. *Annual Review of Genetics* **35:** 589–645.

Sudden Infant Death Syndrome

Adams E.J., Chavez G.F., Steen D., Shah R., Iyasu S., and Krous H.F. 1998. Changes in the epidemiologic profile of sudden infant death syndrome as rates decline among California infants: 1990–1995. *Pediatrics* **102:** 1445–1451.

Carolan P.L. 2002. Sudden infant death syndrome. *EMedicine Journal* 3(5) May 23, 2002. www.emedicine.com/PED/topic2171.htm.

Christiansen M., Larsen L.A., Fosdal I., Svendsen I.H., Andersen P.S., Kanters J.K., et al. Long QT syndrome: Genotype-phenotype relationship and relation to sudden infant death syndrome (SIDS). www.faseb.org/genetics/ashg99/f1618.htm

Cote A., Russo P., and Michaud J. 1999. Sudden unexpected deaths in infancy: What are the causes? *Journal of Pediatrics* **135:** 437–443.

Holton J.B., Allen J.T., Green C.A., Partington S., Gilbert R.E., and Berry P.J. 1991. Inherited metabolic diseases in the sudden infant death syndrome. *Archives of Disease in Childhood* **66:** 1315–1317.

CHILDHOOD

Cerebral Palsy

About UCP—Cerebral Palsy—Facts & Figures www.ucp.org/ucp_generaldoc.cfm/1/3/43-43-43/447y.

American College of Obstetricians and Gynecologists Task Force on Neonatal Encephalopathy and Cerebral Palsy, Neonatal Encephalopathy and Cerebral Palsy, ACOG: Washington D.C. 2003, 94 pages (may be ordered on www.acog.org).

Miller G. 1988. Ataxic cerebral palsy and genetic predisposition. *Archives of Disease in Childhood* **63**: 1260–1261.

Nelson K.B. 2003. Can we prevent cerebral palsy? *New England Journal of Medicine* **349**: 1765–1769.

Shields J.R. and Schifrin B.S. 1988. Perinatal antecedents of cerebral palsy. *Obstetrics and Gynecology* **71**: 899–905.

Mental Retardation

Batshaw M. 1993. Mental retardation. *Pediatric Clinics of North America* **40**: 507–521.

Battaglia A. and Corey J.C. 2003. Diagnostic evaluation of developmental delay/mental retardation: An overview. *American Journal of Medical Genetics* **117C**: 3–4.

Herbst D.S. and Baird P.S. 1982. Sib risks for nonspecific mental retardation in British Columbia. *American Journal of Medical Genetics* **13**: 197–208.

Herbst D.S. and Miller J.R. 1980. Nonspecific x-linked mental retardation II: The frequency in British Columbia. *American Journal of Medical Genetics* **7**: 461–469.

Laxova R., Ridler M.A., and Bowen-Bravery M. 1977. An etiological survey of the severely retarded Hertfordshire children who were born between January 1, 1965 and December 31, 1967. *American Journal of Medical Genetics* **1**: 75–86.

Turner G. and Partington M. 2000. Recurrence risks in undiagnosed mental retardation. *Journal of Medical Genetics* **37**: E45.

Autism

Auranen M., Vanhala R., Varilo T., Ayers K., Kempas E., and Yisaukko-Oja T. et al. 2003. A genome wide screen for autism-spectrum disorders: Evidence for a major susceptibility locus on chromosome 3q25-27. *American Journal of Human Genetics* **71**: 777–790.

Jamain S., Quach H., Betancur C., Rastam M., Colineaux C., Gillberg I.C. et al. 2003. Mutations of the X-linked genes encoding neuroligins NLGN3 and NLGN4 are associated with autism. *Nature Genetics* **34**: 27–28.

Madsen K.M., Lauritsen M.B., Pedersen C.B., Thorsen P., Plesner A.-M., Andersen P.H. et al. 2003. Thimerosal and the occurrence of autism: Negative ecological evidence from Danish population-based data. *Pediatrics* **112**: 604–606.

Rapin I. 2002. The autistic spectrum disorders. *New England Journal of Medicine* **347:** 302–303.

Shao Y., Cuccaro M.L., Hauser E.R., Raiford K.L., Menold M.M., Wolpert C.M. et al. 2003. Fine mapping of autistic disorder to chromosome 15q11-q13 by use of phenotypic subtypes. *American Journal of Human Genetics* **72:** 539–548.

Yonan A.Y., Alarcon M., Cheng R., Magnusson P., Spence S., Palmer A. et al. 2003. A genomewide screen of 345 families for autism-susceptibility loci. *American Journal of Human Genetics* **73:** 886–897.

Developmental Disabilities

Bakker C., van der Meulen E.M., Buitelaar J.K., Sandkujil L.A., Pauls D.L., Monsour A.J. et al. 2003. A whole-genome scan in 164 dutch sib pairs with attention-deficit/hyperactivity disorder: Suggestive evidence for linkage on chromosomes 7p and 15q. *American Journal of Human Genetics* **72:** 1251–1260.

Bartlett C.W., Flax J.F., Logue M.W., Vieland V.J., Bassett A.S.,Tallal P. et al. 2002. A major susceptibility locus for specific language impairment is located on 13q21. *American Journal of Human Genetics* **71:** 45–55.

Fisher S.E., Lai C.S.L., and Monaca A.P. 2003. Deciphering the genetic basis of speech and language disorders. *Annual Review of Neuroscience* **26:** 57–80.

Fisher S., Francks C., MacPhie L., Marlow A., Cardon L., and Monaco A. Genetics of developmental dyslexia. www.well.ox.ac.uk/monaco/dyslexiasimon.html.

Genetics of stuttering project. www.shs.uiuc.edu/research/stuttering/genetics.html.

O'Brien E.K., Zhang X., Nishimura C., Tomblin J.B., and Murray J.C. 2003. Association of specific language impairment (sli) to the region of 7q31. *American Journal of Human Genetics* **72:** 1536–1543.

Epilepsy (Seizures)

Baulac S., Huberfeld G., Gourfinkel-An I., Mitropoulou G., Beranger A., Prud'homme J.F. et al. 2001. First genetic evidence of GABA(A) receptor dysfunction in epilepsy: A mutation in the gamma2-subunit gene. *Nature Genetics* **28:** 46–48.

Chang B.S. and Lowenstein D.H. 2003. Epilepsy. *New England Journal of Medicine* **349:** 1257–1266.

Durner M., Keddache M.A., Tomasini L., Shinnar S., Resor S.R., Cohen J. et al. 2001. Genome scan of idiopathic generalized epilepsy: Evidence for major susceptibility gene and modifying genes influencing the seizure type. *Annals of Neurology* **49:** 328–335.

Noebels J.L. 2003. The biology of epilepsy genes. *Annual Review of Neuroscience* **26:** 599–625.

Pal D.K., Evgrafov O.V., Tabares P., Zhang F., Durner M., and Greenberg D.A. 2003. BRD2 (ring3) is a probable major susceptibility gene for common juvenile myoclonic epilepsy. *American Journal of Human Genetics* **73:** 261–270.

Juvenile Diabetes

Barnett A.H., Eff C., Leslie R.D., and Pyke D.A. 1981. Diabetes in identical twins: A study of 200 pairs. *Diabetologia* **20:** 87–93.

Juvenile Diabetes Research Foundation. www.jdrf.org.

Lie B.A., Todd J.A., Fleming P., Nerup J., Akselsen H.E., Joner G. et al. 2000. The predisposition to type 1 diabetes linked to the human leukocyte antigen complex includes at least one non-class II gene. *American Journal of Human Genetics* **64:** 793–800.

Maclaren N., Riley W., and Skordis N. 1988. Inherited susceptibility to insulin-dependent diabetes is associated with HLA-DR1 (and DR3 and DR4) while DR5 and DR6 are protective. *Autoimmunity* **1:** 197–205.

Rotter J.I. 1981. The modes of inheritance of insulin-dependent diabetes. *American Journal of Human Genetics* **33:** 835–851.

Tisch R. and McDevitt H. 1996. Insulin-dependent diabetes mellitus. *Cell* **85:** 291–297.

Asthma

Collabortive Study on the Genetics of Asthma. 1997. A genome-wide search for asthma susceptibility loci in ethnically diverse populations. *Nature Genetics* **15:** 389–392.

Cookson W. 1999. The alliance of genes and environment in asthma and allergy. *Nature* **25:** B5–B11.

Ghosh B., Sharma S., and Nagarkatti R. 2003. Genetics of asthma: Current research paving the way for development of personalized drugs. *Indian Journal of Medical Research* **117:** 185–197.

Hakonarson H. and Halapi E. 2002. Genetic analysis in asthma: Current concepts and future directions. *American Journal of Pharmacogenetics* **2:** 155–166.

Hakonarson H., Bjornsdottir U.S., Halapi E., Palsson S., Adalsteinsdottir E., Gislason D. et al. 2002. A major susceptibility gene for asthma maps to chromosome 14q24. *American Journal of Human Genetics* **71:** 483–491.

White N.J., Chiano M., Pillai S., Lam R., Brewster S., Ehm M. et al. 2003. A genome scan for asthma and a combined analysis of two asthma collections. *American Journal of Human Genetics* (suppl. to Volume 73, Abstract 1827.)

Zhang Y., Leaves N.I., Anderson G.G., Ponting C.P., Broxholme J., Holt R. et al. 2003. Positional cloning of a quantitative trait locus on chromosome 13q14 that influences immunoglobulin E levels and asthma. *Nature Genetics* **34:** 181–186.

Eczema

Eczema Association of Australasia, Local genetic experts launch national search for siblings suffering eczema. www.eczema.org.au/awareness_2003/.

Forrest S., Dunn K., Elliott K., Fitzpatrick E., Fullerton J., McCarthy M. et al. 1999. Identifying genes predisposing to atopic eczema. *Journal of Allergy and Clinical Immunology* **104:** 1066–1070.

Goldstein B.G. and Goldstein A. 1997. *Practical dermatology*, 2nd edition. Mosby, St. Louis.

MacLean J.A. and Eidelman F.J. 2001. The genetics of atopy and atopic eczema. *Archives of Dermatology* **137**: 1474–1476.

Tanaka K., Sugiura H., Uehara M., Hashimoto Y., Donnelly C., and Montgomery D.S. 2001. Lack of association between atopic eczema and the genetic variants of Interleukin-4 and the Interleukin-4 receptor alpha chain gene: Heterogeneity of genetic background on immunoglobulin E production in atopic eczema patients. *Clinical and Experimental Allergy* **31**: 1522–1527.

Scoliosis

Axenovich T.I., Zaidman A.M., Zorkoltseva I.V., Tregubova I.L., and Borodin P.M. 1999. Segregation analysis of idiopathic scoliosis: Demonstration of a major gene effect. *American Journal of Medical Genetics* **86**: 389–394.

Bashiardes S., Veile R., Wise C.A., Szoppanos L., and Lovett M. 2003. A candidate gene for idiopathic scoliosis. *American Journal of Human Genetics* (suppl. to Volume 73, Abstract 1987).

Kesling K.L. and Reinker A.K. 1997. Scoliosis in twins: A meta-analysis of the literature and report of six cases. *Spine* **22**: 2009–2014.

Robin G.C. and Cohen T. 1975. Familial scoliosis: A clinical report. *Journal of Bone and Joint Surgery in Britain* **57**: 146–147.

Stature

Harvey M.A.S., Smith D.W., and Skinner A.L. 1979. Infant growth standards in relation to parental stature. *Clinical Pediatrics* **18**: 602–603.

Hirschhorn J.N., Lindgren C.M., Daly M.J., Kirby A., Schaffner S., Burtt N.P. et al. 2001. Genomewide linkage analysis of stature in multiple populations reveals several regions with evidence of linkage to adult height. *American Journal of Human Genetics* **69**: 106–116.

Voss L.D. 1999. Short but normal. *Archives of Diseases in Childhood* **81**: 370–371.

Strabismus

Cross H.E. 1975. The heredity of strabismus. *American Orthopics Journal* **25**: 11–17.

Nelson L.B. 1983. Diagnosis and management of strabismus and amblyopia. *Pediatric Clinics of North America* **30**: 1003–1014.

Parikh V., Shugart Y.Y., Doheny K.F., Zhang J., Li L., Williams J. et al. 2003. A strabismus susceptibility locus on chromosome 7p. *Proceedings of the National Academy of Sciences* **100**: 12283–12288.

Paul T.O. and Hardage L.K. 1994. The heritability of strabismus. *Ophthalmalogical Genetics* **15**: 1–18.

Eye Color

Davenport G.C. and Davenport C.B. 1907. Heredity of eye color in man. *Science* **26:** 589–592.

Eiberg H. and Mohr J. 1987. Major genes of eye color and hair color linked to LU and SE. *Clinical Genetics* **31:** 186–191.

Eiberg H. and Mohr J. 1996. Assignment of genes for brown eye color (BEY2) and brown hair colour (HCL3) on chromosome 15q. *European Journal of Human Genetics* **4:** 237–241.

Larsson M., Pedersen N.L., and Statue H. 2003. Importance of genetic effects for characteristics of the human iris. *Twin Research* **6:** 192–200.

Mendelian Inheritance in Man Online; OMIM Entry 227220 Eye Color 3. www.ncbi.nlm.nih.gov/htbin-post/Omim/dispmim?227220.

Handedness

Annett M. 1978. Genetic and nongenetic influences on handedness. *Behavior Genetics* **8:** 227–249.

Francks C., DeLisi L.E., Fisher S.E., Laval S.H., Rue J.E., Stein J.F. et al. 2003. Confirmatory evidence for linkage of relative hand skill to 2p12-q11. *American Journal of Human Genetics* **72:** 499–502.

Francks C., Fisher S.E., MacPhie I.L., Richardson A.J., Marlow A.J., Stein J.F. et al. 2002. A genomewide linkage screen for relative hand skill in sibling pairs. *American Journal of Human Genetics* **70:** 800–805.

ADULTHOOD

Heart Diseases

Coronary Artery Disease (Atherosclerosis)

Arking D.E., Becker S.M., Yanek L.R., Fallin D., Judge D.P., Moy T.F. et al. 2003. KLOTHO allele status and the risk of early-onset occult coronary artery disease. *American Journal of Human Genetics* **72:** 1154–1161.

Becker D.M., Yook R.M., Moy T.F., Blumenthal R.S., and Becker L.C. 1998. Markedly high prevalence of coronary risk factors in apparently healthy African-Americans and white siblings of persons with premature coronary heart disease. *American Journal of Cardiology* **82:** 1046–1051.

Brand F.N., Kiely D.K., Kannel W.B., and Myers R.H. 1992. Family patterns of coronary heart disease mortality: The Framingham Heart Study. *Clinical Epidemiology* **45:**169–174.

Dwyer J.H., Allayee H., Dwyer K.M., Fan J., Wu H., Mar M. et al. 2004. Arachidonate 5-lipoxygenase promoter genotype, dietary arachidonic acid, and atherosclerosis. *New England Journal of Medicine* **350:** 29–39.

Hines L.M., Stamper S.M., Ma J., Gaziano M., Ridker P.M., Hankinson S.E. et al. 2001. Genetic variation in alcohol dehydrogenase and the beneficial effect of moderate alcohol consumption on myocardial infarction. *New England Journal of Medicine* **344:** 549–555.

Nabel E.G. 2003. Genomic medicine: Cardiovascular disease. *New England Journal of Medicine* **349:** 60–72.

Shea S., Ottman R., Gabriele C., Stein Z., and Nichols A. 1983. Family history as an independent risk factor for coronary artery disease. *Journal of the American College of Cardiology* **4:** 793–801.

High Cholesterol

Breslow J.L. 1991. Familial disorders of high density lipoprotein metabolism. In *The metabolic basis of inherited disease* (ed. C. Scriver et al.), pp. 1251–1264. McGraw Hill, New York.

Nabel E.G. 2003. Genomic medicine: Cardiovascular disease. *New England Journal of Medicine* **349:** 60–72.

Pajukanta P., Nuotio I., Terwilliger J.D., Porkka K.V., Ylitalo K., Pihlajamki J. et al. 1998. Linkage of familial combined hyperlipidemia to chromosome 1q21-q23. *Nature Genetics* **18:** 369–373.

Williams R.R., Hunt S.C., Hopkins P.N., Wu L.L., Hasstedt S.J., Berry T.D. et al. 1993. Genetic basis of familial dyslipidemia and hypertension: 15 Year results from Utah. *American Journal of Hypertension* **6:** 319S–327S.

High Blood Pressure

Arnett D.K. Molecular genetics of hypertension and its complications. National Heart Lung and Blood Institute Satellite symposium. www.nhlbi.nih.gov/meetings/ish/arnett.htm.

Hong Y., de Faire U., Heller D.A., McLearn G.E., and Pedersen N. 1994. Genetic and environmental influences on blood pressure in elderly twins. *Hypertension* **24:** 663–670.

Hopkins P.N. and Hunt S.C. 2003. Genetics of hypertension. *Genetics in Medicine* **5:** 413–429.

Lauer R.M., Burns T.L., Clarke W.R., and Mahoney L.T. 1991. Childhood predictors of future blood pressure. *Hypertension* **18:** 74–81.

Levy D., DeStanfano A.L., Larson M.G., O'Donnell C.J., Lifton R.P., Gavras H. et al. 2000. Evidence for a gene influencing blood pressure on chromosome 17: Genome scan linkage results for longitudinal blood pressure phenotypes in subjects from the Framingham Heart Study. *Hypertension* **36:** 477–483.

Tambs K., Moum T., Holmen J., Eaves L.J., Neale M.C., Lund-Larssen G. et al. 1992. Genetic and environmental effects on blood pressure in a Norwegian sample. *Genetic Epidemiology* **9:** 11–26.

Cardiomyopathy

Baylor Heart Clinic, Familial hypertrophic cardiomyopathy. www.bcm.tmc.edu/cardio/bhc/specializations/genetic.html.

Cannon R.O. 2003. Assessing risk in hypertrophic cardiomyopathy. *New England Journal of Medicine* **349:** 1016–1018.

Grunig E., Tasman J.A., Kucherer H., Franz W., Kubler W., and Katus H.A. 1998. Frequency and phenotypes of familial dilated cardiomyopathy. *Journal of the American College of Cardiology* **31:** 186–194.

Michels V.V., Moll P.P., Miller F.A., Tajik A.J., Chu J.S., Driscoll D.J. et al. 1992. The frequency of familial dilated cardiomyopathy in a series of patients with idiopathic dilated cardiomyopathy. *New England Journal of Medicine* **326:** 77–82.

Rampazzo A., Nava A., Malacrida S., Beffagna G., Bauce B., Rossi V. et al. 2002. Mutation in human desmoplakin domain binding to plakoglobin causes a dominant form of arrhythmogenic right ventricular cardiomyopathy. *American Journal of Human Genetics* **71:** 1200–1206.

Pulmonary Embolism

Lee R. 1996. Thromboembolic disease and pregnancy: Are all women equal? *Annals of Internal Medicine* **125:** 1001–1003.

Nizankowska-Mogilnicka E., Adamnek L., Grzanka P., Domagala T.B., Sanaka M., Krzanowski M. et al. 2003. Genetic polymorphisms associated with acute pulmonary embolism and deep venous thrombosis. *European Respiratory Journal* **21:** 25–30.

Ridker P.M., Hennekens C.H., Lindpaintner K., Stampfer M.J., Eisenberg P.R., and Miletich J.P. 1995. Mutation in the gene coding for coagulation factor V and the risk of myocardial infarction, stroke, and venous thrombosis in apparently healthy men. *New England Journal of Medicine* **332:** 912–917.

Wald D.S., Law M., and Morris J.K. 2002. Homocysteine and cardiovascular disease: Evidence on causality from a meta-analysis. *British Medical Journal* **325:** 1202.

Westrich G.H., Weksler B.B., Glueck C.J., Blumenthal B.F., and Salvati E.A. 2002. Correlation of thrombophilia and hypofibrinolysis with pulmonary embolism following total hip arthroplasty. *Journal of Bone and Joint Surgery* **84:** 2161–2167.

Sudden Death

Hodginkinson K., Parfrey P., Stuckless S., Theirfelder L., Dicks E., Bassett A. et al. 2003. Arrhythmogenic right ventricular cardiomyopathy linked to 3p25: Ventricular dysrhythmias and early sudden death, prevented in males with implantable cardioverter defibrillator therapy. *American Journal of Human Genetics* (suppl. to Volume 73 Abstract 578).

Maron B.J. 2003. Sudden death in young athletes. *New England Journal of Medicine* **349:** 1064–1075.

Priori S.G., Schwartz P.J., Napolitano C., Bloise R., Ronchetti E., Grillo M. et al. 2003. Risk stratification in long QT syndrome. *New England Journal of Medicine* **348:** 1866–1874.

Roberts R. and Brugada R. 2003. Genetics and arrhythmias. *Annual Review of Medicine* **54:** 257–267.

Aortic Aneurysms

Boyd C.D. and Tilson M.D. 1996. *The abdominal aortic aneurysm: Etiology, pathophysiology and genetics.* New York Academy of Sciences, New York.

Hasham S.N., Guo P.C., and Milewicz D.M. 2002. Genetic basis of thoracic aortic aneurysms and dissections. *Current Opinion in Cardiology* **17:** 677–683.

Helliker K. and Burton T.M. 2003. Medical ignorance contributes to toll from aortic illness. *Wall Street Journal,* November 4, 2003. p. 1.

Hirose H., Takagi M., Miyagawa N., Hashiyada H., Noguchi M., Tada S. et al. 1998. Genetic risk factor for abdominal aortic aneurysm: HLA_DR2(15), a Japanese study. *Journal of Vascular Surgery* **27:** 500–503.

Milewicz D.M. and Fadulu V.T. 2003. Thoracic aortic aneurysms and aortic dissections. www.genetests.org. Posted February 13, 2003.

Salo J.A., Soisalon-Soininen S., Bondestam S., and Matilla P.S. 1999. Familial occurrence of abdominal aortic aneurysm. *Annals of Internal Medicine* **130:** 637–642.

Wassef M., Baxter B.T., Chisholm R.L., Dalman R.L., Fillinger M.I., Heinecke J. et al. 2001. Pathogenesis of abdominal aortic aneurysms: A multidisciplinary research program supported by the National Heart, Lung and Blood Institute. *Journal of Vascular Surgery* **34:** 730–738.

Atrial Fibrillation

Ellinor P.T. and McCrae C.A. 2003. The genetics of atrial fibrillation. *Journal of Cardiovascular Electrophysiology* **14:** 207–209.

Ellinor P.T., Shin J.T., Moore R.K., Yoerger D.M., and MacRae C.A. 2003. Locus for atrial fibrillation maps to chromosome 6q14-16. *Circulation* **107:** 2880–2883.

Gaudino M., Andreotti F., Zamparelli R., Di Castelnuovo A., Nasso G., Buzotta F. et al. 2003. The –74G/C interleukin-6 polymorphism influences postoperative interleukin-6 levels and postoperative atrial fibrillation. Is atrial fibrillation an inflammatory complication? *Circulation* **108:** 195–199.

Mestroni L. 2003. Genomic medicine and atrial fibrillation. *Journal of the American College of Cardiology* **41:** 2193–2196.

Munich Alliance for Genomic Research in Cardiac Arrhythmias. Functional genomic studies on the pathogenesis and pharmacogenomics of atrial fibrillation. www.rzpd.de/ngfn_en/hk_muen.html.

Yusuf S., Fenske C., Dalageorgou C., Caster N., Alsaady N., Maarouf N. et al. 2003. Modulation of 5-hydroxytryptamine 4 (5ht4) receptor isoform expression predispose to atrial fibrillation after coronary artery bypass surgery. *American Journal of Human Genetics* (suppl. to Volume 73, Abstract 1015).

Mitral Valve Prolapse

Devereux R.B. and Brown W.T. 1983. Genetics of mitral valve prolapse. *Progress in Medical Genetics* **5**: 139–161.

Disse S., Abergel E., Berrebi A., Huout A.-M., and Le Heusey J.-Y. 1999. Mapping of a first locus for autosomal dominant myxomatous mitral-valve prolapse to chromosome 16p11.2-p12.1. *American Journal of Human Genetics* **65**: 1242–1251.

Freed L.A., Acierno J.S. Jr., Dai D., Leyne M., Marshall J.E., Nesta F. et al. 2003. A locus for autosomal dominant mitral valve prolapse on chromosome 11p15.4. *American Journal of Human Genetics* **72**: 1551–1559.

Leyne M., Nesta F., Dai D., Acierno J., Freed L., Levine R. et al. 2003. Examination of the mitral valve prolapse locus on chromosome 11p15.4. *American Journal of Human Genetics* (suppl. to Volume 73, Abstract 2272).

Longevity

Finch C.E. and Ruvkun G. 2001. The genetics of aging. *Annual Review of Genomics and Human Genetics* **2**: 435–462.

Geesaman B.J., Benson E., Brewster S.J., Kunkel L.M., Blanche H., Thomas G. et al. 2003. Haplotype-based identification of a microsomal transfer protein marker associated with human lifespan. *Proceedings of the National Academy of Science* **100**: 14115–14120.

Hall S. 2003. In vino vitalis? Compounds activate life-extending genes. *Science* **301**: 1165.

Martin G.W. 1997. The genetics of aging. *Hospital Practice* February 15: 47–66.

News Focus, 2003. Sardinia's mysterious male methuselahs. *Science* **291**: 2074.

Puca A.A., Daly M.J., Brewster S.J., Matisse T.C., Barrett J., and Shea-Drinkwater K. 2001. A genome wide scan for linkage to human exceptional longevity identifies a locus on chromosome 4. *Proceedings of the National Academy of Sciences* **98**: 10505–10508.

Vaupel J.W., Carey J.R., and Christiansen K. 2003. It's never too late. *Science* **301**: 1679–1682.

Lung Diseases

Chronic Obstructive Pulmonary Disease (COPD, Emphysema)

Hakonarson H., Halapi E., Sigvaldason A., Jonsson H., Gislason T., Laufs J. et al. 2003. A linkage study in heavy smokers suggests the presence of both causative and protective genes for chronic obstructive pulmonary disease (copd). *American Journal of Human Genetics* (suppl. to Volume 73, Abstract 78).

Kueppers F., Miller R.D., Gordon H., Hepper N.G., and Offord K. 1977. Familial prevalence of chronic obstructive pulmonary disease in a matched pair study. *American Journal of Medicine* **63**: 336–342.

Sandford A.J. and Pare P.D. 2000. Genetic risk factors for chronic obstructive pulmonary disease. *Clinics in Chest Medicine* **21**: 633–643.

Sarcoidosis

Berlin M., Fogdell-Hahn A., Olerup O., Ekbund A., and Grunewald J. 1997. HLA-DR predicts the prognosis in Scandinavian patients with pulmonary sarcoidosis. *American Journal of Respiratory and Critical Care Medicine* **156:** 1601–1605.

Du Bois R. 2001. Sarcoidosis: Do our genes really matter? *American Journal of Respiratory and Critical Care* **164:** 725–726.

Grutters J.C., Sato H., Pantelidis P., Lagan A.L., McGrath D.S., Lammers J. et al. 2002. Increased frequency of the uncommon tumor necrosis factor -857T allele in British and Dutch patients with sarcoidosis. *American Journal of Respiratory and Critical Care Medicine* **165:** 1119–1124.

McGrath D.S., Daniil Z., Foley P., duBois J.L., Lympany P.A., Cullinan P. et al. 2000. Epidemiology of familial sarcoidosis in the UK. *Thorax* **55:** 751–754.

Newman L.S., Rose C.S., and Maier A.L. 1997. Sarcoidosis. *New England Journal of Medicine* **336:** 1224–1234.

Rossman M.D., Thompson B., Frederick M., Maliarik M., Iannuzzi M.C., Rybicki B.A. et al. 2003. HLA-DRB1*1101: A significant risk factor for sarcoidosis in blacks and whites. *American Journal of Human Genetics* **73:** 720–735.

Sarcoidosis Genetic Analysis Study. More information on sarcoidosis: background and significance from the NHLBI Grant. www.saga.njc.org/background.html.

Gastrointestinal Diseases

Inflammatory Bowel Disease

Brant S.R., Panhuysen C.I.M., Nicolae D., Reddy M., Bonen K.M., Karaliukas R. et al. 2003. Mdr1 ala893 polymorphism is associated with inflammatory bowel disease. *American Journal of Human Genetics* **73:** 1282–1292.

The IBD International Genetics Consortium. 2001. International collaboration provides convincing linkage replication in complex disease through analysis of a large pooled data set: Crohn disease and chromosome 16. *American Journal of Human Genetics* **68:** 1165–1171.

Podolsky D.K. 2002. Inflammatory bowel disease. *New England Journal of Medicine* **347:** 417–429.

Sugimura K., Taylor K.D., Lin Y.C., Hang T., Wang D., Tang Y.M. et al. 2003. A novel NOD2/CARD15 haplotype conferring risk for Crohn disease in Ashkenazi Jews. *American Journal of Human Genetics* **72:** 509–518.

Yang H. and Rotter J. 2000. The genetics of ulcerative colitis and Crohn's disease. In *Inflammatory bowel disease*, 5th edition (ed. J.B. Kirsner), pp. 250–279. W.B. Saunders, Philadelphia.

Peptic Ulcer Disease

Brenner H., Rothenbacher D., Bode G., and Adler G. 1998. The individual and joint contributions of *Helicobacter pylori* infection and family history to the risk for peptic ulcer disease. *Journal of Infectious Disease* **177:** 1124–1127.

Malaty H.M., Engstrand L., Pedersen N.L., and Graham D.Y. 1994. *Helicobacter pylori* infection: Genetic and environmental influences. A study of twins. *Annals of Internal Medicine* **120:** 982–986.

Malaty H.M., Graham D.Y., Isaksson I., Engstrand L., and Pedersen N.L. 2000. Are genetic influences on peptic ulcer disease dependent or independent of genetic influences for *Helicobacter pylori* infection? *Archives of Internal Medicine* **160:** 105–109.

Otaki Y., Azuma T., Konishi J., Ito S., and Kuriyama M. 1997. Association between genetic polymorphism of the pepsinogen C gene and gastric body ulcer: The genetic predisposition is not associated with *Heliobacter pylori* infection. *Gut* **41:** 469–474.

Rotter J.I., Rimoin D.L., Gursky J.M., Tersaki P., and Sturdevant R.A. 1977. HLA-B5 associated with duodenal ulcer. *Gastroenterology* **73:** 438–440.

Celiac Disease (Gluten-sensitive Enteropathy)

Maki M., Mustalahti K., Kokkonen J., Kulmala P., Haapalahti M., Karttunen T. et al. 2003. Prevalence of celiac disease among children in Finland. *New England Journal of Medicine* **348:** 2517–2524.

McManus R. and Kelleher D. 2003., Celiac disease—The villain unmasked? *New England Journal of Medicine* **348:** 2573–2575.

Naluai A.T., Adamovic S., Louka A.S., Nilsson S., Talseth B., Gudjonstottir A.H. et al. 2003. Celiac disease is associated to a haplotype on 5q in Scandinavian families. *American Journal of Human Genetics* (suppl. to Volume 73, Abstract 1803).

Van Belzen M., Zhernakeva A., Bardoel A., Houwen R., Mulder C., and Wijmenga C. 2003. Identification of a celiac disease gene on chromosome 19. *American Journal of Human Genetics* (supplement of Volume 73, Abstract 2056).

Pancreatitis

Chen J.-M. and Ferec. C. 2000. Molecular basis of hereditary pancreatitis. *European Journal of Human Genetics* **8:** 473–479.

Hirota M., Kuwata K., Ohmuraya M., and Ogawa M. 2003. From acute to chronic pancreatitis: The role of mutations in the pancreatic secretory trypsin inhibitor gene. *Journal of the Pancreas* (Online) **4:** 83–88.

Le Marechal C., Chen J.M., Le Gall C., Plessis G., Chipponi J., Chuzhanova N.A. et al. 2003. Two novel severe mutations in the pancreatic secretory trypsin inhibitor gene (SPINK1) cause familial or/and hereditary pancreatitis. *American Journal of Human Genetics* (suppl. to Volume 73, Abstract 2325).

Lactose Intolerance (Lactase Deficiency)

Jarvela I., Sabri Enattah N., Kokkonen J., Varilo T., Savilahti E., and Peltonnen L. 2002. Assignment of the locus for congenital lactase deficiency to 2q21, in the vicinity of but separate from the lactase-phlorizin hydrolase gene. *American Journal of Human Genetics* **63:** 1078–1085.

Metneki J., Cziezel A., Flatz S.D., and Flatz G. 1984. A study of lactose absorption capacity in twins. *Human Genetics* **67:** 296–300.

Swallow D.M. 2001. Genetics of lactase persistence and lactose intolerance. *Annual Review of Genetics* **37:** 197–219.

Swallow D.M. and Hollox E.J. 2000. The genetic polymorphism of intestinal lactase deficiency in adult humans. In *The metabolic and molecular basis of inherited disease* (ed. C.R. Scriver et al.), pp. 1651–1663. McGraw Hill, New York.

Appendicitis

Andersson N., Griffiths H., Murphy J., Roll J., Serenyi A., Swann I. et al. 1979. Is appendicitis familial? *British Medical Journal* **2:** 697–698.

Basta M., Morton N.E., Mulvihill J.J., Radovanovic Z., Radojicic C., and Marinkovic D. 1990. Inheritance of acute appendicitis: Familial aggregation and evidence of polygenic transmission. *American Journal of Human Genetics* **46:** 377–382.

Holman B.L. 2002. Acute appendicitis in children: The importance of family history. *Journal of Pediatric Surgery* **37:** 1214–1217.

National Digestive Diseases Information Clearinghouse, Appendicitis. www.niddk. nih.gov/health/digest/summary/append/index.htm.

Gallstones (Cholecystitis, Gallbladder Disease)

Kesaniemi Y.A., Koskenvuo M., Vuoristo M., and Miettinen T.A. 1989. Biliary lipid composition in monozygotic and dizygotic pairs of twins. *Gut* **30:** 1750–1756.

Lin J.-P. 1994. Genetic epidemiology of gall bladder disease in Mexican-Americans and cholesterol 7alpha-hydroxylase gene variation. *American Journal of Human Genetics* (suppl. to Volume 55, Abstract 48).

National Digestive Diseases Information Clearinghouse, Gallstones. www.niddk.nih. gov/health/digest/pubs/gallstns/gallstns.htm.

Sama C., Labate A.M., Taroni F., and Barbara L. 1990. Epidemiology and natural history of gallstone disease. *Seminars in Liver Disease* **10:** 149–158.

Endocrine Disorders

Adult-onset Diabetes (NIDDM, Diabetes Type II)

Busfield F., Duffy D.L., Kesting J.B., Walker S.M., Lovelock P.K. et al. 2002. A genomewide search for type diabetes-susceptibility genes in indigenous Australians. *American Journal of Human Genetics* **70:** 349–357.

Ehm M.G., Karnoub M.C., Sakul H., Gottschalk K., Holt D.C. et al. 2000. Genomewide search for type 2 diabetes susceptibility genes in four American populations. *American Journal of Human Genetics* **66:** 1871–1881.

Florez J.C., Hirschhorn J., and Altshuler D.M. 2003. The inherited basis of diabetes mellitus: Implications for the genetic analysis of complex traits. *Annual Review of Genomics and Human Genetics* **4:** 257–292.

Grzeszczak W., Moczulski D.K., Zychma M., Zukowska-Szczechowska E., Trautsolt W., and Szydlowska I. 2001. Role of GLUT1 gene in susceptibility to diabetic nephropathy in type 2 diabetes. *Kidney International 2001* **59:** 631–636.

Reynisdottir I., Thorliefsson G., Benedittsson R., Sigurdsson G., Emilsson V., Einarsdottir A.S. et al. 2003. Localization of a susceptibility gene for type 2 diabetes to chromosome 5q34-q35.2. *American Journal of Human Genetics* **73:** 323–335.

Obesity

Atwood L.D., Heard-Costa N.L., Cupples La, Jaquish C.E., Wilson P.W.F., and D'Agostino R.B. 2002. Genomewide linkage analysis of body mass index across 28 years of the Framingham Heart Study. *American Journal of Human Genetics* **71:** 1044–1050.

Cummings D. and Schwartz M.W. 2003. Genetics and pathophysiology of human obesity. *Annual Review of Medicine* **54:** 453–472.

Hager J. 2003. Targeting obesity through genetics. *Current Drug Discovery.* November: 15–19.

Hager J., Dina C., Francke S., Dubois S., Houari M., Vatin V. et al. 1998. A genomewide scan for human obesity genes reveals a major susceptibility locus on chromosome 10. *Nature Genetics* **20:** 304–308.

List J.F. and Habener J.F. 2003. Defective melanocortin 4 receptors in hyperphagia and morbid obesity. *New England Journal of Medicine* **348:** 1160–1164.

Obesity Gene Map Database. http://obesitygene.pbrc.edu.

Osteoporosis

Arden N.K., Baker J., Hegg C., Baan K., and Spector T.D. 1996. The heritability of bone mineral density, ultrasound of the calcaneus and hip axis length: A study of postmenopausal twins. *Journal of Bone and Mineral Research* **11:** 530–534.

Cardon L.R., Garner C., Bennett S.T., Mackay J.J., Edwards R.M., Cornish J. et al. 2000. Evidence of a major gene for bone mineral density in idiopathic osteoporotic families. *Journal of Bone and Mineral Research* **15:** 1132–1137.

Peacock M., Turner C.H., Econs M.J., and Foroud T. 2002. Genetics of osteoporosis. *Endocrine Reviews* **23:** 303–326.

Prockop D.J. 1998. The genetic trail of osteoporosis. *New England Journal of Medicine* **338:** 1061–1062.

Ralston S.H. 2002. Genetic control of susceptibility to osteoporosis. *Journal of Clinical and Endocrinological Metabolism* **87:** 2460–2467.

Stewart T.L. and Ralston S.H. 2000. Role of genetic factors in the pathogenesis of osteoporosis. *Journal of Endocrinology* **166:** 235–245.

Uitterlinden A.G., Burger S., Huang O., Yue F., McGuigan F.E., and Grant S.F. 1998. Relation of alleles of the collagen type I alpha 1 gene to bone density and the risk of osteoporotic fractures in postmenopausal women. *New England Journal of Medicine* **338:** 1016–1021.

Thyroid Diseases

Alkhaeeb A., Stettler G.L., Old W., Talbert J., Uhlhorn C., Taylor M. et al. 2002. Mapping of an autoimmunity susceptibility locus (A1S1) to chromosome 1p31.3-p32.2. *Human Molecular Genetics* **11:** 661–667.

Imrie H., Vaidya B., Perros P., Kelly W.F., Toft A.D., Young E.T. et al. 2001. Evidence for a Graves' disease susceptibility locus at chromosome Xp11 in a United Kingdom population. *Journal of Clinical Endocrinology and Metabolism* **86:** 626–630.

Pearce E.N., Farwell A.P., and Braverman L.E. 2003. Thyroiditis. *New England Journal of Medicine* **348:** 2646–2655.

Tomer Y., Ban Y., Concepcion E., Barbesino G., Villaneuva R., Greenberg D.A., and Davies T.F. 2003. Common and unique susceptibility loci in Graves' and Hashimoto diseases: Results of whole-genome screening in a data set of 102 multiplex families. *American Journal of Human Genetics* **73:** 736–747.

Infectious Diseases

Susceptibility to Infection

Barnes P.F. and Cave M.D. 2003. Molecular epidemiology of tuberculosis. *New England Journal of Medicine* **349:** 1149–1156.

Bleharski J.R., Li H., Meinken C., Graeber T.G., Ochoa M.-T., Yamamura M. et al. 2003. Use of genetic profiling in leprosy to discriminate clinical forms of the disease. *Science* **301:** 1527–1531.

Bucheton B., Abel L., El-Safi S., Kheir M.M., Pavek S., Lemainque A. et al. 2003. A major susceptibility locus on chromosome 22q12 plays a critical role in the control of kala-azar. *American Journal of Human Genetics* **73:** 1052–1060.

Hill A.V. 2001. The genomics and genetics of human infectious disease susceptibility. *Annual Review of Genomics and Human Genetics* **2:** 373–400.

Omi K., Ohashi J., Patarapotikul J., Hananatachi H., Naka I., Looareesuwan S. et al. 2003. CD36 polymorphism is associated with protection from cerebral malaria. *American Journal of Human Genetics* **72:** 364–374.

HIV/AIDS

Centers for Disease Control and Prevention. 2001. Chances of HIV Infection. *Washington Post* February 9, p. 5.

Majumder P.P. and Dey B. 2001. Absence of the HIV-1 protective delta ccr5 allele in most ethnic populations of India. *European Journal of Human Genetics* **9:** 794–796.

O'Brien S.J. and Dean M. 1997. In search of AIDS resistance genes. *Scientific American* **277:** 44–51.

Paxton W.A. and Kang S. 1998. Chemokine receptor allelic polymorphisms: Relationships to HIV resistance and disease progression. *Seminars in Immunology* **10:** 187–194.

Wiencke J.K., Kelsey K.T., Zuo Z.-F., Weinberg A., and Wrensch M.R. 2001. Genetic resistance factor for HIV-1 and immune response to varicella zoster virus. *Lancet* **357:** 360.

Rheumatological Disorders

Rheumatoid Arthritis

Barrera P., Radstake T.R., Albers J.M., van Riel P.L., van de Putte L.B. et al. 1999. Familial aggregation of rheumatoid arthritis in the Netherlands: A cross-sectional hospital-based survey. *Rheumatology* **38:** 415–422.

Bellamy N., Duffy D., Martin N., and Mathews J. 1992. Rheumatoid arthritis in twins: A study of aetiopathogenesis based on the Australian twin registry. *Annals of Rheumatological Diseases* **51:** 588–593.

Feldman M., Brennan F.M., and Maini R.N. 1996. Rheumatoid arthritis. *Cell* **85:** 307–310.

NIH News Release. Nationwide hunt for rheumatoid arthritis genes launched: National Institutes of Health and Arthritis Foundation announce research partnership. www.nih.gov/news/pr/sept97/niams-o4.htm.

Pascaul M., Lopez-Nevot M.A., Caliz R., Ferrer M.A., Balzo A., Pascual-Salcedo D., and Martin J. 2003. A poly(adp-ribose) polymerase haplotype spanning the promoter region confers susceptibility to rheumatoid arthritis. *Arthritis & Rheumatism* **48:** 638–641.

Remmers E., Balow J., Li W., Aksentijevich I., Lee A.., Damle A. et al. 2003. Possible association of a 14 kb haplotype block from the receptor activator of NF-kappa B (RANK) gene with susceptibility to rheumatoid arthritis. *American Journal of Human Genetics* (suppl. to Volume 73, Abstract 2156).

Osteoarthritis

Aignee T. and Dudhia J. 2003. Genomics of osteoarthritis. *Current Opinion in Rheumatology* **15:** 634–640.

Ingvarsson T.G., Stefansson S.E., Halgrimsdottir I.B., Grigge M.L., Jonsson H. Jr., Gulcher J. et al 2000. The inheritance of hip osteoarthritis in Iceland. *Arthritis and Rheumatism 2000* **43:** 2785–2792.

Jonsson H., Manolescu I., Stefansson S.E., Ingvarsson T., Jonsson H.H., Manolescu A. et al. 2003. The inheritance of hand osteoarthritis in Iceland. *Arthritis & Rheumatism* **48:** 391–395.

MacGregor A.J. and Spector T.D. 1999. Twins and the genetic architecture of osteoarthritis. *Rheumatology* **38:** 583–590.

Gout

Chen S.Y., Chen C.L., Shen M.L., and Kamatani N. 2001. Clinical features of familial gout and effects of probable genetic association between gout and its related disorders. *Metabolism* **50:** 1203–1207.

Klemp P., Stamfield S.A., Castle B., and Robertson M.C. 1997. Gout is on the increase in New Zealand. *Annals of Rheumatological Diseases* **56:** 22–26.

Rich R.L., Nance W.E., Corey L.A., and Boughman J.A. 1978. Evidence for genetic factors influencing serum uric acid levels in man. In *Twin research: Clinical studies* (ed. W.E. Nance), pp. 187–192. Alan R. Liss, New York.

Terkeltaub R.A. 2003. Gout. *New England Journal of Medicine* **349**: 1647–1655.

Lupus

Graham R.R., Ortmann W.A., Langefeld C.D., Jawaheer D., Selby S.A., Rodine P.R. et al. 2002. Visualizing human leukocyte antigen class II risk haplotypes in human systemic lupus erythematosus. *American Journal of Human Genetics* **71**: 543–553.

Johanneson B., Lima G., von Salome J., Alarcon-Segovia D., Alarcon-Riquelme M.E., Collaborative Group on the Genetics of SLE et al. 2002. A major susceptibility locus for systemic lupus erythematosis maps to chromosome 1q31. *American Journal of Human Genetics* **71**: 1060–1071.

Kotzin B.L. 1996. Systemic lupus erythematosus. *Cell* **85**: 303–306.

Lawrence J.S., Martins C.L., and Drake G.L. 1987. A family survey of lupus erythematosis 1. Heritability. *Journal of Rheumatology* **14**: 913–921.

Reichlin M., Harley J.B., and Lockshin M.D. 1992. Serologic studies of monozygotic twins with systemic lupus erythematosus. *Arthritis and Rheumatism* **35**: 457–464.

Fibromyalgia Syndrome

Dudek D.M., Arnold L.M., Iyengar S.K., Khan M.A., Russell I.J., Yunus M.B. et al. 2003. Genetic linkage of fibromyalgia to the serotonin receptor 2A region on chromosome 13 and the HLA region on chromosome 6. *American Journal of Human Genetics* (suppl. to Volume 73, Abstract 1747).

Goldenberg D.L. 2002. *Fibromyalgia*. Penguin Putnam, New York.

Gursoy W., Erdal E., Herken H., Madenci E., Alayehirli B., and Erdel N. 2003. Significance of catechol-O-methyltransferase gene polymorphism in fibromyalgia syndrome. *Rheumatology International* **23**: 104–107.

Pellegrino M.J., Waylonis G.W., and Sommer A. 1989. Familial occurrence of primary fibromyalgia. *Archives of Physical Medicine and Rehabilitation* **70**: 61–63.

Yunus M.B., Khan M.A., Rawlings K.K., Green J.R., Olson J.M., Shah S. et al. 1999. Genetic linkage analysis of multicase families with fibromyalgia syndrome. *Journal of Rheumatology* **26**: 408–412.

Skin Disorders

Atopic Dermatitis

Diepgen T.L. and Blettner M. 1996. Analysis of familial aggregation of atopic eczema and other atopic diseases by odds ratio regression models. *Journal of Investigative Dermatology* **106**: 977–981.

Kuster W., Petersen M., Christophers E., Goos M., and Sterry W. 1990. A family study of atopic dermatitis: Clinical and genetic characteristics of 188 patients and 2151

family members. *Archives of Dermatological Research* **282:** 98–102.
Uehara M. and Kimur A.C. 1993. Descendant family history of atopic dermatitits. *Archives of Dermatology and Venereology* **73:** 62–63.

Psoriasis

Bowcock A.M., Helms C., Cao L., Krueger J.G., Wijsman E.M., Chamian F. et al. 2003. Regulatory variant on chromosome 17q24-q25 associated with psoriasis susceptibility. *American Journal of Human Genetics* (suppl. to Volume 73, Abstract 33).
The International Psoriasis Genetics Consortium. 2003. The international psoriasis genetics study: Assessing linkage to 14 candidate susceptibility loci in a cohort of 942 affected sib pairs. *American Journal of Human Genetics* **73:** 430–437.
Swanbeck G., Inerot A., Martinsson T., Enerback C., Enlund F., Samuelsson L. et al. 1997. Genetic counseling in psoriasis: Empirical data on psoriasis among first-degree relatives of 3095 psoriatic probands. *British Journal of Dermatology* **137:** 939–942.
Veal C.D., Capon F., Allen M.H., Heath E.K., Evans J.C., Jones A. et al. 2002. Family-based analysis using a dense single-nucleotide polymorphism-based map defines genetic variation at PSORS1, the major psoriasis-susceptibility locus. *American Journal of Human Genetics* **71:** 554–566.

Baldness

Ellis J.A. and Harrap S.B. 2001. The genetics of androgenetic alopecia. *Clinical Dermatology* **19:** 149–154.
Ellis J.A., Stebbing M., and Herrap S.B. 1998. Genetic analysis of male pattern baldness and the 5alpha-reductase genes. *Journal of Investigative Dermatology* **110:** 849–853.
Kuster W. and Happle R. 1984. The inheritance of common baldness: Two B or not two B? *Journal of American Academy of Dermatology* **11:** 921–926.
Messenger A.G. and Simpson N.B. 1997. Alopecia areata. In *Diseases of the hair and scalp* (ed. R. Dawber), pp. 338–369. Blackwell, Malden, Massachusetts.

Cancer

Breast Cancer

Meijers-Heijboer H., Wijnen J., Vasen H., Wasielewski M., Wagner A., Hollestelle A. et al. 2003. The CHEK2 1100delC mutation identifies families with a hereditary breast and colorectal cancer phenotype. *American Journal of Human Genetics* **72:** 1308–1314.
National Cancer Institute, Breast Cancer Progress Review Group, The status of breast cancer genetics research. http://.prg.nci.nih.gov/breast/bprggenetics.htm.
The Susan G. Komen Breast Cancer Foundation. Breastcancerinfo.com. www.komen.org/bci/bhealth/html/breast_cancer_genes.asp.
Welsch P.L. and King M.-C. 2001. BRCA1 and BRCA2 and the genetics of breast and ovarian cancer. *Human Molecular Genetics* **10:** 705–713.

Wooster R. and Weber B.L. 2003. Breast and ovarian cancer. *New England Journal of Medicine* **348:** 2339–2347.

Ovarian Cancer

Antoniou A.C., Gayther S.A., Stratton J.F., Ponder B.A., and Easton D.F. 2000. Risk models for familial breast and ovarian cancer. *Genetic Epidemiology* **18:** 173–190.

Antoniou A.C., Pharoah P.D., Narod S., Risch H.A., Eyfjord J.E., Hopper H.L. et al. 2003. Average risks of breast and ovarian cancer associated with brca1 or brca2 mutations detected in case series unselected for family history: A combined analysis of 22 studies. *American Journal of Human Genetics* **72:** 1117–1130.

Cannistra S.A. 1993. Cancer of the ovary. *New England Journal of Medicine* **329:** 1550–1559.

National Cancer Institute, Cancer.gov, Genetics of breast and ovarian cancer. www.nci.nih.gov/cancer_information/doc_pdq.aspx?viewid.

Phelan C.M., Rebbeck T.R., Weber B.L., Devilee P., Ruttledge M.H., and Lynch T. 1996. Ovarian cancer risk in brca1 carriers is modified by the hras1 variable number of tandem repeat (vntr) locus. *Nature Genetics* **12:** 309–311.

Wooster R. and Weber B.L. 2000. Breast and ovarian cancer. *New England Journal of Medicine* **348:** 2339–2347.

Endometrial Cancer

Esteller M., Xercavins J., and Reventes J. 1999. Advances in the molecular genetics of endometrial cancer. *Oncology Reports* **6:** 1377–1382.

Lalloo F. and Evans G. 2001. Molecular genetics and endometrial cancer. *Best Practices Research Clinics in Obstetrics and Gynaecology* **15:** 355–363.

Oehler M.K., Brand A., and Wain G.V. 2003. Molecular genetics of endometrial cancer. *Journal of the British Menopause Society* **9:** 27–31.

Simpkins S.B., Becker T., Swisher E.M., Mutch D.G., Gershell D.J., Koviatich A.J. et al. 1999. MLH1 promoter methylation and gene silencing is the primary cause of microsatellite instabililty in sporadic endometrial cancers. *Human Molecular Genetics* **8:** 661–668.

Watson P. and Lynch H.T. 2001. Cancer risk in mismatch repair gene mutation carriers. *Family Cancer* **1:** 57–60.

Colon Cancer

Chung D.A., Mino M., and Shannon K.M. 2003. Case 34-2003: A 45-year old woman with a family history of colonic polyps and cancer. *New England Journal of Medicine* **349:** 1750–1760.

Fishel R., Lescoe M.K., Rao M.R., Copeland N.G., Jenkins N.A., Garber J. et al. 1993. The human mutator homolog msh2 and its association with hereditary nonpolyposis colon cancer. *Cell* **75:** 1027–1038.

Lynch H. and de la Chapelle A. 2003. Genomic medicine: Hereditary colorectal cancer. *New England Journal of Medicine* **348:** 919–932.

Miyaki M., Konishi M., Tanaka K., Kikuchi-Yanoshita R., Muraoka M., Yasuno M. et al. 1997. Germline mutation of msh6 as the cause of hereditary nonpolyposis colorectal cancer. *Nature Genetics* **17:** 271–272.

Terdiman J.P., Conrad P.G., and Sleisinger M.H. 1999. Genetic testing in hereditary colorectal cancer: Indications and procedures. *American Journal of Gastroenterology* **94:** 2344–2356.

Wagner A., Barrows A., Wijnen J.T., van der Klift H., Franken P.F., Verkuijlen P. et al. 2003. Molecular analysis of hereditary nonpolyposis colorectal cancer in the United States: High mutation detection rate among clinically selected families and characterization of an American founder genomic deletion of the msh2 gene. *American Journal of Human Genetics* **72:** 1088–1100.

Prostate Cancer

Berthon P., Valerie A., Cohen-Akenine A., Drelon E., Paiss T., Wohr G. et al. 1998. Predisposing gene for early-onset prostate cancer, localized on chromosome 1q42.2-43. *American Journal of Human Genetics* **62:** 1416–1424.

Coulibaly A., Long L., Chen W., Panguluri R., Lewis-Smith T., Bonilla C et al. 2003. Germline Bcl-2 snps, haplotypes, and inherited predisposition to prostate cancer. *American Journal of Human Genetic* (suppl. to Volume 73, Abstract 457).

DNA sciences. Genetics of prostate cancer. www.dna.com/diseaseArticle/diseaseARicle.jsp?site+dna&link+ProstaeCancer.htm.

Edwards S.M., Zsofia K.-J., Meitz J., Hamoudi R., Hope Q., Osin P. et al. 2003. Two percent of men with early-onset prostate cancer harbor germline mutations in the brca2 gene. *American Journal of Human Genetics* **72:** 1–12.

Nelson W.G., DeMarzo A.M., and Isaacs W.B. 2003. Prostate cancer. *New England Journal of Medicine* **349:** 366–381.

Kidney Cancer

Bodmer D., Bonne A., Eleveld M., Van Erp F., Schoenmakers E., Gerts van Kessel A. et al. 2003. Molecular analysis of familial cases of renal cell cancer. *American Journal of Human Genetics* (suppl. to Volume 73, Abstract 490).

Gnarra J.R., Tory R., Weng Y., Schmidt L., Weng M.H., Li H. et al. 1994. Mutations of the VHL tumor suppressor gene in renal carcinoma. *Nature Genetics* **7:** 85–90.

Linehan W.M., Walther M.M., and Zbar B. 2003. The genetic basis of kidney cancer. *Journal of Urology* **170:** 2163–2172.

Zbar B., Klausner R., and Linehan W.M. 2003. Studying cancer families to identify kidney cancer genes. *Annual Review of Medicine* **54:** 217–233.

Bladder Cancer

Kaisary A., Smith P., Jaczq E., McCallister C.B., Wilkinson G.R., Ray W.A. et al. 1987. Genetic predisposition to bladder cancer: Ability to hydroxylate debrisoquine and mephenytoin as risk factors. *Cancer Research* **47:** 5488–5493.

The Sidney Kimmell Comprehensive Cancer Center at Johns Hopkins, Bladder cancer. www.hopkinscancercenter.org/types/bladder.cfm.

Wu X., Amos C.I., Zhu Y., Zhao H., Grossman B.H., Shay J.W. et al. 2003. Telomere dysfunction: A potential cancer predisposition factor. *Journal of the National Cancer Institute* **95:** 1211–1218.

Stomach Cancer

Caldas C., Carneiro F., Lynch H.T., Yokota J., Wiesner G.L., Powell S.M. et al. 1999. Familial gastric cancer: An overview and guidelines for management. *Journal of Medical Genetics* **36:** 873–880.

Matloff E.T. and Brierly K.L. Hereditary diffuse gastric cancer (hdgc). Cancer Genetic Counseling Newsletter. http://info.med.yale.edu/ycc/ycc_old/cgtupdate/fall01md. htm.

Torres M.M., Acosta C.P., Sicard D.M., and Groot de Restreppo H. 2003. Genetic susceptibility to gastric cancer in a Colombian population. *American Journal of Human Genetics* (suppl. to Volume 73, Abstract 1306).

Zanghieri G., DiGregorio C., Sacchetti C., Fante R., Sassatelli R., Cannizzio G. et al. 1999. Familial occurrence of gastric cancer in the 2-year experience of a population-based registry. *Cancer* **66:** 2047–2051.

Cancer of the Pancreas

Brand R. and Lynch H. 2000. Hereditary pancreatic adenocarcinoma: A clinical perspective. *Medical Clinics of North America 2000* **84:** 665–675.

Cowgill S.M. and Muscarella P. 2003. The genetics of pancreatic cancer. *American Journal of Surgery* **186:** 279–286.

Hansel D.E., Kern S.E., and Hruban R.H. 2004. Molecular pathogenesis of pancreatic cancer. *Annual Review of Genomics and Human Genetics* **4:** 237–256.

Lynch H.T., Smyrk T., Kern S.E., Hruben R.H., Lightdale C.J., Lemon S.J. et al. 1996. Familial pancreatic cancer: A review. *Seminars in Oncology* **3:** 251–275.

The Johns Hopkins Pancreatic Cancer web site: http://www.pathology.jhu.edu/pancreas.

Warshaw A.L. and Fernandez-Del Castillo C. 1992. Pancreatic carcinoma. *New England Journal of Medicine* **326:** 455–465.

Leukemia

Houlston R.S., Catovsky D., and Yuolle M.R. 2002. Genetic susceptibility to chronic lymphocytic leukemia. *Leukemia* **16:** 1008–1014.

Houlston R.S., Sellick C., Yuolle M., Matutes E., and Catovsky D. 2003. Causation of chronic lymphocytic leukemia—Insights from familial disease. *Leukemia Research* **27:** 871–876.

Kelly L.M. and Gilliland D.G. 2002. Genetics of myeloid leukemias. *Annual Review of Genomics and Human Genetics* **3:** 179–198.

Klitz W., Trachtenberg E., and Maiers M. 2003. The influence of HLA on acute lymphoblastic leukemia of childhood. *American Journal of Human Genetics* (suppl. to Volume 73, Abstract 1255).

Lymphoma

Chakravarti A., Halloron S.L., Bale S.H., and Tucker M.A. 1986. Etiological heterogeneity in Hodgkin's disease: HLA linked and unlinked determinants of susceptibility independent of histological concordance. *Genetic Epidemiology* **3**: 407–415.

Cossman J., Annunziata C.M., Barash S., Staudt L., Dillon P., He W.W. et al. 1999. Reed-Sternberg cell genome expression supports a B cell lineage. *Blood* **94**: 411–416.

Grufferman S., Cole P., Smith P.G., and Lukes R.J. 1977. Hodgkin's disease in siblings. *New England Journal of Medicine* **296**: 248–250.

Robertson S.J., Lowman J.T., Grufferman S., Kostyu D., van der Horst C.M., Matthews T.J. et al. 1987. Familial Hodgkin's disease: A clinical and laboratory investigation *Cancer* **59**: 1314–1319.

Melanoma

Bataille V. 2003. Genetic epidemiology of melanoma. *European Journal of Cancer* **39**: 1341–1347.

Bataille V., Sneider H., MacGregor A.J., Sasieni P., and Spector T.D. 2000. Genetics of risk factors for melanoma: An adult twin study of nevi and freckles. *Journal of the National Cancer Institute* **92**: 457–463.

Chaudru V., Chompret A., Minire A., Laud K., Avril M.F., Bressec de Paillerets B. et al. 2003. MC1R gene, nevus phenotypes and sun-related covariates modify CDKN2A penetrance in French melanoma-prone families. *American Journal of Human Genetics* (suppl. to Volume 73, Abstract 1254).

Gillanders E., HankJuo S.-H., Holland E.A., Jones M.P., Nancarrow D., Freas-Lutz D. et al. 2003. Localization of a novel melanoma susceptibility locus to 1p22. *American Journal of Human Genetics* **73**: 301–313.

Kefford R.F., Newton-Bishop J.A., Bergman W., and Tucker M.A. 1999. Counseling and DNA testing for individuals perceived to be genetically predisposed to melanoma: A consensus statement of the Melanoma Genetics Consortium. *Journal of Clinical Oncology* **17**: 3245–3251.

Piepkorn M. 2000. Melanoma genetics: An update with focus on the CDKN2A (p16)/ARF tumor suppressors. *Journal of the American Academy of Dermatology* **42**: 705–722.

Lung Cancer

Hemminki K., Li X., and Czenc K. 2004. Familial risk of cancer: Data for clinical counseling and cancer genetics. *International Journal of Cancer* **108**: 109–114.

Medical College of Ohio, Family lung cancer study. www.mco.edu/depts/peds/lungstudy.html.

Thorsteinsdottir U., Jonsson S., Jonsson H.H., Kong A., Gudbjartsson D.R., Kristjiansson K. et al. 2003. Familial risk of lung carcinoma in the icelandic population. *American Journal of Human Genetics* (suppl. to Volume 73, Abstract 427.)

Yanamandra K., Rodriguez-Paris J., Smith M., Napper D., Thurmon T.F., and Ursin S.A. 2003. Prothrombin polymorphism and lung cancer. *American Journal of Human Genetics* (suppl. to Volume 73, Abstract 1446).

Yang P., Yokomizo A., Tazelaar H.D., Marks R.S., Lesnick T.G., Miller D. et al. 2002. Genetic determinants of lung cancer short term survival: The role of glutathione-related genes. *Lung Cancer* **35:** 221–229.

BRAIN DISORDERS

Stroke

Bak S., Gaist D., Sindrup S.H., Skytthe A., and Christiansen K. 2002. Genetic liability in stroke: A long-term follow-up study of Danish twins. *Stroke* **33:** 769–774.

Gretarsdottir S., Thorriffson G., Reynisdottir S.T., Manolescu A., Jonsdottir S., Jonsdottir T. et al. 2003. The gene encoding phosphodiesterase 4D confers risk of ischemic stroke. *Nature Genetics* **35:** 131–138.

Hassan A. and Markus H.S. 2000. Genetics and ischaemic stroke. *Brain* **123:** 1784–1812.

Palsdottir A., Abrahamson M., Thorsteinsson L., Amason A., Olaffson I., Grubb A. et al. 1988. Mutation in cystatin C gene causes hereditary brain haemorrhage. *Lancet* **2:** 603–604.

Alzheimer's Disease

Clark R.F. and Goate A.M. 1993. Molecular genetics of Alzheimer's disease. *Archives of Neurology* **50:** 1165–1170.

Meyer M.R., Tschanz J.T., Norton N.C., Welsh-Bohmer K.A., Steffens D.C., Wyse B.W. et al. 1998. APOE genotype predicts when—not whether—one is predisposed to develop Alzheimer disease. *Nature Genetics* **19:** 321–322.

Nussbaum R.L. and Ellis C.E. 2003. Genomic medicine: Alzheimer's disease and Parkinson's disease. *New England Journal of Medicine* **348:** 1356–1364.

Selkoe D. and Podlisny M.B. 2002. Deciphering the genetic basis of Alzheimer's disease. *Annual Review of Genomics and Human Genetics* **3:** 101–128.

Strittmayer W.J. and Roses A.D. 1996. Apolipoprotein E and Alzheimer's disease. *Annual Review of Neuroscience* **19:** 53–77.

Migraine Headaches

Bjornsson A., Gudmundsson G., Gudfinnsson E., Hrafnsdottir M, Benedikz J., Skuladottir S. et al. 2003. Localization of a gene for migraine without aura to chromosome 4q21. *American Journal of Human Genetics* **73:** 986–993.

De Fusco M., Marconi R., Silvestri L., Atorino L., Rampoldi L., Morgante L. et al. 2003. Haploinsufficiency of ATP1A2 encoding the Na+/K+ pump alpha2 subunit associated with familial hemiplegic migraine type 2. *Nature Genetics* **33:** 192–196.

Russell M.B., Ulrich V., Gervil M., and Olesen J. 2002. Migraine without aura and migraine with aura are distinct disorders. A population-based twin survey. *Headache* **42:** 332–336.

Ulrich V., Gervil M., Kyvik K.O., Olesen J., and Russell M.B. 1999. Evidence of a genetic factor in migraine with aura: A population-based Danish twin study. *Annals of Neurology* **45:** 242–246.

Multiple Sclerosis

Barcellos L.F., Oksenberg J.R., Begovich A.B., Martin E.R., Schmidt S., Vittinghoff E. et al. 2003. HLA-DR2 dose effect on susceptibility to multiple sclerosis and influence on disease course. *American Journal of Human Genetics* **72:** 710–716.

Cook S.D. 1996. The epidemiology of multiple sclerosis: Clues to the etiology of a mysterious disease. *The Neuroscientist* **2:** 172–180.

Noseworthy J.H., Lucchinetti C., Rodriquez M., and Weinshenker B.G. 2000. Multiple sclerosis. *New England Journal of Medicine* **343:** 938–952.

Marrosu M.G., Marru R., Murru M.R., Costa G., Zavattari P., Whalen M. et al. 2001. Dissection of the hla association with multiple sclerosis in the founder isolated population of Sardinia. *Human Molecular Genetics* **10:** 2907–2916.

Online Mendelian Inheritance in Man (OMIM). #126200, Multiple sclerosis, susceptibility to. www3.ncbi.nlm.nih.gov/htbin-post/Omim/dispmim?12620.

Sadovick A.D., Baird P.A., and Ward R.H. 1988. Multiple sclerosis: Updated risks for relatives. *American Journal of Medical Genetics* **29:** 533–541.

Parkinson's Disease

Langston J.W. 1998. Epidemiology versus genetics in Parkinson's disease: Progress in resolving an age-old debate. *Annals of Neurology* **1:** S45–S52.

Le W.D., Xu P., Jankovic J., Jiang H., Appel S.H., Smith R.G. et al. 2003. Mutations in NR4A2 associated with familial Parkinson disease. *Nature Genetics* **33:** 85–89.

Nussbaum R.L. and Ellis C.E. 2003. Genomic medicine: Alzheimer's disease and Parkinson's disease. *New England Journal of Medicine* **348:** 1356–1364.

Pankratz N., Nichols W.C., Uniacke S.K., Halter C., Rudolph A., and Shults C. 2003. Significant linkage of Parkinson disease to chromosome 2q36-37. *American Journal of Human Genetics* **72:** 1053–1057.

Amyotrophic Lateral Sclerosis (Lou Gehrig's Disease)

Cleveland J. 2003. A new piece of the ALS puzzle. *Nature Genetics* **34:** 357–358.

Lambrechts D., Storkebaum E., Morimoto M., Del-Favero J., Desmet F., Marklund S.L. et al. 2003. VEGF is a modifier of amyotrophic lateral sclerosis in mice and humans and protects motor neurons against ischemic death. *Nature Genetics* **34:** 383–394.

Ruddy D.M., Parton M.J., Al-Chalabi H., Lewis C.M., Vance C., Smith B.N. et al. 2003. Two families with familial amyotrophic lateral sclerosis are linked to a novel locus on chromosome 16q. *American Journal of Human Genetics* **73:** 390–396.

Sapp P.C., Hosler B.A., McKenna-Yasek D., Chin W., Gann A., Genise H. et al. 2003.

Identification of two novel loci for dominantly inherited familial amyotrophic lateral sclerosis. *American Journal of Human Genetics* **73**: 397–403.
The website of the ALS Therapy Development Foundation. www.als.net.

Eye Disorders

Glaucoma

Abramson K.R., Hauser M.A., Marks O.A., Santiago C., Graham F.L., del Rono E.A. et al. 2003. Investigating candidate genes and novel ests in primary open angle glaucoma. *American Journal of Human Genetics* (suppl. to Volume 73, Abstract 2189).
Armstrong R.A. and Smith S.N. 2001. The genetics of glaucoma. *Optometry Today* November 16.
Duke University Eye Center Newsletters. Uncovering the genetics of glaucoma in Ghana. www.dukeeye.org/newletters/vision14-2/ghana.html.
Friedman J.S. and Walter M.A. 1999. Glaucoma genetics: Present and future. *Clinical Genetics* **55**: 1–79.
Sarfarazi M. 1997. Recent advances in molecular genetics of glaucomas. *Human Molecular Genetics* **6**: 1667–1677.
Sheffield V.C., Stone E.M., Alward W.L., Drack A.V., Johnson A.T., Streb L.M. et al. 1993. Genetic linkage of familial open-angle glaucoma to chromosome 1q21-q31. *Nature Genetics* **4**: 47–50.
WuDunn D. 2002. Genetic basis of glaucoma. *Current Opinion in Ophthalmology* **13**: 55–60.

Macular Degeneration

Majewski J., Schultz D.W., Weleber R.G., Schain M.B., Edwards A.O., Matise T.C. et al. 2003. Age-related macular degeneration—A genome scan in extended families. *American Journal of Human Genetics* **73**: 540–550.
De Jong P.T., Klaver C.C., Wolfs R.C., Assink J.M., and Hofman A. 1997. Familial aggregation of age-related maculopathy. *American Journal of Ophthalmology* **124**: 862–863.
National Eye Institute. Facts about age-related macular degeneration. http://www.nei.nih.gov/health/maculadegen/arnd_facts.htm.
Seddon J.M., Santangelo S.L., Book K., Chong S., and Cote J. 2003. A genomewide scan for age-related macular degeneration provides evidence for linkage to several chromosomal regions. *American Journal of Human Genetics* **73**: 780–790.

Mental Illness

Schizophrenia

Abrams R. and Taylor M.A. 1983. The genetics of schizophrenia: A reassessment using modern criteria. *American Journal of Psychiatry* **140**: 171–175.
Brzustiwicz L.M., Honer W.G., Chow E.W., Little D., Hogan J., Hodgkinson K. et al. 1999. Linkage of familial schizophrenia to chromosome 13q32. *American Journal of Human Genetics* **65**: 1096–1103.

Freedman R. 2003. Drug therapy: Schizophrenia. *New England Journal of Medicine* **349:** 1738–1749.

Levinson D.F. and Mowry B.J. 2000. Genetics of schizophrenia. In *Genetic influences on neural and behavioral functions* (ed. D.W. Pfaff et al.), pp. 47–82. CRC Press, New York.

Lewis C.M., Levinson D.F., Wise L.H., Delisi L.E., Straub R.E., Hovatta I. et al. 2003. Genome scan meta-analysis of schizophrenia and bipolar disorder, part II: Schizophrenia. *American Journal of Human Genetics* **73:** 34–48.

Stefansson H., Sarginson J., Kong A., Yates P., Steinthorsdottir V., Gudfinnsson E. et al. 2003. Association of neuregulin 1 with schizophrenia confirmed in a Scottish population. *American Journal of Human Genetics* **72:** 83–87.

Varma S.L. and Sharma I. 1993. Psychiatric morbidity in the first degree relatives of schizophrenic patients. *British Journal of Psychiatry* **162:** 672–678.

Williams N.M., Norton N., Williams H., Ekholm B., Hamshere M.L., Lindbloom Y. et al. 2003. A systematic genomewide linkage study in 353 sib pairs with schizophrenia. *American Journal of Human Genetics* **73:** 1355–1367.

Affective Disorder (Major Depression, Bipolar Illness)

Abkevich V., Camp N.J., Hensel C.H., Neff C.D., Russell D.L., Hughes D.C. et al. 2003. Predisposition locus for major depression at chromosome 12q22-12q23.2. *American Journal of Human Genetics* **73:** 1271–1281.

Caspi A., Sugden K., Moffitt T.E., Taylor A., Craig I.W., Harrington H. et al. 2003. Influence of life stress on depression: Moderation by a polymorphism in the 5-HTT gene. *Science* **301:** 386–389.

Craddock N. and Jones I. 1999. Genetics of bipolar disorder. *Journal of Medical Genetics* **36:** 585–594.

Lasseter V., Fallin M.D., Wolyniec P.S., McGrath J.A., Nestadt G., Liang K.Y. et al. 2003. A genome-scan for bipolar susceptibility loci among Ashkenazi Jewish families. *American Journal of Human Genetics* (suppl. to Volume 73, Abstract 1810).

Segurado R., Detera-Wadleigh S.D., Levinson D.F., Lewis C.M., Gill M., Nurnberger J.I. Jr. et al. 2003. Genome scan meta-analysis of schizophrenia and bipolar disorder, part III: Bipolar disorder. *American Journal of Human Genetics* **73:** 49–62.

Seong E., Seasholtz A.F., and Burmeister M. 2002. Mouse models of psychiatric disorders. *Trends in Genetics* **18:** 643–650.

Tsuang M.T. and Faraone S.V. 1990. *The genetics of mood disorders.* Johns Hopkins University Press, Baltimore.

Panic Disorder

Gratacos M., Nadal M., Martin-Santos R., Pujana M.A., Gago J., Peral B. et al. 2001. A polymorphic genomic duplication of human chromosome 15 is a susceptibility factor for panic and phobic disorders. *Cell* **106:** 367–379.

Lesch K.P., Bengel D., Heils A., Sabol S.Z., Greenberg B.D., Petri S. et al. 1996. Association of anxiety-related traits with a polymorphism in the serotonin transporter gene regulatory region. *Science* **274:** 1527–1530.

Online Mendelian Inheritance in Man. Entry 167870 Panic disorder. www3.ncbi. nlm.nih.gov.

Pauls D.L., Bucher K.D., Crowe R.R., and Noyes R. 1980. A genetic study of panic disorder pedigrees. *American Journal of Human Genetics* **32:** 639–644.

Thorgeirsson T.E., Oskarsson H., Desnica N., Kostic J.P., Stefansson J.G., Kollbeinsson H. et al. 2003. Anxiety with panic disorder liked to chromosome 9q in Iceland. *American Journal of Human Genetics* **72:** 1221–1230.

Obsessive Compulsive Disorder

Jenike M.A. 2004. Obsessive-compulsive disorder. *New England Journal of Medicine* **350:** 259–264.

Johns Hopkins Department of Psychiatry & Behavioral Sciences, Obsessive-Compulsive Disorder Family Study. www.hopkinsmedicine.org/jhhpsychiatry/ocdstudy. htm.

Hall D., Dhilla A., Charlambous A., Gogos A., and Karayiorgou M. 2003. Sequence variants of the brain-derived neurotrophic factor (bdnf) gene are strongly associated with obsessive-compulsive disorder. *American Journal of Human Genetics* **73:** 370–376.

Rasmussen S.A. and Eisen J.L. 1992. The epidemiology and differential diagnosis of obsessive compulsive disorder. *Journal of Clinical Psychiatry* (suppl.) **53:** 4–10.

Walitza S., Wewetzer C., Warnke A., Gerlach M., Geller F., and Gerber G. 2002. 5-HT2A promoter polymorphism—1438G/A in children and adolescents with obsessive-compulsive disorders. *Molecular Psychiatry* **7:** 1054–1057.

Anorexia Nervosa

Bergen A.W., Yeager M., Welch R., Haque K., Ganjei J.K., Mazzanti C. et al. 2003. Association of the DRD2 -141 Indel polymorphism with anorexia nervosa. *American Journal of Human Genetics* (suppl. to Volume 73, Abstract 1150).

Gorwood P., Kipman A., and Foulon C. 2003. The human genetics of anorexia nervosa. *European Journal of Pharmacology* **480:** 163–170.

Gorwood P., Bouvard M., Mouren-Simeoni M.C., Kipman A., and Ades J. 1998. Genetics and anorexia nervosa: A review of candidate genes. *Psychiatric Genetics* **8:** 1–12.

Holland A.J., Sicotte N., and Treasure J. 1988. Anorexia nervosa: Evidence for a genetic basis. *Journal of Psychosomatic Research* **32:** 561–571.

Wade T.D., Bulik C.M., Neale M., and Kendler K.S. 2000. Anorexia nervosa and major depression: Shared genetic and environmental risk factors. *American Journal of Psychiatry* **15:** 469–471.

Human Behavior

Alcoholism

Foroud T., Dick D., Xuei X., Goate A., Porjesz B., Begleiter H. et al. 2003. Association of SNPS in the ADH gene cluster with alcoholism. *American Journal of Human Genetics* (suppl. to Volume 73, Abstract 2066).

Goate A.M. and Edenberg H.F. 1998. The genetics of alcoholism. *Current Opinion in Genetics & Development* **8:** 282–286.

Lappalainen J., Long J.C., Eggert M., Ozaki N., Robin R.W., Brown G.L. et al. 1998. Linkage of antisocial alcoholism to the serotonin 5-HT1B receptor gene in 2 populations. *Archives of General Psychiatry* **55:** 989–994.

Saccone N.L., Kwon J.M., Corbett J., Goate A., Rochberg N., Edenberg T. et al. 2000. A genome screen of maximum number of drinks as an alcoholism phenotype. *American Journal of Medical Genetics* **96:** 632–637.

Zatz M., Guindalin C., Scivolettos S., Ferreira P.G.M., Breen G., Zilberman M. et al. 2003. Alcohol dehydrogenase 4 polymorphisms as a risk factor for alcoholism in Brazilian patients. *American Journal of Human Genetics* (suppl. to Volume 73, Abstract 2084).

Drug Addiction

Ehringer M.A., Young S., Corley R., Stallings M., Collins A.C., Hewitt J.K. et al. 2003. Investigation of the CHRNA4 gene for a possible role in tobacco use and addiction. *American Journal of Human Genetics* (suppl. to Volume 73, Abstract 2077).

Lerman C., Caporaso N.E., Bush A., Zheng L., Audrain J., Main D. et al. 2001. Tryptophan hydroxylase gene variant and smoking behavior. *American Journal of Medical Genetics* **105:** 518–520.

NIH Guide, Program Announcement, Molecular genetics of drug addiction vulnerability. www.grants.nih.gov/grants/pa-files/PA-00-115.html.

Sabol S.Z., Nelson M.l., Fisher C., Gunzerath L., Brody C.L., Hu S. et al. 1999. A genetic association for cigarette smoking behavior. *Health Psychology* **18:** 7–13.

Shahmoradgoli N., Ohadi M., Valaie F., Riazalhosseini Y., Mohammadbeigi M., and Najmabadi H. 2003. Association of the D2 dopamine receptor gene with opium addiction in Iran. *American Journal of Human Genetics* (suppl. to Volume 73, Abstract 1307).

True W.R., Xian H., Scherrer J.F., Madden P.A., Bucholz K.K., Heath A.C. et al. 1999. Common genetic vulnerability for nicotine and alcohol dependence in men. *Archives of General Psychiatry* **56:** 655–661.

Tyndale R.F. 2003. Genetics of alcohol and tobacco use in humans. *Annals of Medicine* **35:** 94–121.

Homosexuality

Bailey J.M., Dunne M.P., and Martin N.G. 2000. Genetic and environmental influences on sexual orientation and its correlates in an Australian twin sample. *Journal of Personality and Social Psychology* **78:** 524–536.

Hamer D., Hu S., Magnuson V.L., Hu N., and Pattatuci A.M. 1993. A linkage between DNA markers on the X chromosome and male sexual orientation. *Science* **261:** 321–327.

Kallman F.J. 1952. Comparative study on the genetic aspect of male homosexuality. *Journal of Nervous and Mental Disorders* **115:** 283–298.

Mustanki B.S., Chivers M.L., and Bailey J.M. 2002. A critical review of recent biological research on human sexual orientation. *Annual Review of Sexuality Research* **13:** 89–140.

Rice G., Anderson C., Risch N., and Ebers G. 1999. Male homosexuality: Absence of linkage to microsatellite markers at Xq28. *Science* **284:** 665–667.

Index